Mobile Phone and Internet Addiction: Evaluation and Management

Mobile Phone and Internet Addiction: Evaluation and Management

Editor: Ezra Potter

hayle medical

New York

Hayle Medical,
750 Third Avenue, 9th Floor,
New York, NY 10017, USA

Visit us on the World Wide Web at:
www.haylemedical.com

ISBN 978-1-64647-586-5 (Hardback)

Cataloging-in-Publication Data

Mobile phone and internet addiction : evaluation and management / edited by Ezra Potter.
p. cm.
Includes bibliographical references and index.
ISBN 978-1-64647-586-5
1. Nomophobia. 2. Cell phones--Psychological aspects. 3. Internet addiction.
4. Digital media--Psychological aspects. 5. Compulsive behavior--Diagnosis.
6. Compulsive behavior--Treatment. 7. Psychiatry. I. Potter, Ezra.
RC552.N66 M63 2023
616.858 4--dc23

Contents

Preface

This book has been a concerted effort by a group of academicians, researchers and scientists, who have contributed their research works for the realization of the book. This book has materialized in the wake of emerging advancements and innovations in this field. Therefore, the need of the hour was to compile all the required researches and disseminate the knowledge to a broad spectrum of people comprising of students, researchers and specialists of the field.

Mobile phone and Internet addiction refers to a person's inability to control mobile and Internet use. An excessive use of mobile phone and Internet is associated with several complications related to psychological and emotional characteristics such as depression, loneliness, social anxiety and impulsivity. It can lead to an imbalance of chemicals in the brain and can hinder the cognitive capacity of a person. There are several criteria used for diagnosing mobile and Internet addiction. These can be primarily classified as behavioral and functional criteria. The major indicator is the persistent desire and/or unsuccessful attempts to quit or reduce smartphone use. Some of the preventive measures include monitoring the cell mobile phone and Internet use, engaging in mood-boosting activities, counseling, and mental health treatment. This book outlines the evaluation and prevention of mobile phone and Internet addiction in detail. Its extensive content provides the readers with a thorough understanding of the subject.

At the end of the preface, I would like to thank the authors for their brilliant chapters and the publisher for guiding us all-through the making of the book till its final stage. Also, I would like to thank my family for providing the support and encouragement throughout my academic career and research projects.

Editor

1

Problematic Internet Use and Smoking among Chinese Junior Secondary Students: The Mediating Role of Depressive Symptomatology and Family Support

Phoenix Kit-han Mo [1,2,†], Ji-Bin Li [3,†], Hui Jiang [1] and Joseph T. F. Lau [1,2,*]

1 Center for Health Behaviours Research, School of Public Health and Primary Care, The Chinese University of Hong Kong, Hong Kong, China; phoenix.mo@cuhk.edu.hk (P.K.-h.M.); 1155102419@link.cuhk.edu.hk (H.J.)
2 The Chinese University of Hong Kong Shenzhen Research Institute, Shenzhen 518057, China
3 Department of Clinical Research, State Key Laboratory of Oncology in South China, Collaborative Innovation Center for Cancer Medicine, Sun Yat-sen University Cancer Center, Guangzhou 510060, China; lijib@sysucc.org.cn
* Correspondence: jlau@cuhk.edu.hk
† These authors contributed equally to the paper.

Abstract: *Background*: Internet use is significant public health issue and can be a risk factor for other addictive behaviors, such as smoking. The present study examined the association between problematic Internet use (PIU) (i.e., Internet addiction (IA) and social networking addiction (SNA)) and smoking, and the mediating role of depressive symptomatology and family support played in such associations. *Methods*: A cross-sectional study was conducted among 5182 junior secondary students (grade 7 and 8) recruited from nine schools using stratified sampling. *Results*: A total of 3.6% of students had smoked in the past month, and 6.4% of students were identified as IA cases. Adjusted for significant background variables, PIU (ORa = 2.07, 95% CI = 1.48, 2.90 for IA, ORa = 1.26, 95% CI = 1.09, 1.47 for SNA), and probable depression (ORa = 1.33, 95% CI = 1.05, 1.69) were significant risk factors, while family support (ORa = 0.85, 95% CI = 0.77, 0.94) was a significant protective factor of smoking. The mediation effects of lower family support and probable depression on the association between score on IA scale and smoking, and the mediation effect of lower family support on the association between score on SNA scale and smoking were significant, while the mediation effect of probable depression on the association between score on SNA scale and smoking was marginally significant. *Conclusions*: PIU contributed to an increased risk of smoking through depressive symptomatology and decreasing family support among junior school students. Interventions to reduce smoking are warranted; they should seek to reduce problematic Internet use and depressive symptomatology, and promote family support.

Keywords: internet addiction; social networking addiction; smoking; depression; family support; adolescents

---

1. Introduction

Smoking is considered as one of the leading preventable causes of death in the world [1] and is largely initiated and established during adolescence [2]. In China, a lower age of smoking onset has been observed and smoking among adolescents has been commonly reported [3]. One study among vocational high school students found that 45% had initiated smoking and 25% smoked in the past month [4]. Another study among junior high school students has shown that 5.6% have ever smoked in the past month [5]. Starting to smoke in adolescence predicts future smoking patterns [6,7] and also other problem behaviours such as substance use, violent behaviours, dropping out of school, and risky sexual behaviours [8,9]. Adolescent smoking has also been found to be associated with various negative health outcomes, such as sleeping disorders [10] and respiratory infections [11]. It is therefore important to identify factors associated with smoking among adolescents so that effective interventions could be designed.

Factors related to adolescent smoking have been extensively examined and documented. These included background characteristics such as lower socio-economic status [12,13], cognitive factors such as positive attitudes or less negative attitudes towards smoking [5,13], psychological factors such as stress, anxiety and depression [14–16], lower level of self-esteem [13,14], and interpersonal factors such as peer influences [17–19] or low level of parental support [20,21].

With the rapid growth of the Internet and the social media, the emerging issue of problematic Internet use (PIU) might pose additional challenges to the smoking concern among adolescents. A meta-analysis of 31 nations across seven world regions showed that a global prevalence of IA was estimated at 6.0% [22]. In China, one study among 1173 Chinese college students found that 15.2% were classified as having Internet addiction (IA) [23]; another study have reported that 12% of young smart-phone users (mean age = 26) were classified as probable problematic social networking use [24].

As smoking and PIU are both considered addictive behaviors, it might be possible that they share similar underlying roots. It has been shown that that both Internet gaming disorder and nicotine dependence share similar neural mechanisms related to craving and impulsive inhibitions [25]. Similarly, a few studies have documented the association between PIU and smoking. For example, one study investigated the association of smoking and PIU among adolescents reported a dose-dependent relationship between smoking and IA, in which IA tended to increase with current smoking habit or the number of cigarette smoked [26]; a longitudinal study among high school students in China and USA reported a positive predictive relationship between baseline compulsive Internet use and change in substance use (which included smoking) at one-year follow-up among female students [27].

Despite the numerous studies that have reported an association between PIU and smoking, very few studies have explored the mechanisms which PIU might lead to smoking. In the present study, we hypothesized that lower level of support from family and higher level of depressive symptomatology might be the potential mediating factors between PIU and smoking. There is significant concern that adolescents who are frequently exposed to the Internet may substitute the Internet for direct human interactions, leading to decreased level of social support and increased level of depression. Indeed, studies have shown that depression is one of the most common comorbidity of PIU across various populations [28,29]. For instance, a longitudinal study among Chinese adolescents showed that those who have developed IA exhibited increased depression more than that non-addiction group at the one-year follow up [30].

PIU has also found to be significantly associated with parental conflict, social isolation, and low level of social support in various studies [28,29]. One longitudinal study has found that greater use of the Internet was associated with declines in participants' communication with family members in the household, declines in the size of their social circle, and increases in their depression [31]. In China, studies have shown that students who reported poorer parent–child relationships, higher levels of depression, and lower levels of psychosocial competence were more likely to report behaviors indicative of IA [23]. Alternatively, the association between lower level of family support and higher level of depression with smoking has been widely documented [15,16,20,21,32].

Despite the extensive evidence on the association between PIU, family support, and depressive symptomatology, and between family support, depressive symptomatology, and smoking, no studies to date have examined the mediating role of these psychosocial variables on the relationship between PIU and smoking. In addition, most of the evidence reported to date have mainly focused on IA, while relatively less studies have been conducted on the association between social networking addiction (SNA), family support, depressive symptomatology, and smoking. The present study examined the prevalence of smoking, and the association between PIU (as measured by IA and SNA) and smoking among adolescents in China. The potential mediators, including depressive symptomatology and lower level of family support, were also examined.

2. Materials and Methods

2.1. Target Participants

Participants were grade 7–8 students from nine public junior middle schools in Guangzhou, Mainland China. Grade nine students were excluded as they would need to prepare for the high school entrance examination.

2.2. Sampling

A stratified cluster sampling method was applied to recruit participants. First, one district was selected from each of the three regions (core region, suburb region and outer suburb region) of Guangzhou, respectively using convenience sampling. Second, three junior middle schools were selected from each selected district/county using convenience sampling. A total of nine schools were thus selected. All grade 7 and 8 students from the selected schools were invited to take part in the study.

2.3. Participant Recruitment

Consent and permission to administer the survey was obtained by school principals prior to data collection. An anonymous structured questionnaire was administered to the students by trained field workers in the absence of teachers in classroom settings. Information on the study's background and purpose was printed in the cover page of the questionnaire. The voluntary nature and the right of refusal to take part in the study were also highlighted by the field workers. Participants received no incentive and return of the questionnaire implied informed consent. The study was approved by the Survey and Behavioral Research Ethics Committee of the Chinese University of Hong Kong.

A total of 5472 students completed the survey. Only participants who have provided complete data on the studied variables were included for analysis. As a result of this, 290 participants were excluded from the analysis, resulting in a total of 5182 valid responses.

2.4. Measures

Background characteristics. Participants were asked about their gender, grade, and parental educational attainment. They were also asked whether they were social networking users, and to rate their own academic pressure and perceived academic performance.

PIU. PIUs were measured by scores of IA and SNA. IA was measured by the eight-item Young's diagnostic questionnaire (YDQ) [33]. All items involved "yes/no" response categories and participants who provided five or more "yes" answers were classified as cases of IA [34]. The scale has commonly been used in the Chinese student population [35,36]. The Cronbach's α of the scale was 0.66 in the present study. SNA was measured by a modified version of the Facebook addiction scale [37], which included eight items describing addictive symptoms (i.e., cognitive and behavioral salience, conflict with other activities, euphoria, loss of control, withdrawal, and relapse and reinstatement). In the present study, the word "Facebook" was replaced by "online social networking", and translation and back-translation processes were implemented by two bilingual researchers. Response categories rated from 1 = not true to 5 = extremely true. The total score of the scale ranged from 8 to 40, with a higher score indicating a higher level of addictive tendency to social networking. The scale showed good internal reliability in the present study (Cronbach's $\alpha = 0.86$).

Depressive symptomatology. Depressive symptomatology was assessed using the Chinese version of the 20-item Center for Epidemiological Studies-depression scale (CES-D) [38]. The CES-D is one of the most commonly used self-report instruments in screening depressive symptomatology [39]. It has been used in Chinese adolescent population [28,40]. All items were responded on a four-point

Likert scale ranging from 0 = rarely or none of the time (less than 1 day) to 3 = almost or all of the time (5–7 days). The total score ranged from 0 to 60, with a higher score reflecting more depressive symptoms. As suggested by the scale, a score of 16 to 20 was classified as mild depression, 21 to 24 was classified as moderate depression, and 25 or above was classified as severe depression [40]. Based on the suggested cut-off, participants who scored higher than 16 were classified as probable depression in the present study. The scale showed good internal reliability in the present study (Cronbach's $\alpha = 0.86$).

Family support. Family support was measured by the four-item perceived family support subscale of the multidimensional scale of perceived social support (MSPSS) [41]. It has been used on the Chinese adolescent population [42]. Each item was rated on a seven-point Likert scale ranging from 1 = very strongly disagree to 7 = very strongly agree, with higher scores indicating higher level of perceived family support. The scale showed good internal reliability in the present study (Cronbach's $\alpha = 0.90$).

Smoking. Participants were asked to report whether they have smoked in the past month, and the number of cigarettes they smoked per day.

2.5. Data Analysis

Descriptive statistics (e.g., means (M), standard deviation (SD), percentages) were presented. Associations between background characteristics (i.e., socio-demographic variables and variables related to academic issues) and smoking were tested by multilevel logistic regression, with individual students as level 1 and school as level 2; their univariate odds ratios (ORu) and their respective 95% confidence interval (CI) were derived. For IA and depressive symptomology, binary variable was created based on the suggested cut-off. For the continuous variables (i.e., SNA and family support), We standardized the score by its mean and standard deviation to calculate the Z-scores respectively. Multiple multilevel logistic regression models were then fit separately for each of the PIU (i.e., score on IA/SNA scale) and psychosocial (i.e., family support, probable depression) variables on smoking, adjusted for background variables that were significant at the $p < 0.05$. Resulting adjusted odds ratio (ORa) and 95% CI were reported.

Next, based on the procedures proposed by Baron and Kenny, a series of multilevel logistic regressions were conducted to test the mediating role of depressive symptomatology and family support on the association between PIU and smoking. First, the association between the independent variable (i.e., score on IA/SNA scale) and dependent variable (i.e., smoking) was tested after adjusting for significantly background characteristics. Second, the association between the independent variable (i.e., score on IA/SNA scale) and the potential mediators (i.e., family support, probable depression) were examined, adjusting for significant background characteristics. The association between score on IA/SNA scale and family support was calculated using linear regressions (with the Z-score of family support as dependent variable); while the association between IA/SNA and probable depression was calculated using logistic regressions. Third, the independent variable (i.e., the score on the IA/SNA scale) and the potential mediators (i.e., family support, probable depression) were entered into the same model to predict smoking, adjusting for significant background characteristics. The Sobel test was performed to calculate the significance of the mediation, and the proportion of the mediation was calculated based on the procedure set out by Vanderweele et al [43].

3. Results

3.1. Descriptive Statistics

Slightly less than half of the participants were in 7th grade (48.0%), and similar proportion of the participants were female (47.6%). Respectively, 55.4% and 49.2% of the participants reported that their father and mother had senior secondary school level of education of above. About half (47.0%) reported that their family financial situation was very good. In terms of academic-related variables, One-third (34.2%) reported that they had an upper academic performance; and 80.6% perceived they had moderate level of study pressure or above. Most of the participants (92.2%) were social networking users, and 6.4% and 40.5% of the participants scored above the cut-off for IA and probable depression respectively. A total of 184 (3.6%) participants reported they have smoked in the past month, among them 18.5% smoked three cigarettes or more per day (Table 1).

Table 1. Descriptive characteristics of participants (N = 5182).

Variable	No. (%)/M (SD)
Depression	
Score of depression (Center for Epidemiological Studies-Depression Scale, CES-D)	15.17 (9.61)
Probable depression	
CES-D < 16	3085 (59.5)
CES-D 16–20	808 (15.6)
CES-D 21–24	497 (9.6)
CES-D 25 or above	792 (15.3)
Variables related to problematic Internet use	
Social networking user	4779 (92.2)
Score of internet addiction (IA, Young's diagnostic questionnaire)	1.53 (1.65)
Prevalence of IA	332 (6.4)
Score of social network addiction (SNA, modified Facebook addiction scale)	16.85 (5.87)
Variables related to smoking	
Have smoked in the past month	
Yes	184 (3.6)
No	4998 (96.4)
Number of cigarettes smoked per day (among those who have smoked in the past month, N = 184)	
<1	117 (63.6)
1–2	33 (17.9)
3–4	9 (4.9)
>4	25 (13.6)

3.2. Association between Background Characteristics, PIU, Psychosocial Variables and Smoking

Among the background variables, male gender (ORu = 1.47, 95% CI = 1.16, 1.87), having poor or very poor family financial situation (ORu = 2.17, 95% CI = 1.58, 2.96), and having lower level of academic performance (ORu = 1.76, 95% CI = 1.24, 2.50) were positively associated with smoking. These factors were adjusted for in subsequent analyses (Table 2).

Adjusted for significant background variables, both scores on IA and SNA scale (ORa = 2.07, 95% CI = 1.48, 2.90 for IA and ORa = 1.26, 95% CI = 1.09, 1.47 for SNA) were positively associated with smoking. Furthermore, probable depression (ORa = 1.33, 95% CI = 1.05, 1.69) was identified as a significant risk factor while family support was identified as a significant protective factor (ORa = 0.85, 95% CI = 0.77, 0.94) for smoking (Table 2).

Table 2. Association between background characteristics, IA/SNA, psychosocial variables and smoking.

Independent Variable	Odds Ratio (Oru) (95% CI)	ORa (95% CI) †
Socio-demographic background		
Grade		
7th	1	–
8th	1.06 (0.86, 1.32)	–
Gender		
Female	1	–
Male	1.47 (1.16, 1.87) **	–
Father education level		
Primary school or below	1	–
Junior secondary school	0.90 (0.63, 1.30)	–
Senior secondary school	0.71 (0.47, 1.09)	–
College or above	0.70 (0.49, 1.02)	–
Do not know	0.80 (0.40, 1.58)	–
Mother education level		
Primary school or below	1	–
Junior secondary school	1.01 (0.81, 1.26)	–
Senior secondary school	1.10 (0.83, 1.46)	–
College or above	0.98 (0.80, 1.21)	–
Do not know	1.04 (0.65, 1.65)	–
Family financial situation		
Very good/good	1	–
Average	0.99 (0.91, 1.09)	–
Poor/very poor	2.17 (1.58, 2.96) ***	–
Academic issues		
Academic performance		
Upper	1	–
Medium	1.20 (0.98, 1.47)	–
Lower	1.76 (1.24, 2.50) **	–
Perceived study pressure		
Nil/mild	1	–
Moderate	0.86 (0.66, 1.11)	–
Heavy/very heavy	1.24 (0.87, 1.76)	–
Variables related to problematic Internet use		
IA		
No	1	
Yes	2.30 (1.63, 3.24) ***	2.07 (1.48, 2.90) ***
Z-score of SNA	1.31 (1.12, 1.54) **	1.26 (1.09, 1.47) **
Psychosocial variables		
Z-score of family support	0.83 (0.75, 0.90) ***	0.85 (0.77, 0.94) **
Probable depression (CES-D ≥ 16)		
No	1	
Yes	1.38 (1.11, 1.73) **	1.33 (1.05, 1.69) *

* $p < 0.05$, ** $p < 0.01$, *** $p < 0.001$. †: Odds ratio obtained by two-level multilevel logistic regression (level 1: student; level 2: school) adjusted by gender, family financial situation and academic performance.

3.3. Testing the Mediation Effects

Adjusting for significant background variables, both scores on IA and SNA scale were significantly associated with probable depression (OR = 4.06, 95% CI = 3.16, 5.23 for IA and OR = 1.86, 95% CI = 1.74, 1.98 for SNA) and family support ($\beta = -0.41$, 95% CI = −0.52, −0.30 for IA and $\beta = -0.17$, 95% CI = −0.20, −0.14 for SNA) (Table 3). Therefore, the requirements for testing mediation effects were fulfilled. The mediation hypothesis was then tested by entering each of the two potential mediators (i.e., family support and probable depression) individually into the regression model plus score on IA/SNA scale (Model 2 and 3 for IA and Model 5 and 6 for SNA, Table 4). Each of these models contained a single mediator plus score on IA/SNA scale, and was compared against the model of score on IA/SNA scale alone (Model 1 for IA and Model 4 for SNA, Table 4). The odds ratio of score on IA/SNA scale diminished though remained significant. For the model of association between SNA and smoking, the odds ratio of probable depression on smoking become marginally significant (Model 6, Table 4). Results of the Sobel test revealed that the mediation effects of family support and probable depression on the association between score on IA scale and smoking, and the mediation effect of family support on the association between score on SNA scale and smoking were significant ($p < 0.05$, proportion of mediation ranged from 11% to 43%, Table 5), while the mediation effect of probable depression on the association between score on SNA scale and smoking was marginally significant ($p = 0.07$, proportion of mediation 36%, Table 5).

Table 3. Association between problematic Internet use (PIU), family support and probable depression.

Independent Variable	Z-Score on Family Support	Probable Depression (CES-D ≥ 16)
	β (95% CI) †	OR (95% CI) §
IA	−0.41 (−0.52, −0.30) ***	4.06 (3.16, 5.23) ***
Z-score of SNA	−0.17 (−0.20, −0.14) ***	1.86 (1.74, 1.98) ***

*** $p < 0.001$; †: Obtained by two-level linear regression (level 1: student; level 2: school) adjusted by gender, family financial situation and academic performance; §: obtained by two-level logistic regression (level 1: student; level 2: school) adjusted by gender, family financial situation and academic performance.

Table 4. Testing mediation effect of family support and probable depression on the association between PIU and smoking.

Independent Variable	Model 1	Model 2	Model 3
	ORa (95% CI) †	ORa (95% CI) †	ORa (95% CI) †
IA	2.07 (1.48, 2.90) ***	1.96 (1.46, 2.64) ***	1.93 (1.44, 2.59) ***
Z-score of family support		0.87 (0.80, 0.95) **	
Probable depression			1.25 (1.01, 1.55) *
Independent Variable	**Model 4**	**Model 5**	**Model 6**
	ORa (95% CI) †	ORa (95% CI) †	ORa (95% CI) †
Z-score of SNA	1.26 (1.09, 1.47) **	1.24 (1.07, 1.44) **	1.23 (1.07, 1.43) **
Z-score of family support		0.89 (0.81, 0.97) *	
Probable depression			1.18 (0.99, 1.42)

* $p < 0.05$, ** $p < 0.01$, *** $p < 0.001$ †: Odds ratio obtained by two-level multilevel logistic regression (level 1: student; level 2: school) adjusted by gender, family financial situation and academic performance.

Table 5. Coefficients, significance and proportion of mediation effect of family support and probable depression on the association between PIU and smoking.

Independent Variable	a	*SE*a	b	*SE*b	c′	Sobel	*p*	Proportion
IA								
Z-score of family support	−0.414	0.056	−0.140	0.046	0.674	2.81	0.005	0.11
Probable depression	1.402	0.129	0.224	0.108	0.656	2.04	0.041	0.43
SNA								
Z-score of family support	−0.171	0.015	−0.118	0.046	0.215	2.50	0.01	0.10
Probable depression	0.618	0.034	0.167	0.092	0.210	1.81	0.07	0.36

a: regression coefficient between independent variable (i.e., IA, Z-score of SNA) and the mediator (i.e., Z-score of family support, probable depression). b: coefficient between the mediator (i.e., Z-score of family support, probable depression) and the dependent variable (i.e., smoking) when both mediator and independent variable were included in the same model. c′: coefficient between independent variable (i.e., IA, Z-score of SNA) and the dependent variable (i.e., smoking) when both mediator and independent variable were included in the same model. *SE*a, *SE*b: standard errors of the corresponding coefficients.

4. Discussion

Both PIU and smoking are important public health concerns among adolescents. The present study examined the association between PIU and smoking, and elucidated the mechanism underlying such an association. It is first important to point out that 3.6% of our sampled students had smoked over the past month. The prevalence was similar to those reported among junior secondary school students in China [5].

Our findings show that PIU is a potential significant risk factor of smoking. Results corroborate with those previous studies showing a significant association between IA and smoking [26,27] and extend the knowledge that smoking is also associated with SNA. Addiction with the Internet may interfere with normal, adaptive functioning, leading to engagement in risky behaviors. It is important to note that nearly all participants in the present study were social networking users and about 6.5% of them had IA. The figures are alarming given that the sampled students are at a very young age. Findings highlight the importance of investigating the effect of addictions to specific Internet platform (i.e., social network) and the need to designing interventions to reduce PIU, which might possibly reduce the risk of smoking among adolescents.

The present study also suggests that 40.5% of the sample scored above the cut-off for probable depression. Using the same scale (CES-D) with the same cut-off, the prevalence of probable depression was lower than those reported among secondary school students in Hong Kong (53.2% among male and 62.1% among female) [28]. In the present study, probable depression was also shown to be a potential significant risk factor to smoking. Findings support the literature that depression is associated with an increased frequency of smoking [44–46], and that depressive symptomatology is more common among smokers [45]. The self-medication hypothesis, which individuals with depression might use smoking as an emotion regulation strategy to cope with their depressive mood or reduce their negative affect, might explain such association [47]. Alternatively, depressive symptomatology may leave adolescents more vulnerable to peer smoking influences, which increase their chance of smoking [47,48]. Findings suggest that improving adolescents' mental state may be a useful strategy for smoking cessation for adolescents.

To effectively combat adolescent smoking, it is important to promote protective factors and the same time, reduce the risk factors associated with smoking. Our findings revealed that family support was a potential protective factor to smoking, results which are consistent with the extant literature [49,50]. Adolescence represents an important period when young people strive for independence in order to establish their self-identify. During this period, family remains an important source of support and influence on their development. Support from parents is important and consequential for them in coping with stressors, and establishing a positive personal development. Adolescents with higher level of parental support might have better problem solving skills such that they would be less likely to turn to maladaptive behaviors (such as smoking) when they encounter adversities.

Currently there is a dearth of studies looking at the mechanism between PIU and smoking. Examining the association between PIU and smoking and its underlying mechanism would help us elucidate specific factors for PIU and smoking. Such information would be useful for health care professionals to design appropriate interventions to reduce smoking among the adolescents. Findings suggest that PIU was associated with lower level of family support and higher levels of depressive symptomatology, which in turn, associated with a higher likelihood to smoke. Adolescents with PIU might prefer to turn to the Internet for communication, which ultimately lead to decreased time spend in face-to-face interactions, decreased level of support from family and increased level of depressive symptoms, and subsequently increased chance of smoking. PIU might also weaken the protective effect of family support, which increased one's vulnerability to smoke. Interventions for smoking should not only reduce PIU but promote family support and reduce depressive symptomatology in order to lower the potential negative impact of PIU on smoking.

4.1. Implications for Practice

Given the prevalence of PIU and its potential positive association with smoking, evidence-based interventions to reduce smoking are warranted. Findings of the present study suggest that reducing PIU could possibly be a useful way to combat adolescent smoking problem. A few evidence-based interventions to reduce PIU among the adolescences have been reported in the literature. For example, it has been shown that school-based group using cognitive behavioral theory (CBT) was effective in reducing IA [51]. Other studies also reported that reality therapy counselling [52], reality therapy combined with mindfulness mediation [53], and motivational interviewing [54,55] were effective in reducing PIU. Findings also suggest that reducing participants' depressive symptoms may be a useful strategy for reducing smoking. Indeed, evidence has suggested that psychological interventions are effective in reducing smoking [56]. To develop effective interventions for reducing smoking, it is important to enhance protective factors of smoking, besides reducing risk factors. Findings of the present study suggest that interventions to increase family support may have the potential to reduce smoking. There is a need for health care professionals to understand the context of family support and the way in which adolescents obtain support from the family. Family-based approaches that focuses on improving the parent–child relationship, increasing communication and understanding among family members can be a direction for increasing family support of adolescents. Review studies have suggested that family-based interventions were effective in reducing the onset of smoking among children and adolescents [57].

4.2. Limitations of the Study

There are several limitations of the study that should be noted. First, the study is limited by its cross-sectional nature, therefore the association between PIU, depressive symptomatology, lower levels of family support and smoking are only suggestive. It might also be plausible that smoking leads to depressive symptomatology and lower levels of family support, which in turn lead to PIU. Longitudinal studies are warranted to elucidate the prospective relationship between the variables. Second, all data were self-reported so the levels of IA and smoking might have been underestimated. Third, due to the lack of an established cut-off point for SNA, the extent of SNA of the sample was unclear. Fourth, the association between PIU and smoking could have been mediated by other individual factors, such as individual differences in circadian rhythm [58]. Future studies should explore other potential mediators of such association. Fifth, written consent was not obtained from the students, and their return of the questionnaire implied informed consent. We have been advised by the schools that written consent was not necessary, but students needed to be briefed very thoroughly and the participation should be completely voluntary. We have taken careful steps to make sure that a very detailed briefing was provided to ensure confidentiality, anonymity, and voluntariness. Sixth, the internal reliability of YDQ was low in the present study. We were aware that other validated scales for IA (e.g., the Internet addiction test, IAT [59]) were available but due to concern about length of the questionnaire, YDQ was chosen over other validated scales. Finally, the current sample was collected from nine secondary schools in Guangzhou, generalization to other secondary school students might be limited.

5. Conclusions

To conclude, findings of the present study call for a need to reduce PIU and smoking among junior secondary school students in China and provide insights on the variables that could be targeted when designing anti-smoking interventions targeting this population. In particular, findings show that PIU was associated with smoking among junior secondary school students in China and such associations were mediated by depressive symptomatology and lower levels of family support. Results provide important implications that interventions to reduce smoking among the current sample should target not only to reduce PIU, but also to reduce depression and promote family support.

Author Contributions: J.-B.L., J.T.F.L., P.K.-h.M. designed the research; J.-B.L. performed the data collection; J.-B.L. and H.J. analyzed data; all authors interpreted results; P.K.-h.M. wrote the manuscript. All authors read and approved the final manuscript.

Acknowledgments: This study was supported by the Jockey Club School of Public Health and Primary Care research. Postgraduate Students' research Grants and CUHK research Postgraduate Student Grants for Overseas

Academic Activities in the Chinese University of Hong Kong, it was also partially supported by National Science Foundation of China (No.: 81373021). The funders had no role in study design, data collection and analysis, decision to publish, or preparation of the manuscript. The authors would like to give great appreciation to all participants and schools.

References

1. World Health Organization. *Global Health Risks: Mortality and Burden of Disease Attributable to Selected Major Risks*; WHO: Geneva, Switzerland, 2009.
2. US Department of Health and Human Services. *Preventing Tobacco Use Among Young People: A Report of the Surgeon General*; US Department of Health and Human Services: Washington, DC, USA, 1994.
3. Wang, M.; Luo, X.; Xu, S.; Liu, W.; Ding, F.; Zhang, X.; Wang, L.; Liu, J.; Hu, J.; Wang, W. Trends in smoking prevalence and implication for chronic diseases in China: Serial national cross-sectional surveys from 2003 to 2013. *Lancet Respir Med.* **2019**, *7*, 35–45. [CrossRef]
4. Yan, Y.; Jacques-Tiura, A.J.; Chen, X.; Xie, N.; Chen, J.; Yang, N.; Gong, J.; MacDonell, K.K. Application of the Protection Motivation Theory in predicting cigarette smoking among adolescents in China. *Addict. Behav.* **2014**, *39*, 181–188. [CrossRef] [PubMed]
5. Su, X.; Li, L.; Griffiths, S.M.; Gao, Y.; Lau, J.T.F.; Mo, P.K.H. Smoking behaviors and intentions among adolescents in rural China: The application of the Theory of Planned Behavior and the role of social influence. *Addict. Behav.* **2015**, *48*, 44–51. [CrossRef] [PubMed]
6. Hu, M.-C.; Davies, M.; Kandel, D.B. Epidemiology and Correlates of Daily Smoking and Nicotine Dependence Among Young Adults in the United States. *Am. J. Public Health* **2006**, *96*, 299–308. [CrossRef]
7. Reidpath, D.D.; Ling, M.-L.; Wellington, E.; Al-Sadat, N.; Yasin, S. The Relationship Between Age of Smoking Initiation and Current Smoking: An Analysis of School Surveys in Three European Countries. *Nicotine Tob. Res.* **2013**, *15*, 729–733. [CrossRef]
8. Ellickson, P.L.; Saner, H.; McGuigan, K.A. Profiles of violent youth: Substance use and other concurrent problems. *Am. J. Public Health* **1997**, *87*, 985–991. [CrossRef]
9. Ellickson, P.L.; Tucker, J.S.; Klein, D.J. High-risk behaviors associated with early smoking: Results from a 5-year follow-up. *J. Adolesc. Health* **2001**, *28*, 465–473. [CrossRef]
10. Mak, K.K.; Ho, S.Y.; Thomas, G.N.; Lo, W.S.; Cheuk, D.K.L.; Lai, Y.K.; Lam, T.H. Smoking and sleep disorders in Chinese adolescents. *Sleep Med.* **2010**, *11*, 268–273. [CrossRef]
11. Lai, H.K.; Ho, S.Y.; Wang, M.P.; Lam, T.H. Secondhand Smoke and Respiratory Symptoms Among Adolescent Current Smokers. *Pediatrics* **2009**, *124*, 1306. [CrossRef]
12. Hanson, M.D.; Chen, E. Socioeconomic Status and Health Behaviors in Adolescence: A Review of the Literature. *J. Behav. Med.* **2007**, *30*, 263. [CrossRef]
13. Joffer, J.; Burell, G.; Bergström, E.; Stenlund, H.; Sjörs, L.; Jerdén, L. Predictors of smoking among Swedish adolescents. *BMC Public Health* **2014**, *14*, 1296. [CrossRef] [PubMed]
14. Byrne, D.G.; Mazanov, J. Self-esteem, stress and cigarette smoking in adolescents. *Stress Health J. Int. Soc. Investig. Stress* **2001**, *17*, 105–110. [CrossRef]
15. Diego, M.A.; Field, T.M.; Sanders, C.E. Academic perforamce, popularity, and depression predict adolescent substance use. *Adolescence* **2003**, *38*, 35.
16. Leventhal, A.M.; Zvolensky, M.J. Anxiety, depression, and cigarette smoking: A transdiagnostic vulnerability framework to understanding emotion–smoking comorbidity. *Psychol. Bull.* **2015**, *141*, 176–212. [CrossRef]
17. Leonardi-Bee, J.; Jere, M.L.; Britton, J. Exposure to parental and sibling smoking and the risk of smoking uptake in childhood and adolescence: A systematic review and meta-analysis. *Thorax* **2011**, *66*, 847–855. [CrossRef]
18. Huang, G.C.; Unger, J.B.; Soto, D.; Fujimoto, K.; Pentz, M.A.; Jordan-Marsh, M.; Valente, T.W. Peer Influences: The Impact of Online and Offline Friendship Networks on Adolescent Smoking and Alcohol Use. *J. Adolesc. Health* **2014**, *54*, 508–514. [CrossRef]
19. Lakon, C.M.; Wang, C.; Butts, C.T.; Jose, R.; Timberlake, D.S.; Hipp, J.R. A Dynamic Model of Adolescent Friendship Networks, Parental Influences, and Smoking. *J. Youth Adolesc.* **2015**, *44*, 1767–1786. [CrossRef]

20. Maggi, S.; Lovato, C.Y.; Hill, E.M.; Johnson, J.L.; Ratner, P.A.; Shoveller, J.A. Adolescents' Perceptions of Parental Influences on Their Smoking Behavior. *Youth Soc.* **2014**, *46*, 132–149. [CrossRef]
21. Zaborskis, A.; Sirvyte, D. Familial determinants of current smoking among adolescents of Lithuania: A cross-sectional survey 2014. *BMC Public Health* **2015**, *15*, 889. [CrossRef]
22. Cheng, C.; Li, A.Y.-L. Internet Addiction Prevalence and Quality of (Real) Life: A Meta-Analysis of 31 Nations Across Seven World Regions. *Cyberpsychol. Behav. Soc. Netw.* **2014**, *17*, 755–760. [CrossRef]
23. Chi, X.; Lin, L.; Zhang, P. Internet Addiction Among College Students in China: Prevalence and Psychosocial Correlates. *Cyberpsychol. Behav. Soc. Netw.* **2016**, *19*, 567–573. [CrossRef] [PubMed]
24. Wu, A.M.; Cheung, V.I.; Ku, L.; Hung, E.P. Psychological risk factors of addiction to social networking sites among Chinese smartphone users. *J. Behav. Addict.* **2013**, *2*, 160–166. [CrossRef] [PubMed]
25. Ge, X.; Sun, Y.; Han, X.; Wang, Y.; Ding, W.; Cao, M.; Du, Y.; Xu, J.; Zhou, Y. Difference in the functional connectivity of the dorsolateral prefrontal cortex between smokers with nicotine dependence and individuals with internet gaming disorder. *BMC Neurosci.* **2017**, *18*, 54. [CrossRef] [PubMed]
26. Morioka, H.; Itani, O.; Osaki, Y.; Higuchi, S.; Jike, M.; Kaneita, Y.; Kanda, H.; Nakagome, S.; Ohida, T. Association Between Smoking and Problematic Internet Use Among Japanese Adolescents: Large-Scale Nationwide Epidemiological Study. *Cyberpsychol. Behav. Soc. Netw.* **2016**, *19*, 557–561. [CrossRef]
27. Sun, P.; Johnson, C.A.; Palmer, P.; Arpawong, T.E.; Unger, J.B.; Xie, B.; Rohrbach, L.A.; Spruijt-Metz, D.; Sussman, S. Concurrent and Predictive Relationships Between Compulsive Internet Use and Substance Use: Findings from Vocational High School Students in China and the USA. *Int. J. Environ. Res. Public Health* **2012**, *9*, 660–673. [CrossRef]
28. Wu, A.M.S.; Li, J.; Lau, J.T.F.; Mo, P.K.H.; Lau, M.M.C. Potential impact of internet addiction and protective psychosocial factors onto depression among Hong Kong Chinese adolescents–Direct, mediation and moderation effects. *Compr. Psychiatry* **2016**, *70*, 41–52. [CrossRef]
29. Wu, X.S.; Zhang, Z.H.; Zhao, F.; Wang, W.J.; Li, Y.F.; Bi, L.; Qian, Z.Z.; Lu, S.S.; Feng, F.; Hu, C.Y.; et al. Prevalence of Internet addiction and its association with social support and other related factors among adolescents in China. *J. Adolesc.* **2016**, *52*, 103–111. [CrossRef]
30. Ko, C.-H.; Liu, T.-L.; Wang, P.-W.; Chen, C.-S.; Yen, C.-F.; Yen, J.-Y. The exacerbation of depression, hostility, and social anxiety in the course of Internet addiction among adolescents: A prospective study. *Compr. Psychiatry* **2014**, *55*, 1377–1384. [CrossRef]
31. Kraut, R.; Patterson, M.; Lundmark, V.; Kiesler, S.; Mukopadhyay, T.; Scherlis, W. Internet paradox. A social technology that reduces social involvement and psychological well-being? *Am. Psychol.* **1998**, *53*, 1017–1031. [CrossRef]
32. Piko, B. Perceived Social Support from Parents and Peers: Which Is the Stronger Predictor of Adolescent Substance Use? *Subst. Use Misuse* **2000**, *35*, 617–630. [CrossRef]
33. Young, K.S. Internet Addiction: The Emergence of a New Clinical Disorder. *CyberPsychol. Behav.* **1998**, *1*, 237–244. [CrossRef]
34. Aboujaoude, E. Problematic Internet use: An overview. *World Psychiatry* **2010**, *9*, 85–90. [CrossRef] [PubMed]
35. Fu, K.W.; Chan, W.S.; Wong, P.W.; Yip, P.S. Internet addiction: Prevalence, discriminant validity and correlates among adolescents in Hong Kong. *Br. J. Psychiatry J. Ment. Sci.* **2010**, *196*, 486–492. [CrossRef] [PubMed]
36. Li, Y.; Zhang, X.; Lu, F.; Zhang, Q.; Wang, Y. Internet addiction among elementary and middle school students in China: A nationally representative sample study. *Cyberpsychol. Behav. Soc. Netw.* **2014**, *17*, 111–116. [CrossRef]
37. Koc, M.; Gulyagci, S. Facebook addiction among Turkish college students: The role of psychological health, demographic, and usage characteristics. *Cyberpsychol. Behav. Soc. Netw.* **2013**, *16*, 279–284. [CrossRef]
38. Radloff, L.S. The CES-D Scale: A self-report depression scale for research in the general population. *Appl. Psychol. Meas.* **1977**, *1*, 385–401. [CrossRef]
39. Beekman, A.T.F.; Deeg, D.J.H.; Van Limbeek, J.; Braam, A.W.; De Veries, M.Z.; Van Tilburg, W. Criterion validity of the Center for Epidemiologic Studies Depression scale (CES-D): Results from a community-based sample of older subjects in the Netherlands. *Psychol. Med.* **1997**, *27*, 231–235. [CrossRef]
40. Song, Y.; Huang, Y.; Liu, D.; Kwan, J.S.; Zhang, F.; Sham, P.C.; Tang, S.W. Depression in college: Depressive symptoms and personality factors in Beijing and Hong Kong college freshmen. *Compr. Psychiatry* **2008**, *49*, 496–502. [CrossRef]

41. Zimet, G.D.; Dahlem, N.W.; Zimet, S.G.; Farley, G.K. The Multidimensional Scale of Perceived Social Support. *J. Personal. Assess.* **1988**, *52*, 30–41. [CrossRef]
42. Chou, K.-L. Assessing Chinese adolescents' social support: The multidimensional scale of perceived social support. *Personal. Individ. Differ.* **2000**, *28*, 299–307. [CrossRef]
43. Vanderweele, T.J.; Vansteelandt, S. Odds ratios for mediation analysis for a dichotomous outcome. *Am. J. Epidemiol.* **2010**, *172*, 1339–1348. [CrossRef] [PubMed]
44. Patton, G.C.; Carlin, J.B.; Coffey, C.; Wolfe, R.; Hibbert, M.; Bowes, G. Depression, anxiety, and smoking initiation: A prospective study over 3 years. *Am. J. Public Health* **1998**, *88*, 1518–1522. [CrossRef] [PubMed]
45. Murphy, J.M.; Horton, N.J.; Monson, R.R.; Laird, N.M.; Sobol, A.M.; Leighton, A.H. Cigarette smoking in relation to depression: Historical trends from the Stirling County Study. *Am. J. Psychiatry* **2003**, *160*, 1663–1669. [CrossRef] [PubMed]
46. Nezami, E.; Unger, J.; Tan, S.; Mahaffey, C.; Ritt-Olson, A.; Sussman, S.; Nguyen-Michel, S.; Baezconde-Garbanati, L.; Azen, S.; Johnson, C.A. The influence of depressive symptoms on experimental smoking and intention to smoke in a diverse youth sample. *Nicotine Tob. Res.* **2005**, *7*, 243–248. [CrossRef]
47. Audrain-McGovern, J.; Rodriguez, D.; Kassel, J.D. Adolescent smoking and depression: Evidence for self-medication and peer smoking mediation. *Addiction (Abingdon England)* **2009**, *104*, 1743–1756. [CrossRef]
48. Ritt-Olson, A.; Unger, J.; Valente, T.; Nezami, E.; Chou, C.P.; Trinidad, D.; Milam, J.; Earleywine, M.; Tan, S.; Johnson, C.A. Exploring peers as a mediator of the association between depression and smoking in young adolescents. *Subst. Use Misuse* **2005**, *40*, 77–98. [CrossRef]
49. Borca, G.; Rabaglietti, E.; Roggero, A.; Keller, P.; Haak, E.; Begotti, T. Personal Values as a Mediator of Relations Between Perceived Parental Support and Control and Youth Substance Use. *Subst Use Misuse* **2017**, *52*, 1589–1601. [CrossRef]
50. Hill, K.G.; Hawkins, J.D.; Catalano, R.F.; Abbott, R.D.; Guo, J. Family influences on the risk of daily smoking initiation. *J. Adolesc. Health* **2005**, *37*, 202–210. [CrossRef]
51. Du, Y.-s.; Jiang, W.; Vance, A. Longer term effect of randomized, controlled group cognitive behavioural therapy for Internet addiction in adolescent students in Shanghai. *Aust. N. Z. J. Psychiatry* **2010**, *44*, 129–134. [CrossRef]
52. Kim, J.-U. The Effect of a R/T Group Counseling Program on The Internet Addiction Level and Self-Esteem of Internet Addiction University Students. *Int. J. Real. Ther.* **2008**, *27*, 4–12.
53. Yao, Y.-W.; Chen, P.-R.; Li, C.-s.R.; Hare, T.A.; Li, S.; Zhang, J.-T.; Liu, L.; Ma, S.-S.; Fang, X.-Y. Combined reality therapy and mindfulness meditation decrease intertemporal decisional impulsivity in young adults with Internet gaming disorder. *Comput. Hum. Behav.* **2017**, *68*, 210–216. [CrossRef]
54. Orzack, M.H.; Voluse, A.C.; Wolf, D.; Hennen, J. An ongoing study of group treatment for men involved in problematic Internet-enabled sexual behavior. *Cyberpsychol. Behav.* **2006**, *9*, 348–360. [CrossRef] [PubMed]
55. Shek, D.T.; Tang, V.M.; Lo, C.Y. Evaluation of an Internet addiction treatment program for Chinese adolescents in Hong Kong. *Adolescence* **2009**, *44*, 359–373. [PubMed]
56. Hall, S.M.; Humfleet, G.L.; Reus, V.I.; Muñoz, R.F.; Hartz, D.T.; Maude-Griffin, R. Psychological intervention and antidepressant treatment in smoking cessation. *Arch. Gen. Psychiatry* **2002**, *59*, 930–936. [CrossRef]
57. Thomas, R.E.; Baker, P.R.A.; Thomas, B.C.; Lorenzetti, D.L. Family-based programmes for preventing smoking by children and adolescents. *Cochrane Database Syst. Rev.* **2015**, *27*, CD004493. [CrossRef]
58. Adan, A. A chronobiological approach to addiction. *J. Subst. Use* **2013**, *18*, 171–183. [CrossRef]
59. Young, K. *Caught in the Net*; John Wiley & Sons: New York, NY, USA, 1998.

2

The Association of Problematic Internet Shopping with Dissociation among South Korean Internet Users

Young-Mi Ko [1], Sungwon Roh [2] and Tae Kyung Lee [3,*]

1 Mental Health Research Institute, National Center for Mental Health, Seoul 04933, Korea; daquin07@korea.kr
2 Department of Psychiatry, Hanyang University, College of Medicine, Seoul 04763, Korea; swroh@hanyang.ac.kr
3 Department of Mental Health, ChunCheon National Hospital, ChunCheon City 24409, Korea
* Correspondence: TKLeeMD@gmail.com

Abstract: *Background*: This study examined patterns of problematic shopping behavior by South Korean internet users to investigate the association between problematic internet shopping (PIS) and dissociative experiences.; *Methods*: Five hundred and ninety eight participants from 20–69 years old were recruited through an online panel survey. We gathered information about sociodemographic characteristics, alcohol use, caffeine intake, and online shopping behaviors. Psychopathological assessments included Korean version of dissociative experience scale (DES-K), Canadian Problem Gambling Index (CPGI-K), the modified Stress Response Inventory (SRI-MF), the Barratt Impulsive Scale-11-Revised (BIS-K). We used multiple logistic regression analysis with the Richmond compulsive buying scale (RCBS-K) as the dependent variable.; *Results*: The prevalence of shoppers with internet-based problem shopping was 12.5%. The amount of time spent on online shopping was correlated with PIS severity (OR = 1.008, $p < 0.01$). The risk of PIS was related to an increased tendency toward dissociation (OR = 1.044, $p < 0.001$) and impulsivity (OR = 1.046, $p < 0.05$). *Conclusions*: PIS participants with dissociation showed higher levels of perceived stress, gambling problems, and impulsivity than did PIS participants without dissociation. This study suggests that dissociation was associated with a higher burden of PIS as it was connected to poor mental health problems.

Keywords: compulsive buying; addictive shopping; impulsivity; online shopping; dissociation

---

1. Introduction

With the spread of the internet, online shopping is also showing steady growth. The convenience offered by the internet contributes to its popularity. The internet provides a huge diversity of shopping information and simultaneous access to many online stores, thereby living up to expectations for immediate rewards and emotional enhancement.

South Korea is one of the best-connected countries in the world. In 2018, the internet penetration rate was at around 96 percent, while the internet usage rate was at 91.6 percent [1]. The South Korean government reported that online or internet-based shopping transaction value was 9.926 billion USD in July 2019, rising by 15.4% from July 2018 [2]. Because of an increase in high-speed internet access connections, lower connection costs, and increasing consumer competence, e-commerce activity has been rising.

For most people, buying is a normal and routine part of everyday life. Today, shopping is considered both a utilitarian and social or leisure activity with hedonistic features [3]. However, excessive shopping leads to distress or impairment. Compulsive and excessive spending is controversial, and such consumption and buying behaviors have been researched in both the business and medical literature.

The phenomenon of compulsive buying or an uncontrolled shopping spree has been described for 100 years in the literature [4,5]. Still, the phenomenon has not been included as a formal mental health disorder in the most recent, 5th edition of the Diagnostic and Statistical Manual of Mental Disorders (DSM-5) and the recently released 11th revision of the International Classification of Diseases (ICD-11) [6–8]. Uncontrolled buying behavior has been referred to in the literature as uncontrolled buying [9], compulsive buying [10], compulsive shopping [11], addictive buying [12], excessive buying [13], and pathological buying [14].

Given the rapid growth of online shopping, researchers have concerns about issues surrounding repetitive problematic behaviors associated with internet-based shopping. According to Rose and Dhandayudham [15], addictive online shopping may negatively influence not only an individual's daily and social life but also their economic status. Zhao et al. [16] described a tendency to engage in excessive, compulsive, and problematic shopping behavior via the internet that results in consequences associated with economic, social, and emotional problems such as online shopping addiction. Müller et al. use the term "online buying-shopping disorder" [17]. In the current paper, we use "Problematic Internet Shopping (PIS)", a more neutral expression in accordance with Lam and Lam [18].

Investigating the clinical characteristics of PISis of great importance as it will provide insights for developing diagnostic criteria. Improvement of understanding for PIS will enhance our capacity to recognize and define their presence. However, PIS is a complex and highly debated concept. Previous studies suggest that compulsive or pathological forms of buying behavior fit well into the behavioral addiction spectrum [19–21]. Disordered gambling, the only behavioral addiction being included in the main section of DSM-5 [6], is associated with problematic shopping [22,23]. Problematic shopping is associated with comorbid psychiatric conditions, such as mood disorders, and other behavioral addictions [14,24].

Behavioral addictions have been hypothesized as having similarities to substance addictions. Substance use disorders (SUD) co-occur with behavioral addictions. Higher caffeine intake has been associated with impulsivity and gambling [25]. In the case of Compulsive Buying, the co-morbidity rate with SUD was estimated as 21–46% [26]. Maraz et al. reported that Compulsive Buyers showed high impulsivity, high levels of distress, and substance use (alcohol, smoking, and illicit drug) in their shopping mall visitor sample [27]. These findings suggest that behavioral addictions share a common pathophysiology with SUD.

Some research has noted a correlation between behavioral addiction and dissociation [20,21]. Berancy and colleagues (2013) suggested that addiction is an absorbent relation established with an object that determines a person's cognitive, emotional, and behavioral states, causing significant damage in different areas of life [28].

Ludwig [29] said, "Dissociation represents a process whereby certain mental functions which are ordinarily integrated with other functions presumably operate in a more compartmentalized or automatic way, usually outside the sphere of conscious awareness or memory recall."

Maldonado and Spiegel [30] and DSM-5 [6] defines dissociation as the "disruption of and/or discontinuity in the normal integration of consciousness, memory, identity, emotion, perception, body representation, motor control, and behavior. Dissociative symptoms in mental disorders are of high clinical relevance".

Researchers have reported that symptoms of dissociation have been linked to maladaptive functioning, symptom severity, and poor treatment response in substance-related and addictive disorders [30,31].

The importance of dissociation in the psychopathology of addiction has been confirmed [32–34]. Somer [35] found that levels of dissociation negatively contributed to the prediction of abstinence. Craparo et al. [32] reported that addictive behaviors have a dissociative nature that allows individuals to manage negative and unregulated emotions. They suggested that dissociation is a predictor of addiction.

Thus, the present exploratory study examined clinical characteristics and psychological aspects of PIS among South Korean Internet users. Based on the extant literature, we expected that PIS would be associated with elevated impulsivity, emotional distress, depression, more severe gambling problems, and substance abuse (alcohol and caffeine). Secondly, we investigate the relationship between PIS and dissociative symptoms. We hypothesized that dissociation would be positively associated with higher PIS severity and mental health problems.

2. Methods

2.1. Participants

The total number of participants was 598, and we applied random sampling through proportionate allocation in accordance with the sex and age distribution of South Korea. Participants from 20–69 years were recruited through an online research service, ZINNOS R&C (ZINNOS R&C Co. Ltd., Seoul, Korea). The cross-sectional study was performed from August to September 2015. As this study aimed to collect research materials from dedicated, internet-based shoppers, this study was done through an online panel survey conducted by ZINNOS R&C, which, at the time of the survey, had 75,000 or more members.

Email invitations to complete an online survey were sent out to a random sample of potential respondents in the ZINNOS R&C panel. Of the 8977 Korean internet users who received an invitation, 598 (6.66%) visited the survey webpage. Participants completed a self-administered questionnaire that gathered information about sociodemographic characteristics, alcohol and caffeine use, online shopping behaviors, problematic buying, dissociation experiences, gambling problems, depression, stress perception, and impulsivity. Problematic shopping was measured with the Korean version of the Richmond Compulsive Buying Scale (RCBS). This study was approved by the National Center for Mental Health Institutional Review Board (NCMH 2015-06) and adhered to ethical policies.

2.2. Measures

2.2.1. Sociodemographic Characteristics

We examined the subjects' sex, age, and marital status. Participants aged 20–69 years were recruited, and for analysis were divided into age groups by decade: 20–29, 30–39, 40–49, 50–59, and 60–69. Marital status was divided into three groups: married, separated/widowed/divorced, and single.

2.2.2. Internet Shopping Behaviors

The total time that participants had spent internet shopping, the amount of money they had spent on internet shopping in the past month, the time spent on activities related to shopping during the day, and the average number of days per week they engaged in activities related to shopping in the past month were surveyed and measured as continuous variables. Additionally, participants were asked whether they had the experience of making an online purchase in excess of their income.

2.2.3. Alcohol and Caffeine Use

Alcohol use was assessed with the question: "How many glasses do you drink?" For the question, "How many times have you drunk four or more glasses of an alcoholic beverage in the past year?" answers of "not at all," "once a month," "twice a month," "once a week," and "two or three times a week" were given. The question, "How many caffeine drinks (including coffee) do you drink a day on average?" was asked, and the answers were measured as a continuous variable.

2.2.4. The Korean Version of the Richmond Compulsive Buying Scale (RCBS-K)

The scale was developed by Ridgway et al. [36] and was used to measure the severity of PIS in this study. The scale consists of six questions that use a seven-point Likert scale. A score of 25 points or higher indicates that a respondent's online shopping is a source of significant problems [36]. The RCBS has been reported to have high internal consistency, with a Cronbach's alpha coefficient of 0.84, and evidence of validity [36]. For this study, the Cronbach's alpha coefficient of RCBS-K was 0.906.

2.2.5. The Korean Version of the Dissociative Experiences Scale (DES-K)

The Dissociative Experiences Scale (DES) is a 28-item self-report instrument. The DES was developed by Bernstein and Putman [37] and has adequate test-retest reliability, good split-half reliability, and good clinical validity. It can be completed in 10 min and scored in less than 5 min. It is easy to understand, and the questions are framed in a normative way that does not stigmatize the respondent for positive responses. The respondent clicks along a line anchored at 0% on the left and 100% on the right to show how often they have this experience. The overall DES score is obtained by adding up the answers of the 28 items and then dividing by 28; this yields an overall score ranging from 0 to 100. Scores higher than 20 on the Korean version of the DES (DES-K) may indicate the presence of a dissociative disorder. The DES-K has good validity and reliability, and overall good psychometric properties, exhibiting a Cronbach's alpha coefficient of 0.94 [38]. The Cronbach's alpha of DES-K for this study was 0.985.

2.2.6. The Korean Version of the Canadian Problem Gambling Index (CPGI-K)

This scale was developed by Ferris and Wynne [39] to measure participant degree of gambling addiction. Scores for a total of nine questions are measured on a 4-point Likert-type scale (0: never, 1: sometimes, 2: frequently, 3: always). The range of the total score is from 0–27. According to the total score, the degree of gambling addiction is divided into nonproblematic gambling (0 points), low-danger gambling (1–2 points), mid-danger gambling (3–7 points), and problematic gambling (8 points or higher). The Korean version of the scale was standardized by Kim et al. [40], and the Cronbach's alpha coefficient was 0.94. The Cronbach's alpha of CPGI-K for this study was 0.947.

2.2.7. The Korean Version of the Zung Self-Rating Depression Scale (ZDS-K)

The ZDS is a 20-item self-report measure of the symptoms associated with depression. Subjects rate each item with regard to how they have felt during the preceding week using a four-point Likert scale, with 4 representing the most unfavorable response. The sum of the 20 items, after transposing the 10 items that are reverse-scored, produces a raw score from 20–80. Previous studies have pointed out that scores are not meant to offer strict diagnostic criteria but rather denote levels of depressive symptoms that might be clinically significant [41,42]. The Korean version of the ZDS (ZDS-K) was used in this study and has high internal consistency (i.e., Cronbach's alpha for the SDS = 0.79) [43]. The Cronbach's alpha coefficient for ZDS-K in this study was 0.876

2.2.8. The Modified Form of the Stress Response Inventory (SRI-MF)

SRI-MF is the short form of the Stress Response Inventory (SRI) was developed by Choi and colleagues [44] to score mental and physical symptoms occurring during the previous two weeks that might influence the current status of mental stress levels [45]. SRI scores can be categorized into seven stress factors: tension, aggression, somatization, anger, depression, fatigue, and frustration. The SRI assesses stress severity based on the stress symptoms or the effects of stressors. The SRI consists of 39 items that focus on emotional, somatic, cognitive, and behavioral stress responses. The SRI-MF consists of 22 items employing three factors: somatization, depression, and anger. The SRI-MF has good validity and reliability, exhibiting a Cronbach's alpha coefficient of 0.93 [44]. The Cronbach's alpha coefficient for SRI-MF in this study was 0.958.

2.2.9. The Barratt Impulsive Scale-11-Revised (BIS-K).

The Barratt Impulsive Scale was developed to evaluate the degree of impulsiveness [46]. Sora Lee et al. [47] conducted a study on the reliability and validity of the Korean version of the scale. The scale has a total of 30 questions that are scored based on a four-point Likert scale. Sora Lee et al.'s (2012) study analyzed three sub-factors (cognitive impulsiveness, motor impulsiveness, and unplanned impulsiveness). Cronbach's alpha for all questions was 0.78 (for cognitive impulsiveness: 0.623, for motor impulsiveness: 0.626, for unplanned impulsiveness: 0.580) [47]. For this study, the Cronbach's alpha coefficient was 0.855.

2.3. *Data Analysis*

Investigators classified the participants into two groups (i.e., PIS and NPIS) based on their RCBS score. Byeon et al. [48] suggested that a score of 25 points or higher on the Korean version of the RCBS indicates a problematic shopper. We classified those whose RCBS score was 25 or more as the PIS group. Those whose RCBS-K score was below 25 were assigned to the non-PIS group (NPIS).

Chi-square tests of independence were employed to analyze the sociodemographic differences between the PIS and NPIS groups. For continuous variables, we used two-tailed t-tests to compare group mean differences. Mann–Whitney U test was adapted for non-normal distributed data. Pearson correlation analysis was used for data analysis. A multiple logistic regression analysis was used for four models. We estimated odds ratios (OR), adjusting for sex, age, and marital status (Model 1); adjusting for online shopping duration, online shopping amount, online shopping time, online shopping days, and experience of buying in excess of income (Model 2); adjusting for drinking and caffeine (Model 3); and adjusting for DES-K, CPGI-K, ZDS-K, SRI-MF, BIS-K (Model 4).

Model 4 is a full model. We considered statistical tests to be significant at an alpha level of 0.05 using a two-tailed test. We performed our data analyses using IBM SPSS Statistics version 21.0 (SPSS Inc., Chicago, IL, USA).

3. Results

Descriptive Statistics

The sample size of the online panel survey was 598 adults. Their sociodemographic characteristics included 50.7% (n = 303) men and 49.3% (n = 295) women. Seventyfive (12.5%) participants were classified as PIS. Thirty-four (45.3%) men and 41 (54.7%) women scored 25 or above, with no difference between them.

By age group, there was no statistically significant difference between PIS and non-PIS (NPIS) participants. As for marital status, the PIS participants were more often married than NPIS participants (Table 1). The PIS participants spent more money on shopping than did NPIS participants in the previous month. The PIS participants reported that they bought things more often in excess of their income than did NPIS participants.

With respect to shopping behaviors, PIS participants spent more money on shopping, more of their time on shopping-related activities, and had more buying experiences in excess of their income than did NPIS participants (Table 2).

Compared to the NPIS participants, the PIS participants reported higher alcohol use. The PIS group also had higher scores on measures of dissociation, gambling severity, depression, perceived stress, and impulsivity (Table 3). Pearson's correlation analysis revealed that the RCBS-K scores were positively related to DES-K, CPGI-K, ZDS-K, SRI-MF, and BIS-K ($p < 0.01$) (Table 4).

Table 1. Comparison of online shopper with and without problematic shopping behavior.

Variable		Demographics			Group Difference	
		PIS $n = 75$ (%), Mean (± SD)	NPIS $n = 523$ (%), Mean (± SD)	Total $n = 598$ (%), Mean (± SD)	χ2 /t	*p* Value
Gender	Male	34 (45.3)	269 (51.4)	303 (50.7)	0.977	0.323
	Female	41 (54.7)	254 (48.6)	295 (49.3)		
Age (years)	20–29	18 (24.0)	87 (16.6)	105 (17.6)	3.090	0.543
	30–39	16 (21.3)	114 (21.8)	130 (21.7)		
	40–49	17 (22.7)	131 (25.0)	148 (24.7)		
	50–59	17 (22.7)	120 (22.9)	137 (22.9)		
	60–69	7 (9.3)	71 (13.6)	78 (13.0)		
Marital status	Married	41 (54.7)	329 (62.9)	370 (61.9)	6.476	0.039
	Separated/ widowed/divorced	2 (2.7)	39 (7.5)	41 (6.9)		
	single	32 (42.7)	155 (29.6)	187 (31.3)		

PIS, Problematic Internet Shopping; NPIS, Non-Problematic Internet Shopping.

Table 2. Comparisons of online shopping pattern between PIS and NPIS participants.

		Shopping Pattern			Group Differences	
		PIS Mean or *n* (*SD or %*)	NPIS Mean or *n* (*SD or %*)	Total Mean or *n* (SD or %)	χ2 /t	*p* Value
Online shopping duration	year	11.06 (5.19)	10.37 (4.56)	10.46 (4.64)	1.202	0.230
Online shopping amount of budget	10k Won	46.69 (56.30)	27.84 (44.96)	30.21 (46.90)	2.776	0.007
Time spent shopping per day	minutes	109.84 (91.10)	47.26 (55.49)	55.12 (64.43)	5.796	0.000
The number of days shopping per week	days	4.37 (1.92)	3.33 (1.87)	3.46 (1.91)	4.477	0.000
Buying in the excess over the income	No	37 (49.3)	427 (81.6)	464 (77.6)	39.386	0.000
	Yes	38 (50.7)	96 (18.4)	134 (22.4)		

PIS, Problematic Internet Shopping; NPIS, Non-Problematic Internet Shopping.

Table 3. Mental health problems in participants with and without PIS.

Variables		Mental Health			Group Difference	
		PIS Mean or *n* (SD)	NPIS Mean or *n* (SD)	Total	χ2 /t	*p* Value
Alcohol use	Not at all	8 (10.7)	96 (18.4)	104 (17.4)	11.968	0.018
	Once a month	10 (13.3)	134 (25.6)	144 (24.1)		
	Twice a month	16 (21.3)	99 (18.9)	115 (19.2)		
	Once a week	17 (22.7)	88 (16.8)	105 (17.6)		
	Two or three times a week	24 (32.0)	106 (20.3)	130 (21.7)		
Caffeine use	cups	2.71 (1.84)	2.66 (2.01)	2.66 (1.98)	0.199	0.842
DES-K		41.78 (24.43)	14.30 (14.50)	17.75 (18.46)	9.502	0.000
CPGI-K		6.16 (6.79)	1.14 (2.96)	1.77 (4.02)	6.319	0.000
ZDS-K		50.47 (8.09)	42.33 (9.13)	43.35 (9.39)	8.017	0.000
SRI-MF		41.24 (17.09)	21.84 (15.57)	24.27 (17.02)	9.963	0.000
BIS-K		69.69 (10.30)	58.46 (9.14)	59.87 (10.00)	9.791	0.000

DES-K, The Korean version of the Dissociative Experiences Scale; CPGI-K, The Korean version of the Canadian Problem Gambling Index; ZDS-K, The Korean version of ZungSelf-Rating Depression Scale; SRI-MF, The modified form of the Stress Response Inventory; BIS-K, The Korean version of The Barratt Impulsive Scale-11-Revised.

Table 4. Reliabilities and Correlation between RCBS-K and other psychological scales.

Psychological Scales	Cronbach's Alpha	95% CI	r(*p*)
RCBS-K	0.906	0.894–0.917	1
DES-K	0.985	0.984–0.987	0.559 **
CPGI-K	0.947	0.941–0.954	0.422 **
ZDS-K	0.876	0.861–0.890	0.356 **
SRI-MF	0.958	0.953–0.963	0.461 **
BIS-K	0.855	0.837–0.871	0.484 **

** $p < 0.01$. RCBS-K, The Korean version of the Richmond Compulsive Buying Scale; DES-K, The Korean version of the Dissociative Experiences Scale; CPGI-K, The Korean version of the Canadian Problem Gambling Index; ZDS-K, The Korean version of Zung Self-Rating Depression Scale; SRI-MF, The modified form of the Stress Response Inventory; BIS-K, The Korean version of the Barratt Impulsive Scale-11-Revised.

Table 5 presents the result of the multivariate logistic regression analysis. The dependent variable was the RCBS-K, and the reference group was NPIS. The OR was calculated from Model 1 with explanatory variables of sex, age, and marital status that are sociodemographic aspects, but no variable was statistically significant. The variable of online shopping behaviors was added to Model 2, while the variables of Model 1 were controlled. Among them, the OR value for the time spent on shopping-related activities was 1.010, showing a tendency toward an increased risk of PIS following an increase in the time spent on shopping-related activities ($p < 0.001$). Those reporting the experience of buying in excess of their income showed a tendency toward a greater risk for PIS than those who did not report such an experience (OR = 2.961, $p < 0.001$). Model 3 evaluated the impact of alcohol and caffeine consumption. The risk of PIS rose by frequency of alcohol consumption. Notably, those who consumed alcohol two or three times a week showed a higher OR of 2.88 than those who did not consume alcohol at all, and the value was statistically significant ($p < 0.05$). However, there is not significant relation for the amount of caffeine consumption with PIS.

Model 3 showed statistical significance between the time spent on shopping-related activities during a day (OR = 1.010, $p< 0.001$) and the experience of buying in excess of income (OR = 2.860, $p < 0.001$), both of which were still variables that were associated with PIS. Model 4 was a full model that assessed the impact of DES-K, CPGI-K, ZDS-K, SRI-MF, and BIS-K while all the variables of Model 3 were controlled. The result showed that the risk of PIS increased when the tendency toward pathological dissociation was higher (OR = 1.044, $p < 0.001$) and that the risk of PIS was higher when the level of impulsiveness was higher (OR = 1.046, $p < 0.05$). In addition, time spent on shopping-related activities was correlated with PIS severity (OR = 1.008, $p < 0.01$), as well as with the duration of online shopping, indicating that the higher the online shopping duration was, the higher the risk of PIS (OR = 1.093, $p < 0.05$).

When we compared mental health problems between PIS participants with dissociation and without dissociation, PIS participants with dissociation showed higher levels of perceived stress, gambling problems, and impulsivity than did PIS participants without dissociation (Table 6).

Table 5. Contributing factors to RCBS-K identified in the multiple logistic regression.

Variable	Model 1				Model 2				Model 3				Model 4			
	B	S.E.	OR	*p* Value	B	S.E.	OR	*p* Value	B	S.E.	OR	*p*-Value	B	S.E.	OR	*p* Value
Gender (ref:male)																
female	0.253	0.250	1.288	0.310	−0.168	0.285	0.845	0.555	0.111	0.304	1.118	0.714	0.090	0.387	1.094	0.817
Age (ref:60~69)																
20~29	0.138	0.580	1.148	0.813	0.092	0.655	1.096	0.889	−0.002	0.658	0.998	0.997	−0.539	0.844	0.584	0.523
30~39	0.027	0.512	1.028	0.958	−0.436	0.574	0.647	0.448	−0.694	0.582	0.499	0.233	−1.116	0.753	0.328	0.138
40~49	0.121	0.482	1.128	0.802	0.266	0.531	1.304	0.617	0.048	0.536	1.050	0.928	−0.253	0.676	0.777	0.709
50~59	0.333	0.476	1.395	0.484	0.385	0.527	1.470	0.465	0.295	0.525	1.343	0.574	0.093	0.668	1.098	0.889
Marital status(ref:married)																
seperated/widowed/divorced	−0.915	0.747	0.400	0.221	−1.098	0.795	0.333	0.167	−1.097	0.790	0.334	0.165	−1.245	0.892	0.288	0.163
single	0.552	0.361	1.737	0.126	0.478	0.385	1.613	0.214	0.628	0.396	1.874	0.113	0.980	0.499	2.664	0.050
Online shopping duration					0.039	0.034	1.039	0.253	0.054	0.035	1.055	0.119	0.089	0.040	1.093	0.026
Online shopping amount					0.003	0.002	1.003	0.177	0.002	0.002	1.002	0.336	0.000	0.003	1.000	0.964
Time spent shopping per day					0.010	0.002	1.010	0.000	0.010	0.002	1.010	0.000	0.008	0.002	1.008	0.001
The number of days shopping per week					0.099	0.079	1.104	0.210	0.101	0.080	1.106	0.211	0.180	0.097	1.197	0.063
Buying exceeding the income (ref:No)																
Yes					1.086	0.287	2.961	0.000	1.051	0.294	2.860	0.000	0.608	0.372	1.837	0.102
Alcohol use (ref:Not at all)																
Once a month									−0.293	0.539	0.746	0.586	−0.275	0.601	0.759	0.647
Twice a month									0.552	0.505	1.737	0.274	0.111	0.617	1.117	0.858
Once a week									0.972	0.505	2.643	0.054	0.614	0.636	1.847	0.335
Two or three times a week									1.058	0.488	2.880	0.030	1.017	0.579	2.765	0.079
Caffeine consumption									−0.042	0.073	0.959	0.569	−0.018	0.100	0.982	0.854
DES-K													0.043	0.010	1.044	0.000
CPGI-K													0.075	0.042	1.078	0.073
ZDS-K													0.006	0.029	1.006	0.829
SRI-MF													0.021	0.014	1.021	0.131
BIS-K													0.045	0.022	1.046	0.035
-2LL	442.969				371.731				359.010				247.218			

RCBS-K, The Korean version of the Richmond Compulsive Buying Scale; DES-K, The Korean version of the Dissociative Experiences Scale; CPGI-K, The Korean version of the Canadian Problem Gambling Index; ZDS-K, The Korean version of ZungSelf-Rating Depression Scale; SRI-MF, The modified form of the Stress Response Inventory; BIS-K, The Korean version of the Barratt Impulsive Scale-11-Revise.

Table 6. Comparison of mental health problems in PIS participants with and without dissociation.

Variables	Mental Health		Group Difference	
	Normal (n = 19) Mean Rank	Dissociation (n = 56) Mean Rank	M-W U	p Value
CPGI-K	25.24	42.33	289.50	0.003
SRI-MF	25.42	42.27	293.00	0.004
BIS-K	26.18	42.01	307.50	0.006

PIS, Problematic Internet Shopping, CPGI-K, The Korean version of the Canadian Problem Gambling Index; SRI-MF, The modified form of the Stress Response Inventory; BIS-K, The Korean version of the Barratt Impulsive Scale-11-Revised; M-W U Mann–Whitney U.

4. Discussion

In line with the rapid increase in e-commerce activities, there have been growing concerns about PIS. However, little is known about the clinical and psychopathological aspects of PIS. In this cross-sectional study, we found out a significant prevalence rate (12.5%) of PIS among South Korean internet users. The number was lower than in those reported in previous studies (17.7% [49] and 33.6% [17]). This rate difference might be due to the use of a different survey method: The participants in the Kukar-Kinney et al. [49] study were women. Muller et al. [17] analyzed the pooled data of treatment-seeking patients with shopping disorders.

Contrary to previous findings which indicating that young people and women were more prone to manifest PIS [17,50], the results indicated no link between PIS and gender, age, and monthly income. Of the demographic variables, only marital status distinguished between the group, with PIS participants were more often single than NPIS members. The result is not consistent with past findings regarding link between online buying disorder and partnership status [17]. Some studies have argued that loneliness is an important reason why people are developing addictive behaviors. Andreassen et al. (2017) suggested that individuals who were no in a personal relationship were more prone to developing addictive social media use than people who had partners [51]. Elton-Marshall et al. (2018) presented that gambling to escape feeling of loneliness was linked with problem gambling severity. They suggested that being married was a protective factor against problem gambling severity [52].

The results showed that PIS participants connected to online shopping sites longer and more frequently, and they spent more money when online shopping. This result was consistent with previous studies [53,54]. Increasing the time spent using the internet has been considered an index of problematic use and possible addiction. Lemmens and Hendriks [55] indicated that the time spent playing online games was strongly related to internet addiction.

Although the amount of coffee intake did not distinguish PIS from NPIS, the results showed that individuals with PIS had more mental health predicaments as they presented with an increase in depression, perceived stress, impulsiveness, gambling, alcohol use, and dissociative experiences than the NPIS group. This result provides support for PIS as a behavioral addiction requiring clinical recognition and treatment.

In the current study, PIS participants' gambling severity was higher than NPIS participants. Although disordered gambling is the only behavioral addiction classified in DSM-5, problematic gambling was categorized into the Impulse-Control Disorder section in DSM-IV. In this regard, the association of PIS with gambling indicates that PIS is a behavioral addiction.

The relationship of PIS with impulsivity was consistent with previous studies. Impulsivity has been found to play an important role in the occurrence of addiction-related disorders [56,57]. Billieux et al. [58] reported that compulsive buying was positively correlated with impulsivity, and impulsivity was the most significant predictor of compulsive buying. Black [4] argued that pathological or compulsive buying should be classified as an impulse control disorder.

The key finding here was that the best-fit logistic regression model identified dissociation and impulsivity as being associated with PIS. The importance of dissociation in the psychopathology of addiction has been confirmed [32–34]. The literature indicates that symptoms of dissociation are present in a variety of mental disorders and connect to higher-burden illnesses and poorer treatment response [31,33,59–61].

As hypothesized, participants with PIS and dissociation exhibited poorer mental health, including higher stress levels, gambling, and impulsivity. According to Jacobs [34], dissociative symptoms resemble detachment states accompanying the acting-out phase of impulse control disorder. Maldonado and Spiegel (2019) indicated that dissociation represents more a disturbance in the organization or structure of mental contents than a disturbance in the mental contents themselves [30]. Lyssenko et al. (2018) suggested that the experience of dissociation can induce stress itself because it not only disrupts neurocognitive functioning but can also be perceived as losing control [31]. Kianpoor and Bakhshani (2012) reported that dissociation related with high-risk behaviors such as violence, heavy drinking, the use of illicit drugs, and dangerous driving [62]. From a clinical perspective, this finding underlines the importance of careful evaluation of dissociation symptoms. It will help health professionals to have recognition of people prone to high-risk behaviors as well as implement more effective strategies to prevent high-risk behaviors among at-risk populations.

The current research has important implications for the prevention of problematic internet shopping. As the results were reviewed, our data pointed to the importance of interventions aimed at helping internet-using shoppers increase their level of awareness to prevent dissociation. For example, introducing a time or monetary limit pop-up reminder into the internet-based shopping mall sites might help control impulsiveness. Stewart and Wohl [63] suggested that a monetary limit pop-up reminder was effective for internet gamblers to facilitate adherence to monetary limits.

Limitations

Despite this being one of the first studies to explore the clinical and psychopathological characteristics of PIS, this study has several limitations that might influence the generalizability of the findings. First, the use of cross-sectional, self-reported data in this study might have influenced our results through common method bias (e.g., causality problems; a prevalence-incidence bias) [64]. Second, because we used self-report measures instead of structured interviews, we cannot make a clinical diagnosis of dissociative disorders or clinically assess the relationship of PIS with different types of dissociative disorders (e.g., dissociative identity disorder, dissociative amnesia, depersonalization/derealization disorder). Third, we did not screen participants for the presence of traumatic psychological experiences, which can play an important role as the cause of dissociative disorders. Hence, we could not evaluate whether the dissociative disorder is a consequence of psychological trauma-related dissociative disorders. Finally, it is worth noting that we recruited participants through an online research service, ZINNOS R&C, which operates its own independent consumer panel in which participants are preregistered. The sample might not be representative of South Korean internet-based online shoppers or the general public. Besides, the response rate of this online panel study was 6.6%. The low rate may reflect the fact that only the panel members who have interested in the topic may have answered the invitation. Callegaro et al. [65] indicated that completion rates of online panel studies had a large variability going from 3%–91% with an average of 18%.

5. Conclusions

This study suggests that increasing awareness to prevent dissociation is important for addressing PIS. Individuals with PIS and dissociation showed a more severe mental health status than the PIS participants without dissociation. PIS participants with dissociation showed higher levels of perceived stress, gambling problems, and impulsivity than did PIS participants without dissociation. Introducing measures to prevent PIS and triggering of the state of detachment might increase a person's ability to tolerate negative affect.

Author Contributions: Writing—original draft, Y.-M.K. and T.K.L.; Writing—review & editing, Y.-M.K., S.R. and T.K.L. All authors have read and agreed to the published version of the manuscript.

References

1. Statistical Research Department. Internet Usage in South Korea-Statistics & Facts. Available online: https://www.statista.com/topics/2230/internet-usage-in-south-korea/ (accessed on 16 February 2020).
2. Statistics Korea. Online Shopping in July 2019. Available online: http://kostat.go.kr/portal/eng/pressReleases/1/index.board?bmode=read&aSeq=377546 (accessed on 4 September 2019).
3. Hirschman, E.C.; Holbrook, M.B. Hedonic consumption: Emerging concepts, methods and propositions. *J. Mark.* **1982**, *46*, 92–101. [CrossRef]
4. Black, D.W. A review of compulsive buying disorder. *World Psychiatry* **2007**, *6*, 14–18. [PubMed]
5. Müller, A.; Brand, M.; Claes, L.; Demetrovics, Z.; de Zwaan, M.; Fernández-Aranda, F.; Frost, R.O.; Jimenez-Murcia, S.; Lejoyeux, M.; Steins-Loeber, S. Buying-shopping disorder—is there enough evidence to support its inclusion in ICD-11? *CNS Spectr.* **2019**, 1–6. [CrossRef] [PubMed]
6. American Psychiatric Association. *Diagnostic and statistical manual of mental disorders (DSM-5®)*; American Psychiatric Pub: Arlington, VA, USA, 2013.
7. WHO. ICD-11 for Mortality and Morbidity Statistics. Available online: https://icd.who.int/browse11/l-m/en#/http%3a%2f%2fid.who.int%2ficd%2fentity%2f826065555 (accessed on 21 April 2020).
8. Gaebel, W.; Zielasek, J.; Reed, G.M. Mental and behavioural disorders in the ICD-11: Concepts, methodologies, and current status. *Psychiatr. Pol.* **2017**, *51*, 169–195. [CrossRef] [PubMed]
9. McElroy, S.L.; Keck, P.E., Jr.; Pope, H.G., Jr.; Smith, J.M.; Strakowski, S.M. Compulsive buying: A report of 20 cases. *J. Clin. Psychiatry* **1994**, *55*, 242–248.
10. O'Guinn, T.C.; Faber, R.J. Compulsive buying: A phenomenological exploration. *J. Consum. Res.* **1989**, *16*, 147–157. [CrossRef]
11. Black, D.W. Compulsive shopping. In *Clinical Manual of Impulse-control Disorders*; Hollander, E., Stein, D.J., Eds.; American Psychiatric Pub: Washington, DC, USA, 2006; pp. 203–228.
12. Scherhorn, G.; Reisch, L.A.; Raab, G. Addictive buying in West Germany: An empirical study. *J. Consum. Policy* **1990**, *13*, 355–387. [CrossRef]
13. Dittmar, H.; Beattie, J. Impulsive and excessive buying behaviour. In *Choice and public policy: The limits to welfare markets*; Taylor-Gooby, P., Ed.; Macmillan: London, UK, 1998; pp. 123–144.
14. Muller, A.; Mitchell, J.E.; de Zwaan, M. Compulsive buying. *Am. J. Addict.* **2015**, *24*, 132–137. [CrossRef]
15. Rose, S.; Dhandayudham, A. Towards an understanding of Internet-based problem shopping behaviour: The concept of online shopping addiction and its proposed predictors. *J. Behav. Addict.* **2014**, *3*, 83–89. [CrossRef]
16. Zhao, H.; Tian, W.; Xin, T. The Development and Validation of the Online Shopping Addiction Scale. *Front. Psychol* **2017**, *8*, 735. [CrossRef]
17. Muller, A.; Steins-Loeber, S.; Trotzke, P.; Vogel, B.; Georgiadou, E.; de Zwaan, M. Online shopping in treatment-seeking patients with buying-shopping disorder. *Compr. Psychiatry* **2019**, *94*, 152120. [CrossRef] [PubMed]
18. Lam, L.T.; Lam, M.K. The association between financial literacy and Problematic Internet Shopping in a multinational sample. *Addict. Behav. Rep.* **2017**, *6*, 123–127. [CrossRef] [PubMed]
19. Brewer, J.A.; Potenza, M.N. The neurobiology and genetics of impulse control disorders: Relationships to drug addictions. *Biochem. Pharmacol.* **2008**, *75*, 63–75. [CrossRef] [PubMed]
20. Granero, R.; Fernandez-Aranda, F.; Mestre-Bach, G.; Steward, T.; Bano, M.; Del Pino-Gutierrez, A.; Moragas, L.; Mallorqui-Bague, N.; Aymami, N.; Gomez-Pena, M.; et al. Compulsive Buying Behavior: Clinical Comparison with Other Behavioral Addictions. *Front. Psychol* **2016**, *7*, 914. [CrossRef] [PubMed]
21. Brand, M.; Wegmann, E.; Stark, R.; Muller, A.; Wolfling, K.; Robbins, T.W.; Potenza, M.N. The Interaction of Person-Affect-Cognition-Execution (I-PACE) model for addictive behaviors: Update, generalization to addictive behaviors beyond internet-use disorders, and specification of the process character of addictive behaviors. *Neurosci. Biobehav. Rev.* **2019**, *104*, 1–10. [CrossRef]
22. Ford, M.; Hakansson, A. Problem gambling, associations with comorbid health conditions, substance use, and behavioural addictions: Opportunities for pathways to treatment. *PLoS ONE* **2020**, *15*, e0227644. [CrossRef]
23. Moore, T.J.; Glenmullen, J.; Mattison, D.R. Reports of pathological gambling, hypersexuality, and compulsive shopping associated with dopamine receptor agonist drugs. *JAMA Intern. Med.* **2014**, *174*, 1930–1933. [CrossRef]
24. Aboujaoude, E. Compulsive buying disorder: A review and update. *Curr. Pharm. Des.* **2014**, *20*, 4021–4025. [CrossRef]

25. Grant, J.E.; Chamberlain, S.R. Caffeine's influence on gambling behavior and other types of impulsivity. *Addict. Behav.* **2018**, *76*, 156–160. [CrossRef]
26. Grant, J.E.; Potenza, M.N.; Weinstein, A.; Gorelick, D.A. Introduction to behavioral addictions. *Am. J. Drug Alcohol Abuse* **2010**, *36*, 233–241. [CrossRef]
27. Maraz, A.; van den Brink, W.; Demetrovics, Z. Prevalence and construct validity of compulsive buying disorder in shopping mall visitors. *Psychiatry Res.* **2015**, *228*, 918–924. [CrossRef] [PubMed]
28. Beranuy, M.; Carbonell, X.; Griffiths, M.D. A qualitative analysis of online gaming addicts in treatment. *Int. J. Ment. Health Addict.* **2013**, *11*, 149–161. [CrossRef]
29. Ludwig, A.M. The psychobiological functions of dissociation. *Am. J. Clin. Hypn.* **1983**, *26*, 93–99. [CrossRef] [PubMed]
30. Maldonado, J.R.; Spiegel, D. Dissociative disorders. In *The American Psychiatic Association Publishing Textbook of Psychiatry*, 7th ed.; Roberts, L.W., Ed.; American Psychiatric Association Publishing: Washington DC, USA, 2019; pp. 437–474.
31. Lyssenko, L.; Schmahl, C.; Bockhacker, L.; Vonderlin, R.; Bohus, M.; Kleindienst, N. Dissociation in Psychiatric Disorders: A Meta-Analysis of Studies Using the Dissociative Experiences Scale. *Am. J. Psychiatry* **2018**, *175*, 37–46. [CrossRef] [PubMed]
32. Craparo, G.; Ardino, V.; Gori, A.; Caretti, V. The relationships between early trauma, dissociation, and alexithymia in alcohol addiction. *Psychiatry Investig.* **2014**, *11*, 330–335. [CrossRef]
33. Karadag, F.; Sar, V.; Tamar-Gurol, D.; Evren, C.; Karagoz, M.; Erkiran, M. Dissociative disorders among inpatients with drug or alcohol dependency. *J. Clin. Psychiatry* **2005**, *66*, 1247–1253. [CrossRef]
34. Jacobs, D.F. Evidence for a common dissociative-like reaction among addicts. *J. Gambl. Behav.* **1988**, *4*, 27–37. [CrossRef]
35. Somer, E. Prediction of abstinence from heroin addiction by childhood trauma, dissociation, and extent of psychosocial treatment. *Addict. Res. Theory* **2003**, *11*, 339–348. [CrossRef]
36. Ridgway, N.M.; Kukar-Kinney, M.; Monroe, K.B. An expanded conceptualization and a new measure of compulsive buying. *J. Consum. Res.* **2008**, *35*, 622–639. [CrossRef]
37. Bernstein, E.M.; Putnam, F.W. Development, reliability, and validity of a dissociation scale. *J. Nerv. Ment. Dis.* **1986**, *174*, 727–735. [CrossRef]
38. Park, J.; Choe, B.; Kim, M.; Han, H.; Yoo, S.; Kim, S. Standardization of dissociative experiences scale-Korean version. *Korean J. Psychopathol* **1995**, *4*, 105–125.
39. Ferris, J.A.; Wynne, H.J. *The Canadian problem gambling index*; Final report; Canadian Centre on Substance Abuse: Ottawa, Canada, 2001.
40. Kim, A.Y.; Cha, J.E.; Kwon, S.J.; Lee, S.M. Construction and Validation of Korean Version of CPGI. *Korean J. Psychol. Gen.* **2011**, *30*, 1011–1038.
41. Zung, W.W. A self-rating depression scale. *Arch. Gen. Psychiatry* **1965**, *12*, 63–70. [CrossRef] [PubMed]
42. Passik, S.D.; Kirsh, K.L.; Donaghy, K.B.; Theobald, D.E.; Lundberg, J.C.; Holtsclaw, E.; Dugan, W.M., Jr. An attempt to employ the Zung Self-Rating Depression Scale as a "lab test" to trigger follow-up in ambulatory oncology clinics: Criterion validity and detection. *J. Pain Symptom Manag.* **2001**, *21*, 273–281. [CrossRef]
43. Lee, Y.H.; Song, J.Y. A study of the reliability and the validity of the BDI, SDS, and MMPI-D scales. *Korean J. Clin. Psychol.* **1991**, *10*, 98–113.
44. Choi, S.-M.; Kang, T.-Y.; Woo, J.-M. Development and validation of a modified form of the stress response inventory for workers. *J. Korean Neuropsychiatr. Assoc.* **2006**, *45*, 541–553.
45. Koh, K.B.; Park, J.K.; Kim, C.H.; Cho, S. Development of the stress response inventory and its application in clinical practice. *Psychosom. Med.* **2001**, *63*, 668–678. [CrossRef]
46. Patton, J.H.; Stanford, M.S.; Barratt, E.S. Factor structure of the Barratt impulsiveness scale. *J. Clin. Psychol.* **1995**, *51*, 768–774. [CrossRef]
47. Lee, S.-R.; Lee, W.-H.; Park, J.-S.; Kim, S.-M.; Kim, J.-W.; Shim, J.-H. The Study on Reliability and Validity of Korean Version of the Barratt Impulsiveness Scale-11-Revised in Nonclinical Adult Subjects. *J. Korean Neuropsychiat. Assoc.* **2012**, *51*, 378–386. [CrossRef]
48. Byeon, G.H.; Kim, R.; Han, J.H.; Ko, Y.M.; Roh, S.; Lee, T.K. Reliability and validity of the Korean version of Richmond Compulsive Buying Scale. *J. Korean Neuropsychiatr. Assoc.* **2017**, *56*, 35–44. [CrossRef]
49. Kukar-Kinney, M.; Ridgway, N.M.; Monroe, K.B. The relationship between consumers' tendencies to buy compulsively and their motivations to shop and buy on the Internet. *J. Retail.* **2009**, *85*, 298–307. [CrossRef]

50. Sorce, P.; Perotti, V.; Widrick, S. Attitude and age differences in online buying. *Int. J. Retail. Distrib. Manag.* **2005**, *33*, 122–132. [CrossRef]
51. Andreassen, C.S.; Pallesen, S.; Griffiths, M.D. The relationship between addictive use of social media, narcissism, and self-esteem: Findings from a large national survey. *Addict. Behav.* **2017**, *64*, 287–293. [CrossRef] [PubMed]
52. Elton-Marshall, T.; Wijesingha, R.; Sendzik, T.; Mock, S.E.; van der Maas, M.; McCready, J.; Mann, R.E.; Turner, N.E. Marital Status and Problem Gambling among Older Adults: An Examination of Social Context and Social Motivations. *Can. J. Aging* **2018**, *37*, 318–332. [CrossRef]
53. Lejoyeux, M.; Mathieu, K.; Embouazza, H.; Huet, F.; Lequen, V. Prevalence of compulsive buying among customers of a Parisian general store. *Compr. Psychiatry* **2007**, *48*, 42–46. [CrossRef]
54. Duroy, D.; Gorse, P.; Lejoyeux, M. Characteristics of online compulsive buying in Parisian students. *Addict.Behav* **2014**, *39*, 1827–1830. [CrossRef]
55. Leeman, R.F.; Potenza, M.N. A targeted review of the neurobiology and genetics of behavioural addictions: An emerging area of research. *Can. J. Psychiatry* **2013**, *58*, 260–273. [CrossRef]
56. Cudo, A.; Toroj, M.; Demczuk, M.; Francuz, P. Dysfunction of Self-Control in Facebook Addiction: Impulsivity Is the Key. *Psychiatr. Q.* **2019**, *91*, 91–101. [CrossRef]
57. Rømer Thomsen, K.; Callesen, M.B.; Hesse, M.; Kvamme, T.L.; Pedersen, M.M.; Pedersen, M.U.; Voon, V. Impulsivity traits and addiction-related behaviors in youth. *J. Behav. Addict.* **2018**, *7*, 317–330. [CrossRef]
58. Billieux, J.; Rochat, L.; Rebetez, M.M.L.; Van der Linden, M. Are all facets of impulsivity related to self-reported compulsive buying behavior? *Personal. Individ. Differ.* **2008**, *44*, 1432–1442. [CrossRef]
59. Schimmenti, A.; Bifulco, A. Toward a Better Understanding of the Relationship between Childhood Trauma and Psychiatric Disorders: Measurement and Impact on Addictive Behaviors. *Psychiatry Investig.* **2015**, *12*, 415–416. [CrossRef] [PubMed]
60. Schimmenti, A.; Guglielmucci, F.; Barbasio, C.P.; Granieri, A. Attachment disorganization and dissociation in virtual worlds: A study on problematic Internet use among players of online role playing games. *Clin. Neuropsychiatry* **2012**, *9*, 195–202.
61. Moskowitz, A. Dissociation and violence: A review of the literature. *Trauma Violence Abus.* **2004**, *5*, 21–46. [CrossRef] [PubMed]
62. Kianpoor, M.; Bakhshani, N.M. Trauma, dissociation, and high-risk behaviors. *Int. J. High. Risk Behav. Addict.* **2012**, *1*, 9–13. [CrossRef]
63. Stewart, M.J.; Wohl, M.J. Pop-up messages, dissociation, and craving: How monetary limit reminders facilitate adherence in a session of slot machine gambling. *Psychol. Addict. Behav.* **2013**, *27*, 268–273. [CrossRef]
64. Carlson, M.D.; Morrison, R.S. Study design, precision, and validity in observational studies. *J. Palliat. Med.* **2009**, *12*, 77–82. [CrossRef]
65. Callegaro, M.; Baker, R.P.; Bethlehem, J.; Göritz, A.S.; Krosnick, J.A.; Lavrakas, P.J. *Online panel research: A data quality perspective*; John Wiley & Sons: Hoboken, NJ, USA, 2014.

3

Problematic Social-Networks-Use in German Children and Adolescents—The Interaction of Need to Belong, Online Self-Regulative Competences, and Age

Sina Ostendorf [1], Elisa Wegmann [1] and Matthias Brand [1,2,*]

[1] Department of General Psychology: Cognition and Center for Behavioral Addiction Research (CeBAR), University of Duisburg-Essen, 47057 Duisburg, Germany; sina.ostendorf@uni-due.de (S.O.); elisa.wegmann@uni-due.de (E.W.)

[2] Erwin L. Hahn Institute for Magnetic Resonance Imaging, 45141 Essen, Germany

* Correspondence: matthias.brand@uni-due.de

Abstract: Adolescents nowadays spend much time communicating via social networks. Recent investigations also report a noticeable proportion showing a problematic usage behavior, underlining the importance of better understanding its development and maintenance in young individuals. Theoretical views on Internet-use disorders assume that specific predispositions and needs can contribute to addictive behaviors in interaction with further aspects including Internet-related cognitive biases. This study focuses on vulnerable individuals due to their age and investigates interactions between possible risk (need to belong, NTB) and protective factors (online self-regulative competences, OSRC). Participants (N = 466) between 10 and 17 years answered questionnaires assessing social-networks-use disorder symptoms, NTB, and OSRC. Moderated regression analysis revealed significant effects of age, NTB, and OSRC. Three-way interaction was also significant (potentially mainly caused by females), with highest social-networks-use disorder symptoms found for individuals with high NTB and low OSRC, especially when older. With high OSRC, symptoms were significantly lower for both younger and older individuals having high NTB. However, even if NTB was low, older individuals showed high social-networks-use disorder symptoms if their OSRC were low. The results highlight the importance of improving specific competences to prevent problematic usage behaviors, which should be considered in youth-tailored prevention and intervention programs.

Keywords: social-networks-use disorder; internet addiction; social media use; social networking sites; protective competences; self-regulation; social needs; behavioral addiction

---

1. Introduction

Given the easy and almost unrestricted access to social media applications including social networking sites such as Facebook, video/photo sharing platforms such as Instagram or TikTok, and instant messengers such as WhatsApp [1,2], social interactions are largely taking place online. By sharing personally relevant information via text, voicemails, photos, and videos, individuals can communicate with others, express and present themselves, build and maintain relationships, or perceive social support and connectedness [3–6]. Especially, young people seem to value the possibilities to socially interact via online applications as this can strengthen their sense of belonging [3,7]. Following research on media use of more than 1200 German children and adolescents between 12 and 19 years, 95% stated that they owned a smartphone [8]. In the new reports of EU Kids Online [9], the authors also point out that the majority of young people state that they use the smartphone almost all the time, with adolescents aged between 15 and 16 years spending about twice as much time online as children aged between nine and 11 years. Furthermore, during their leisure time, the usage of the Internet in general, the usage of the smartphone and listening to music were the most important media activities stated by German adolescents in 2018 [8]. Regarding the Internet-usage time, communication accounted for the largest share, followed by entertainment and games, whereby the most frequently used communication applications were WhatsApp, Instagram, and Snapchat [8]. Communicating and staying in contact with others is generally an important motive for using social networks, as highlighted by several authors [10–15]. Following Pertegal, Oliva, and Rodríguez-Meirinhos [16], research also identified two important motives for very young individuals: on the one hand obtaining social recognition, and on the other hand belonging to an online community.

Besides several advantages of such applications, research has also critically pointed out that the use of social networks can have undesired and disadvantageous consequences as well. These include, for example, becoming a cyberbullying victim, being threatened by other people, or experiencing problems in everyday life due to an uncontrolled usage [17–19]. Based on recent developments in the International Classification of Diseases (11th revision; ICD-11) including the classification of gaming disorder as a disorder due to addictive behaviors, researchers also discuss the problematic use of social networks as potential addictive behavior [20,21]. We therefore use the term social-networks-use disorder (although this term has not been included in classification systems, so far) for the definition of an uncontrolled, problematic use of online-communication applications. This describes the experiences of negative consequences due to, and the diminished control over the use of, social networks, whereby the communicative and social aspect is considered as the key element the users are addicted to rather than a certain device or platform [21,22].

With respect to age, being younger was associated with a more problematic social-networks-use [23] and an addictive/problematic smartphone behavior [24,25]. A recent study with a representative sample of German adolescents reported an estimated prevalence of 2.6% for a problematic social-networks-use [26], which is in line with the European-wide prevalence rates ranging from 0% to 2.1% [9]. The results emphasize the relevance of investigating this phenomenon in children and adolescents. They also highlight the importance of investigating potential mechanisms that contribute to the development and maintenance of such behaviors especially in younger ages in order to derive possible implications for prevention measures. Brand and colleagues [27,28] proposed a theoretical model (Interaction of Person-Affect-Cognition-Execution; I-PACE) to specify mechanisms involved in addictive behaviors, such as the problematic use of social networks. The I-PACE model is based on the assumption that specific motives, needs and further personal predispositions including social deficiencies interact with affective and cognitive processes (e.g., Internet-related cognitive biases such as specific expectancies) as well as executive components (e.g., reduced inhibitory control) and experiences of gratification and compensation in the development and maintenance of addictive behaviors. Considering the development of a (potential) social-networks-use disorder, the aforementioned processes may lead individuals to use specific social network services, resulting in experienced gratification and/or compensation (supposedly depending on individual's addiction stage) and possible reinforcement processes, potentially intensifying a problematic/addictive usage [28]. As one further extension of the development and maintenance of a social-networks-use disorder, Wegmann and Brand [22] specify the addiction process and assume that especially individuals with specific needs (e.g., high need to belong) or social deficits may be vulnerable to developing a problematic use of social networks, since the experience of gratified social needs may reinforce specific expectancies and coping styles, and may lead to the recurring decision to use those applications to strengthen a sense of belonging.

Need to belong in general is considered as a fundamental human motivation [29] and was previously assumed to be a driving motivator for the use of social networks, such as Facebook [5]. The authors propose a dual-factor model of Facebook use including two primary social needs: the need to belong, representing an intrinsic drive to get in touch and connect with others, and the need for self-presentation, corresponding to impression management processes [5]. A study by Beyens, Frison, and Eggermont [30] confirmed the proposed role of need to belong and found that it is associated with an increased Facebook usage. Besides, Martin [31] reported a positive correlation between individual's need to belong and the frequency of checking social media applications as well as intensity of social-networks-use. Wang and colleagues [32] even found that the need to belong depicts a positive predictor for what the authors called "adolescent smartphone addiction" (note that this term has been criticized recently [33]), and it further moderated the relation between self-esteem and addiction. The results show that the effect of need to belong as a risk factor interacts with further variables, which is consistent with the I-PACE model by Brand and colleagues [28]. Brand and colleagues [28] also highlight that the relevance of predisposing variables, such as usage motives, on the tendency of an additive behavior is related to further affective and cognitive responses such as Internet-related cognitive biases (e.g., specific Internet use expectancies, Internet-related competences). Several studies have already shown that the interaction of those Internet-related cognitive biases and predisposing variables is related to addictive behavior online [2,34].

Focusing on the relevance of Internet-related competences, Wegmann, Stodt, and Brand [35], for example, found that self-regulative competences as a subdomain of Internet literacy had a negative effect on the symptom severity of a social-networks-use disorder and, moreover, partially mediated the relationship between psychopathological symptoms and symptom severity. The authors conclude that the ability to regulate one's own online behavior and to be able to manage time online might be a preventive factor for developing a social-networks-use disorder [35]. This conclusion is consistent with further studies, since Stodt, Wegmann, and Brand [36] also found a preventive effect of self-regulation when considering an unspecific Internet-use disorder. Additionally, Błachnio and Przepiorka [37] concluded that a dysfunction of self-regulation and self-control might be a risk factor for a problematic social-networks-use and van Deursen, Bolle, Hegner, and Kommers [24] found a negative effect of general self-regulation on addictive usage behaviors, but a positive effect of age on self-regulation. This underlines, on the one hand, that self-regulation can be considered as a protective factor preventing a problematic usage, and, on the other hand, implies that especially young individuals seem to have a low level of general self-regulation. Going one step further, online-specific self-regulative competences could play an even more relevant role when investigating problematic social-networks-use in children and adolescents.

Based on the aforementioned studies and theoretical assumptions, we argue that there is strong need for investigating not only possible factors in isolation, but especially their interactions in order to better understand the development and maintenance of a problematic social-networks-use. This appears particularly important in order to support prevention and intervention measures especially for young individuals. We hypothesize that the effect of need to belong on symptoms of a social-networks-use disorder is moderated by the ability to self-regulate one's own online behavior. However, when keeping in mind that the online behavior of children and adolescents is notably changing during childhood and adolescence [9], the interaction effects have to be controlled for a possible age effect. This means that we include age as first predictor to investigate the effect age may have on symptoms of a social-networks-use disorder. We then include need to belong and online self-regulative competences to examine their incremental validity beyond age. Overall, we aim at gaining deeper insights into the protective power of online self-regulative competences by focusing on individuals at risk due to their age and specific needs. Our hypothesized model is depicted in Figure 1.

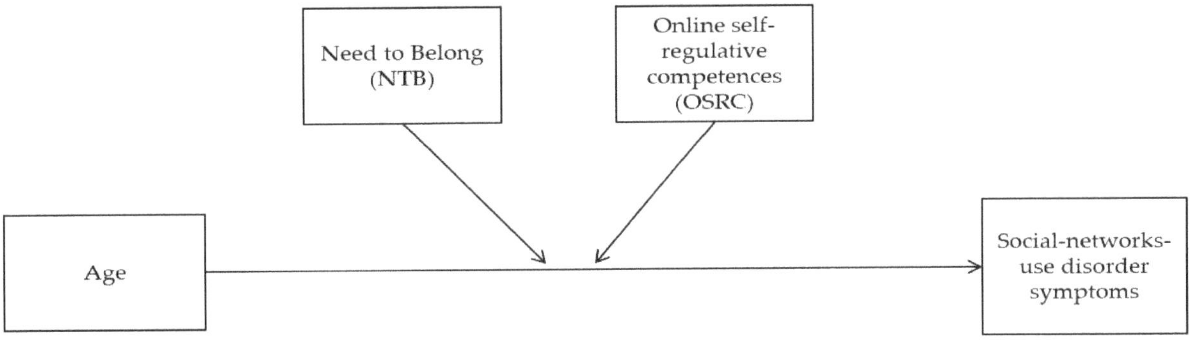

Figure 1. Hypothesized moderated regression model with age, need to belong (NTB), and online self-regulative competences (OSRC) as (moderating) predictors for a social-networks-use disorder.

2. Materials and Methods

2.1. Participants and Recruitment

In total, 466 children and adolescents between 10 and 17 years (M = 13.05, SD = 1.99) took part in the current study. Of these, 239 were female and 227 were male. The frequency of individual ages was as follows: 10.5% (49 participants) were 10 years old, 18.2% (85) 11 years, 12.2% (57) 12 years, 18.9% (88) 13 years, 13.1% (61) 14 years, 11.4% (53) 15 years, 13.5% (63) 16 years, and 2.2% (10) 17 years. The modal value and the median are both 13 years. Of all participants, 85 stated that they used the Internet actively up to one hour a day, 186 between two and three hours, 105 participants four to five hours, 79 more than five hours a day, and 11 did not report their daily Internet usage time. All participants used at least one social media application including social networking sites, instant messaging services, and photo/video sharing platforms. The most frequently mentioned app was WhatsApp (used by 99.4% of all participants), followed by Instagram (55.4%) and Snapchat (55.2%). Facebook was used by 18.7% of all participants, the Facebook Messenger by 12.9% and Twitter by 15.7%. Besides, 37.1% of the participants mentioned that they used further services, for example Musical.ly (now known as TikTok), YouTube, or Threema. Of all 466 participants, 463 stated to have either their own or a shared smartphone and/or computer. Another three participants reported to not have their own or a shared device but stated that they used at least one social media application. Since the usage of specific applications is the more relevant condition, we decided to include these three participants as well.

The current sample was recruited in 2017 at a local secondary school in a large city in Western Germany within a period of two weeks. Parents and legal guardians gave their informed consent before children and adolescents voluntarily took part. All persons involved (including parents/legal guardians, teaching staff, school administration, and pupils) were informed about the purpose of the study and participants were surveyed in the school premises. The processing of all questionnaires (including those that are not relevant for the current manuscript) took about 40 to 60 min. The study was conducted in accordance with the Declaration of Helsinki and was approved by the local ethics committee of the University of Duisburg-Essen (date: 21st March, 2017).

2.2. Instruments

2.2.1. Short Internet Addiction Test Modified for Social-Networks-Use Disorder

In order to measure tendencies of a social-networks-use disorder, a modified version [35] of the short Internet Addiction Test [38] was answered by the participants. This modified version measures subjectively perceived problems in an individual's everyday life due to the use of online-communication applications, including active (e.g., creating posts/content) and passive use (e.g., browsing/reading content) of social networking sites, (micro-)blogs, and instant messengers. In the course of this study, 4 out of originally 12 items were applied in order to keep the study as short as possible. These four items are considered as key items to represent the scale's two factors: loss of control/time management and social problems/craving [39,40]. In detail, these were "How often do you find that you spend more time with online-communication applications than you intended?" and "How often do you neglect household chores to spend more time with online-communication applications?" for the subscale loss of control/time management and "How often do you feel preoccupied with online-communication applications when offline, or fantasize about online-communication applications?" and "How often do you choose to spend more time with online-communication applications over going out with others?" for social problems/craving. All items were rated from 1 = "never" to 5 = "very often". The sum score for the four items ranges from 4 to 20. The overall internal consistency was $\alpha = 0.844$.

2.2.2. Single-Item Need to Belong Scale

The extent of participants' need to belong was assessed by applying the Single-Item Need to Belong Scale by Nichols and Webster [41], to which a good reliability and validity is attributed. Here, participants are asked to rate from 1 = "disagree" to 4 = "agree" to what extent the statement "I have a strong need to belong" applies to them. Thus, higher scores indicate a higher need to belong.

2.2.3. Internet Literacy Questionnaire

To measure online self-regulative competences we used the Internet Literacy Questionnaire developed by Stodt and colleagues [42]. The scale assesses four dimensions of individuals' competences in using the Internet in an adequate way, namely technical expertise, reflection and critical analysis, production and interaction, and self-regulation. The subscale self-regulation consists of five items, which are answered on a 6-point Likert scale ranging from 0 = "strongly disagree" to 5 = "strongly agree". For the purpose of this manuscript, we only used the subscale self-regulation with an internal consistency of $\alpha = 0.752$. A mean score was used to test the hypothesis.

2.3. *Statistical Analyses*

We used SPSS 24.0 for Windows [43] for the statistical analyses. To test for bivariate correlations, we calculated Pearson's correlations, with $|r| \geq 0.10$ indicating a small, $|r| \geq 0.30$ a medium, and $|r| \geq 0.50$ a large effect [44]. To test our hypothesis, we calculated a hierarchical moderated regression analysis with age as first predictor, need to belong in the second step, and online self-regulative competences in the third step, followed by the respective interactions and the three-way interaction in the last step. All independent variables were Fisher's z-transformed beforehand. Here, standardized beta-coefficients serve as measure of the effect sizes (with similar indicators for a small, medium, and large effect as for correlations). Simple Slopes analyses are calculated for significant three-way interactions.

3. Results

3.1. *Descriptive Values and Multivariate Statistics*

Mean values with corresponding standard deviations of all variables are depicted in Table 1. Table 1 also shows bivariate correlations between symptoms of a social-networks-use disorder, age, need to belong, and online self-regulative competences. Social-networks-use disorder symptoms were significantly positively correlated with need to belong and age, and significantly negatively with online self-regulative competences. Need to belong was not significantly correlated with both age and online self-regulative competences, whereas age and online self-regulative competences were significantly negatively correlated. Moreover, age correlated significantly positively with participants' Internet usage time ($r = 0.369$, $p < 0.001$; $n = 455$ due to missing data) and social-networks-use disorder symptoms also correlated significantly positively with Internet usage time ($r = 0.465$, $p < 0.001$, $n = 455$).

Table 1. Mean values, standard deviations, range, and bivariate correlations between the study's variables.

Variables	*M*	*SD*	Range	1	2	3
1. Social-networks-use disorder symptoms	7.56	3.55	4–20			
2. Age	13.05	1.98	10–17	0.310 ***		
3. NTB	2.58	0.89	1–4	0.202 ***	−0.073	
4. OSRC	3.02	1.20	0–5	−0.374 ***	−0.136 **	−0.077

Note. NTB = Need to belong; OSRC = Online self-regulative competences. $^{**}p < 0.01$; $^{***}p < 0.001$.

3.2. Hypothesis Testing

In accordance with our hypothesized model, we calculated a hierarchical moderated regression analysis including age, need to belong (NTB), and online self-regulative competences (OSRC), corresponding interactions and the three-way interaction, in the order as stated. The results revealed significant main effects for age, NTB, and OSRC in the prediction of social-networks-use disorder symptoms (see Figure 2). Furthermore, the interaction effect of age and OSRC was significant ($\Delta R^2 = 0.011$, $\Delta F = 6.88$, $p = 0.009$), as well as the three-way interaction ($\Delta R^2 = 0.009$, $\Delta F = 5.36$, $p = 0.021$). The overall model also proved to be significant, explaining 27.1% of the criterion's variance ($R^2 = 0.271$, F (7, 458) = 24.35, $p < 0.001$) and supporting our assumptions. Investigating the interaction effects in more detail, simple slopes analyses were calculated. The results showed that, especially when older, individuals with high NTB and low OSRC showed the highest tendency towards a social-networks-use disorder (grey line, Figure 3). With higher OSRC, social-network-use disorder tendency was significantly lower in both younger and older individuals with high NTB (yellow line, Figure 3), whereby younger individuals showed even less a social-networks-use disorder tendency than older ones. However, older individuals even had a high social-networks-use disorder tendency when their NTB was low, if they also had low OSRC (blue line, Figure 3). Finally, especially older individuals showed the lowest social-networks-use disorder tendency when they had a low NTB level and also high OSRC. Corresponding statistical values including beta-coefficients are depicted in Table 2.

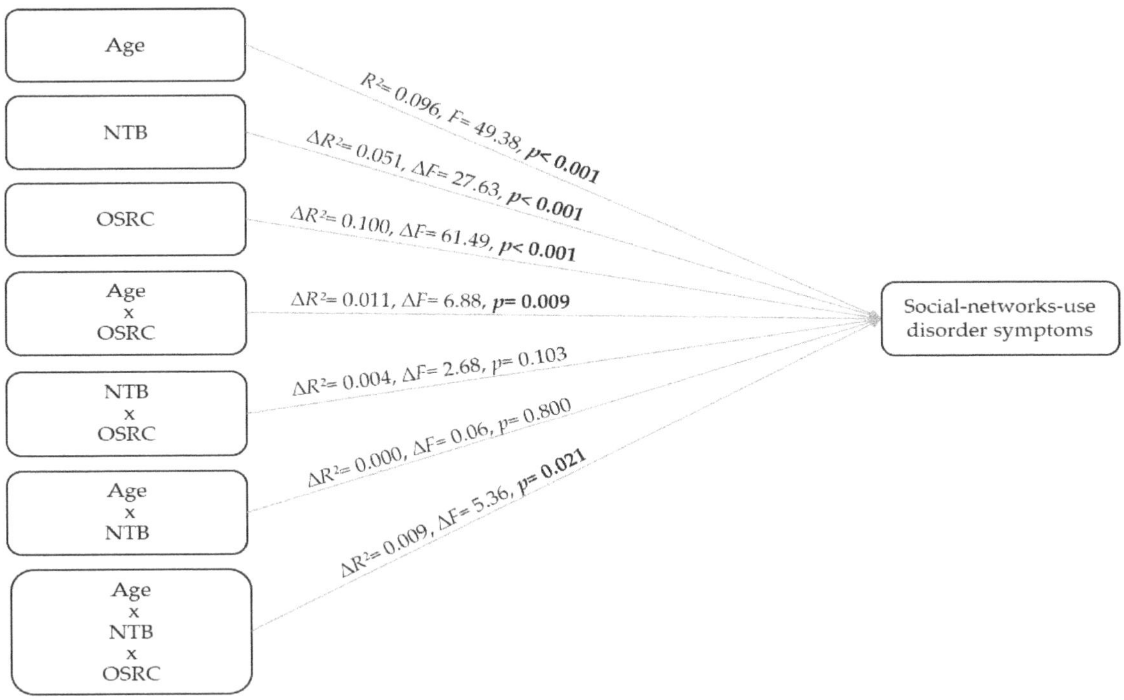

Figure 2. Results of the hierarchical moderated regression analysis with symptoms of a social-networks-use disorder as dependent variable and age, need to belong (NTB), and online self-regulative competences (OSRC) as well as their respective interactions as predictors.

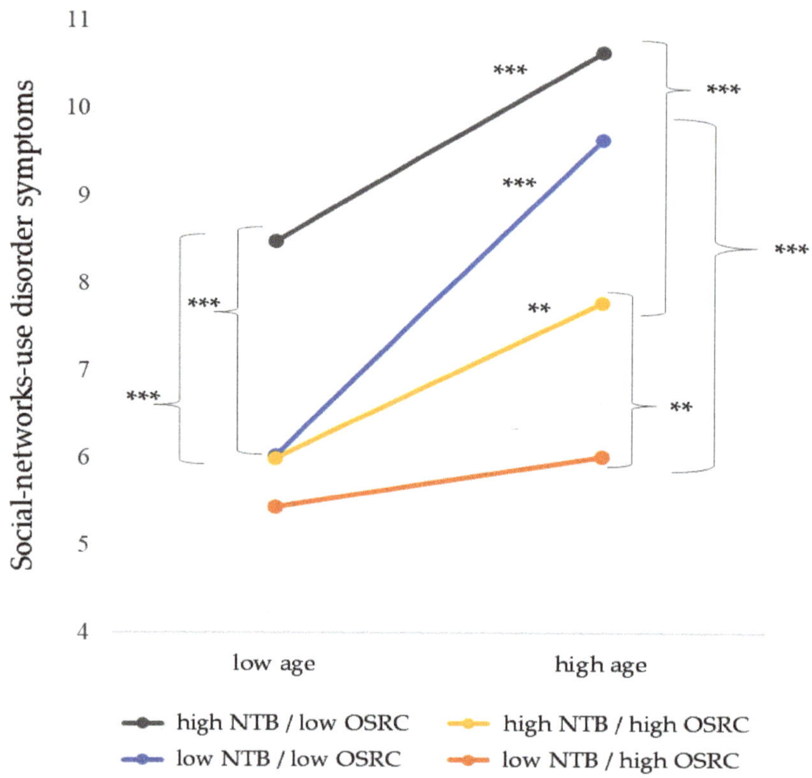

Figure 3. Simple Slopes visualizing the significant three-way interaction between age, need to belong (NTB), and online self-regulative competences (OSRC) in the prediction of social-networks-use disorder symptoms with ** $p < 0.01$, *** $p < 0.001$ and for all significant t: $2.65 \leq t \leq 6.78$.

Table 2. Regression coefficients of the hierarchical moderated regression analysis with age, need to belong (NTB), and online self-regulative competences (OSRC) predicting symptoms of a social-networks-use disorder.

Predictors	*B*	*SE (B)*	ß	*t*	*p*
Age	0.51	0.07	0.287	7.00	<0.001
NTB	0.81	0.16	0.203	4.98	<0.001
OSRC	−1.00	0.12	−0.337	−8.11	<0.001
Age × OSRC	−0.18	0.06	−0.115	−2.81	0.005
NTB × OSRC	−0.14	0.13	−0.044	−1.05	0.295
Age × NTB	−0.02	0.09	−0.009	−0.21	0.834
Age × NTB × OSRC	0.17	0.07	0.097	2.32	0.021

Note. Significant values depicted in bold.

3.3. Additional Analyses

As an additional analysis, we controlled our results for a potential gender effect. We firstly calculated t-tests for independent samples. We found no significant differences between male and female participants for NTB, OSRC, and age (all $p \geq 0.768$). For tendencies towards a social-networks-use disorder, we found a significant difference (males: $M = 6.62$, $SD = 3.14$; females: $M = 8.45$, $SD = 3.68$; t (458.76) $= -5.77$, $p < 0.001$, $d = -0.54$). We therefore calculated our hierarchical moderated regression analysis in a second step again separately for male and female participants. For female participants, the effects of age ($\beta = 0.403$, $p < 0.001$), NTB ($\beta = 0.214$, $p < 0.001$), and OSRC ($\beta = -0.418$, $p < 0.001$) on symptoms of a social-networks-use disorder remained significant, as well as the interaction effect of age and OSRC ($\beta = -0.180$, $p < 0.001$) and the three-way interaction ($\beta = 0.151$, $p = 0.003$). The overall model also proved to be significant and explained 46.0% of the criterion's variance ($R^2 = 0.460$, $F(7, 231)$

= 28.11, $p < 0.001$). For male participants we also found significant effects of age (β = 0.197, $p = 0.003$), NTB (β = 0.188, $p = 0.004$), and OSRC (β = −0.244, $p < 0.001$), but no significant interaction effect of age and OSRC (β = −0.045, $p = 0.488$) and no significant three-way interaction (β = 0.052, $p = 0.440$). The overall model remained significant, explaining 14.4% of the criterion's variance ($R^2 = 0.144$, F (7, 219) = 5.25, $p < 0.001$). The subsequently calculated Chow Test comparing both hierarchical moderated regression analyses yielded a significant difference (F (8, 450) = 9.37, $p < 0.001$).

4. Discussion

In this study, we aimed at contributing to a better understanding of a social-networks-use disorder by considering on the one hand specific needs that can increase the risk of developing a problematic use and on the other hand Internet-related cognitive biases (i.e., self-regulative competences) that may play a protective role. Further, we focused on a specific group of individuals that can be particularly vulnerable to developing a social-networks-use disorder due to their young age (here individuals between 10 and 17 years) and investigated interaction effects between the respective variables. The calculated hierarchical moderated regression analysis revealed that 27.1% of the variance of social-networks-use disorder symptoms were explained by the included variables: age, need to belong, and online self-regulative competences. All variables showed a significant main effect and the three-way interaction was significant as well. Controlling for possible gender effects, the results illustrate that female participants showed higher symptoms of social-networks-use disorder compared to male participants, which is in line with previous studies [45,46]. When calculating the hierarchical moderated regression analysis separately for male and female participants, we found significant main effects of age, need to belong, and online self-regulative competences for both males and females, but the interaction effects only remained significant for females.

The results illustrate that high need to belong may be a vulnerability factor for the development and maintenance of a problematic social-networks-use. The findings support previous reports regarding the important role of need to belong [32] and further strengthen that this fundamental social need is also an important factor for both female and male children and adolescents as potentially contributing to a problematic use of social networks. The findings therefore extend current research, illustrating the relevance of specific needs and motives for using social networks for children and adolescents. It can be assumed that online social networks are perceived as a possible means to feel socially integrated and to gratify individual's need for belonging [22]. Especially, young individuals may perceive a strong desire to fulfill their need to belong, since they find themselves in an important developmental part of life, in which their respective peer group occupies an important place [30,47,48] and depicts an essential source of experiencing social support [49]. Thus, particularly younger individuals seem to be a vulnerable group that might use social networks in an intense and potentially critical way to gratify their need to be socially connected and accepted. This is in line with the I-PACE model [27,28], assuming that the aim to fulfill personal needs and motives can lead individuals to use specific applications, resulting in gratification and reinforcement processes, which potentially ends up in an uncontrolled or even problematic usage.

The current results also indicate that high online self-regulative competences are associated with significantly lower symptoms of a problematic use of social-networks in both males and females, underlining the protective power of specific competences and abilities [24,35,36]. These results strengthen previously found empirical results and again broaden current research since the ability to regulate one's own online behavior appears to be an important competence for very young individuals too.

When investigating the interaction between both factors (need to belong and online self-regulative competences), we found no significant effect on the symptom severity of a social-networks-use disorder, neither for females, males, nor when taking both together. This result appears unexpected at first sight, but when considering that age had a significantly positive direct effect (for both males and females), and the interaction between online self-regulative competences and age was (except for males) also significant, it becomes apparent that the investigation of interactions between potential risk and protective factors for individuals, and especially for females, in such a young phase of life additionally needs to consider age. As the three-way interaction illustrates, children and adolescents with a high need to belong and low online self-regulative competences had a high problematic usage behavior, especially when older within the age range of 10 to 17 years. Higher online self-regulative competences, in contrast, were related to significantly lower social-networks-use disorder symptoms. Moreover, especially younger adolescents seem to benefit from online self-regulative competences when having a high need to belong level, as they showed even fewer symptoms of a social-networks-use disorder compared to older ones. However, even if the need to belong is low, particularly older individuals seem to need good self-regulative competences in order to reduce the risk of developing social-networks-use disorder symptoms. Since these interaction effects have been observed in the overall sample and in the female sample, but not in the male sample, they may be mainly caused by female participants. However, in accordance with the I-PACE model, interactions between different variables are assumed to contribute to the development and maintenance of problematic behavior generally for both men and women [28]. Thus, theoretically assumed interactions may be valid for both genders, although gender-specific differences can occur. Regarding the for females significant interaction between online self-regulative competences and age, which was not significant for males, one possible explanation could be that female participants reported higher symptoms of problematic behavior compared to male participants and thus the interaction effect may mainly occur along with a certain symptom severity. Moreover, the development of specific competences in such a young phase of life could be assumed to proceed differentially in females and males and thus potential mechanisms may also be different at this age [50]. The development of these competences with regard to age and gender and their relevance as protective mechanisms for a problematic behavior must specifically be addressed in further, preferably longitudinal studies.

Overall, the current results emphasize the importance of improving specific competences, particularly the ability to regulate oneself when using social networks, in order to prevent problematic usage behaviors. They further underline that in a time span of only seven years, young individuals undergo many changes, and that specific needs and also competences can vary in their importance for the development and maintenance of a social-networks-use disorder depending on the respective age. Since we, moreover, found that age and symptoms of a social-networks-use disorder were positively correlated with Internet usage time within our sample, it seems that using the Internet is rapidly increasing in a relatively short age span and is additionally related to the risk of a problematic social-networks-use. This is also in line with the investigation of Smahel and colleagues [9], illustrating that time online is significantly higher in young adults aged between 15 and 16 years, compared to children aged between nine and 11 years.

Based on the current results and statistics, it appears important to investigate the developmental trends of specific needs as well as competences and strategies especially in youths, in order to better understand respective problematic and uncontrolled behaviors. Self-regulation is likely to be learnable and research has previously pointed out that, when growing older, not only personal interests or goals change, but individuals also seem to be more settled [24,51]. However, loneliness and the need to be socially integrated can also increase over lifetime, probably leading people to use media even more [24,52]. Thus, possible changes and developments over time need to be considered more strongly when investigating the interplay of different factors in the context of problematic online behaviors. In addition, possible differences between male and female children and adolescents should also be kept in mind. Along with changes in people's communicative behavior, future research also needs to continue addressing the question of when the usage of social networks in order to fulfill personal needs becomes a significant problem. Using specific applications to keep social contact might in general be beneficial, but if individuals, and particularly youths, for example, lose control over their usage and perceive those applications as the only way to feel socially integrated, this might increase negative consequences in their everyday lives.

To sum up, we strongly recommend that prevention programs should focus specifically on the improvement in self-regulative competences from early on, including children and adolescents, to sensitize for a more functional use of social networks. Individuals should be supported in developing competence to better evaluate an appropriate extent of their social-networks-use, which is meant as an individually suitable amount not causing problems in everyday life. Teaching specific competences in school could help individuals not to satisfy their personal needs exclusively online, but to focus on a more purposeful behavior. Totally restricting youths' access to the Internet and its various platforms to communicate is certainly not an effective strategy [53], particularly since young individuals use social networks not only to avoid parental control, but also to handle their friendships and to explore new identities in an important stage of life [54,55]. In contrast, finding ways to empower users, especially children and adolescents, seems to be a promising approach, which is also noted by other authors [56]. Besides the communication context, specific competences and needs might also play an important role in other specific Internet-use disorders since there is, at least for German youths, a slow but noticeable increase in using social networks for entertainment and gaming purposes [8]. Thus, the interplay between potential risk and protective factors should also be further investigated in other specific Internet-use disorders.

For the current study, some limitations have to be mentioned. The current sample only includes children and adolescents aged between 10 and 17 years from one school in Germany and is not representative for the whole German population in this age range. The information given is based on self-reports, which did not include questions on participants' primary time of day to use social networks and other applications. However, this information can be very important for prevention and intervention measures and should be included in future studies [57]. Furthermore, we were not able to assess epidemiological characteristics, such as social class or rural/urban area, but since these aspects can give valuable insights, they should be considered in future studies. Overall, it should be noted that conclusions about possible changes in self-regulation or other specific competences over lifespan from childhood to adolescence are only based on the cross-sectional investigation and should be examined with a longitudinal study. However, the results are a first hint about the relevance of specific needs, specific competences such as online self-regulation, and age on a problematic use of social networks. In addition, younger individuals should also be taken further into account, since certain needs and the use of the smartphone have already been observed in even younger ages. In order to be able to generalize the results, future studies are still needed.

5. Conclusions

Childhood and adolescence depict an important phase of life in which communicating and socializing is increasingly realized via social networks. The current study revealed that in particular female children and adolescents aged between 10 and 17 years with high need to belong and low online self-regulative competences showed a high tendency towards a social-networks-use disorder, especially when they were older. High online self-regulative competences were associated with significantly lower symptom severity. Moreover, even if the need to belong was low, older individuals were found to need high online self-regulative competences in order to prevent a problematic usage. Accordingly, prevention and intervention programs should try to improve individuals' competences, in particular self-regulation, to support individuals in using social networks in a purposeful and appropriate way.

Author Contributions: Conceptualization, S.O., E.W. and M.B.; Formal analysis, S.O.; Methodology, S.O. and E.W.; Project administration, M.B.; Supervision, M.B.; Visualization, S.O.; Writing – original draft, S.O.; Writing – review & editing, S.O., E.W. and M.B. All authors have read and agreed to the published version of the manuscript.

Acknowledgments: We thank Marco Fileccia for actively supporting us in conducting this study. Additionally, we thank Benjamin Stodt for the assistance regarding the administrative support and study design as well as Lydia Harbarth and Dario Stolze for the assistance regarding data preparation.

References

1. Aichner, T.; Jacob, F. Measuring the degree of corporate social media use. *Int. J. Mark. Res.* **2015**, *57*, 257–275. [CrossRef]
2. Wegmann, E.; Ostendorf, S.; Brand, M. Is it beneficial to use Internet-communication for escaping from boredom? Boredom proneness interacts with cue-induced craving and avoidance expectancies in explaining symptoms of Internet-communication disorder. *PLoS ONE* **2018**, *13*, e0195742. [CrossRef]
3. Allen, K.A.; Ryan, T.; Gray, D.L.; McInerney, D.M.; Waters, L. Social media use and social connectedness in adolescents: The positives and the potential pitfalls. *Aust. Educ. Dev. Psychol.* **2014**, *31*, 18–31. [CrossRef]
4. Cheung, C.; Lee, Z.W.Y.; Chan, T.K.H. Self-disclosure in social networking sites: The role of perceived cost, perceived benefits and social influence. *Internet Res.* **2015**, *25*, 279–299. [CrossRef]
5. Nadkarni, A.; Hofmann, S.G. Why do people use Facebook. *Pers. Individ. Dif.* **2012**, *52*, 243–249. [CrossRef] [PubMed]
6. Taddicken, M.; Jers, C. The uses of privacy online: Trading a loss of privacy for social web gratifications? In *Privacy Online*; Trepte, S., Reinecke, L., Eds.; Springer: Berlin, Germany, 2011; pp. 143–156.
7. Davis, K. Friendship 2.0: Adolescents' experiences of belonging and self-disclosure online. *J. Adolesc.* **2012**, *35*, 1527–1536. [CrossRef]
8. Feierabend, S.; Rathgeb, T.; Reutter, T. *JIM-Studie 2018—Jugend, Information, Medien—Basisuntersuchung zum Medienumgang 12- 19-Jähriger*; Medienpädagogischer Forschungsverbund Südwest (LFK, LMK): Stuttgart, Germany, 2018; pp. 1–80.
9. Smahel, D.; Machackova, H.; Mascheroni, G.; Dedkova, L.; Staksrud, E.; Ólafsson, K.; Livingstone, S.; Hasebrink, U. *EU Kids Online 2020: Survey Results from 19 Countries*; EU Kids Online: London, UK, 2020; pp. 1–156.
10. Guedes, E.; Sancassiani, F.; Carta, M.G.; Campos, C.; Machado, S.; King, A.L.S.; Nardi, A.E. Internet addiction and excessive social networks use: What about Facebook? *Clin. Pract. Epidemiol. Ment. Heal.* **2016**, *12*, 43–48. [CrossRef]
11. Ryan, T.; Chester, A.; Reece, J.; Xenos, S. The uses and abuses of Facebook: A review of Facebook addiction. *J. Behav. Addict.* **2014**, *3*, 133–148. [CrossRef]
12. Giannakos, M.N.; Chorianopoulos, K.; Giotopoulos, K.; Vlamos, P. Using Facebook out of habit. *Behav. Inf. Technol.* **2013**, *32*, 594–602. [CrossRef]
13. Lee, E.; Lee, J.A.; Moon, J.H.; Sung, Y. Pictures speak louder than words: Motivations for using Instagram. *Cyberpsychology Behav. Soc. Netw.* **2015**, *18*, 553–556. [CrossRef]
14. Alzougool, B. The impact of motives for Facebook use on Facebook addiction among ordinary users in Jordan. *Int. J. Soc. Psychiatry* **2018**, *64*, 528–535. [CrossRef] [PubMed]
15. Pertegal-Vega, M.A.; Oliva-Delgado, A.; Rodríguez-Meirinhos, A. Systematic review of the current state of research on online social networks: Taxonomy on experience of use. *Communicar* **2019**, *27*, 81–91. [CrossRef]
16. Pertegal, M.A.; Oliva, A.; Rodríguez-Meirinhos, A. Development and validation of the Scale of Motives for Using Social Networking Sites (SMU-SNS) for adolescents and youths. *PLoS ONE* **2019**, *14*, 1–21. [CrossRef] [PubMed]
17. Aharony, N. Relationships among attachment theory, social capital perspective, personality characteristics, and Facebook self-disclosure. *Aslib J. Inf. Manag.* **2016**, *68*, 362–386. [CrossRef]
18. Debatin, B.; Lovejoy, J.P.; Horn, A.K.; Hughes, B.N. Facebook and online privacy: Attitudes, behaviors, and unintended consequences. *J. Comput. Commun.* **2009**, *15*, 83–108. [CrossRef]
19. Andreassen, C.S. Online social network site addiction: A comprehensive review. *Curr. Addict. Reports* **2015**, *2*, 175–184. [CrossRef]
20. Kuss, D.J.; Griffiths, M.D. Social networking sites and addiction: Ten lessons learned. *Int. J. Environ. Res. Public Health* **2017**, *14*, 311. [CrossRef]

21. Wegmann, E.; Müller, S.M.; Ostendorf, S.; Brand, M. Highlighting Internet-communication disorder as further Internet-use disorder when considering neuroimaging studies. *Curr. Behav. Neurosci. Reports* **2018**, *5*, 295–301. [CrossRef]
22. Wegmann, E.; Brand, M. A narrative overview about psychosocial characteristics as risk factors of a problematic social networks use. *Curr. Addict. Reports* **2019**, *6*, 402–409. [CrossRef]
23. Andreassen, C.S.; Billieux, J.; Griffiths, M.D.; Kuss, D.J.; Demetrovics, Z.; Mazzoni, E.; Pallesen, S. The relationship between addictive use of social media and video games and symptoms of psychiatric disorders: A large-scale cross-sectional study. *Psychol. Addict. Behav.* **2016**, *30*, 252–262. [CrossRef]
24. Van Deursen, A.J.A.M.; Bolle, C.L.; Hegner, S.M.; Kommers, P.A.M. Modeling habitual and addictive smartphone behavior: The role of smartphone usage types, emotional intelligence, social stress, self-regulation, age, and gender. *Comput. Human Behav.* **2015**, *45*, 411–420. [CrossRef]
25. Lopez-Fernandez, O.; Honrubia-Serrano, L.; Freixa-Blanxart, M.; Gibson, W. Prevalence of problematic mobile phone use in British adolescents. *Cyberpsychology Behav. Soc. Netw.* **2014**, *17*, 91–98. [CrossRef] [PubMed]
26. Wartberg, L.; Kriston, L.; Thomasius, R. Internet gaming disorder and problematic social media use in a representative sample of German adolescents: Prevalence estimates, comorbid depressive symptoms and related psychosocial aspects. *Comput. Human Behav.* **2020**, *103*, 31–36. [CrossRef]
27. Brand, M.; Young, K.S.; Laier, C.; Wölfling, K.; Potenza, M.N. Integrating psychological and neurobiological considerations regarding the development and maintenance of specific Internet-use disorders: An Interaction of Person-Affect-Cognition-Execution (I-PACE) model. *Neurosci. Biobehav. Rev.* **2016**, *71*, 252–266. [CrossRef] [PubMed]
28. Brand, M.; Wegmann, E.; Stark, R.; Müller, A.; Wölfling, K.; Robbins, T.W.; Potenza, M.N. The Interaction of Person-Affect-Cognition-Execution (I-PACE) model for addictive behaviors: Update, generalization to addictive behaviors beyond internet-use disorders, and specification of the process character of addictive behaviors. *Neurosci. Biobehav. Rev.* **2019**, *104*, 1–10. [CrossRef]
29. Baumeister, R.F.; Leary, M.R. The need to belong: Desire for interpersonal attachments as a fundamental human motivation. *Psychol. Bull.* **1995**, *117*, 497–529. [CrossRef]
30. Beyens, I.; Frison, E.; Eggermont, S. 'I don't want to miss a thing': Adolescents' fear of missing out and its relationship to adolescents' social needs, Facebook use, and Facebook related stress. *Comput. Human Behav.* **2016**, *64*, 1–8. [CrossRef]
31. Martin, P. *Social Media and the Need to Belong: Self-Esteem, Narcissism and Life Satisfaction on Facebook and Instagram*; Higher Diploma Final Year Project, Dublin Business School: Dublin, Ireland, 2018.
32. Wang, P.; Zhao, M.; Wang, X.; Xie, X.; Wang, Y.; Lei, L. Peer relationship and adolescent smartphone addiction: The mediating role of self-esteem and the moderating role of the need to belong. *J. Behav. Addict.* **2017**, *6*, 708–717. [CrossRef]
33. Montag, C.; Wegmann, E.; Sariyska, R.; Demetrovics, Z.; Brand, M. How to overcome taxonomical problems in the study of Internet use disorders and what to do with 'smartphone addiction'? *J. Behav. Addict.* **2019**, 1–7. [CrossRef]
34. Laier, C.; Wegmann, E.; Brand, M. Personality and cognition in gamers: Avoidance expectancies mediate the relationship between maladaptive personality traits and symptoms of Internet-gaming disorder. *Front. Psychiatry* **2018**, *9*, 304. [CrossRef]
35. Wegmann, E.; Stodt, B.; Brand, M. Addictive use of social networking sites can be explained by the interaction of Internet use expectancies, Internet literacy, and psychopathological symptoms. *J. Behav. Addict.* **2015**, *4*, 155–162. [CrossRef] [PubMed]
36. Stodt, B.; Wegmann, E.; Brand, M. Predicting dysfunctional Internet use: The role of age, conscientiousness, and Internet literacy in Internet addiction and cyberbullying. *Int. J. Cyber Behav. Psychol. Learn.* **2016**, *6*, 28–43. [CrossRef]
37. Błachnio, A.; Przepiorka, A. Dysfunction of self-regulation and self-control in Facebook addiction. *Psychiatr. Q.* **2016**, *87*, 493–500. [CrossRef]
38. Pawlikowski, M.; Altstötter-Gleich, C.; Brand, M. Validation and psychometric properties of a short version of Young' s Internet Addiction Test. *Comput. Human Behav.* **2013**, *29*, 1212–1223. [CrossRef]
39. Müller, M.; Brand, M.; Mies, J.; Lachmann, B.; Sariyska, R.Y.; Montag, C. The 2D:4D marker and different forms of Internet use disorder. *Front. Psychiatry* **2017**, *8*, 213. [CrossRef]

40. Wegmann, E.; Oberst, U.; Stodt, B.; Brand, M. Online-specific fear of missing out and Internet-use expectancies contribute to symptoms of Internet-communication disorder. *Addict. Behav. Reports* **2017**, *5*, 33–42. [CrossRef] [PubMed]
41. Nichols, L.; Webster, G.D. The single-item need to belong scale. *Pers. Individ. Dif.* **2013**, *55*, 189–192. [CrossRef]
42. Stodt, B.; Brand, M.; Sindermann, C.; Wegmann, E.; Li, M.; Zhou, M.; Sha, P.; Montag, C. Investigating the effect of personality, Internet literacy, and use expectancies in Internet-use disorder: A comparative study between China and Germany. *Int. J. Environ. Res. Public Health* **2018**, *15*, 579. [CrossRef]
43. IBM. *SPSS Statistics*; IBM: Armonk, NY, USA, 2017.
44. Cohen, J. *Statistical Power Analysis for the Behavioral Sciences*; Lawrence Erlbaum Associates: Hillsdale, MI, USA, 1988.
45. Cudo, M.; Torój, M.; Demczuk, M.; Francuz, P. Dysfunction of self-control in Facebook addiction: Impulsivity is the key. *Psychiatr. Q.* **2020**, *91*, 91–101. [CrossRef]
46. Xie, W.; Karan, K. Predicting Facebook addiction and state anxiety without Facebook by gender, trait anxiety, Facebook intensity, and different Facebook activities. *J. Behav. Addict.* **2019**, *8*, 79–87. [CrossRef]
47. Brown, B.B.; Larson, J. Peer relationships in adolescence. In *Handbook of Adolescent Psychology*; Lerner, R.M., Steinberg, L., Eds.; Wiley: New York, NY, USA, 2009; pp. 74–103.
48. Pombeni, M.L.; Kirchler, E.; Palmonari, A. Identification with peers as a strategy to muddle through the troubles of the adolescent years. *J. Adolesc.* **1990**, *13*, 351–369. [CrossRef]
49. Bokhorst, C.L.; Sumter, S.R.; Westenberg, P.M. Social support from parents, friends, classmates, and teachers in children and adolescents aged 9 to 18 years: Who is perceived as most supportive? *Soc. Dev.* **2010**, *19*, 417–426. [CrossRef]
50. Montroy, J.J.; Bowles, R.B.; Skibbe, L.E.; McClelland, M.M.; Morrison, F.J. The development of self-regulation across early childhood. *Dev. Psychol.* **2016**, *52*, 1744–1762. [CrossRef]
51. Diehl, M.; Semegon, A.B.; Schwarzer, R. Assessing attention control in goal pursuit: A component of dispositional self-regulation. *J. Pers. Assess.* **2006**, *86*, 306–317. [CrossRef] [PubMed]
52. Pearson, J.C.; Carmon, A.; Tobola, C.; Fowler, M. Motives for communication: Why the millennial generation uses electronic devices. *J. Commun. Speech Theatr. Assoc. North Dakota* **2010**, *22*, 45–56.
53. Staksrud, E.; Ólafsson, K.; Livingstone, S. Does the use of social networking sites increase children's risk of harm? *Comput. Human Behav.* **2013**, *29*, 40–50. [CrossRef]
54. Boyd, D. *It's Complicated: The Social Lives of Networked Teens*; Yale University Press: New Haven, CT, USA, 2014; pp. 1–281.
55. Jöckel, S.; Wilhelm, C. Everything under control? The role of habit strength, deficient self-regulation and media literacy for the use of social network sites among children and adolescents. In *Youth and Media: Current Perspectives on Media Use and Effects*, 1st ed.; Kühne, R., Baumgartner, S.E., Koch, T., Hofer, M., Eds.; Nomos: Baden-Baden, Germany, 2018; pp. 55–74.
56. Livingstone, S.; Ólafsson, K.; Staksrud, E. Risky social networking practices among 'underage' users: Lessons for evidence-based policy. *J. Comput. Commun.* **2013**, *18*, 303–320. [CrossRef]
57. Adan, A. A chronobiological approach to addiction. *J. Subst. Use* **2013**, *18*, 171–183. [CrossRef]

4

Relationship between Self-Identity Confusion and Internet Addiction among College Students: The Mediating Effects of Psychological Inflexibility and Experiential Avoidance

Kuan-Ying Hsieh [1,2], Ray C. Hsiao [3,4], Yi-Hsin Yang [2,5], Kun-Hua Lee [6,*] and Cheng-Fang Yen [2,7,*]

1 Department of Child and Adolescent Psychiatry, Kaohsiung Municipal Kai-Syuan Psychiatric Hospital, Kaohsiung 80276, Taiwan
2 Graduate Institute of Medicine, College of Medicine, Kaohsiung Medical University, Kaohsiung 80708, Taiwan
3 Department of Psychiatry and Behavioral Sciences, University of Washington School of Medicine, Seattle, WA 98195, USA
4 Department of Psychiatry, Children's Hospital and Regional Medical Center, Seattle, WA 98195, USA
5 School of Pharmacy, Kaohsiung Medical University, Kaohsiung 80708, Taiwan
6 Department of Educational Psychology and Counseling, National Tsing Hua University, Hsin-Chu City 30013, Taiwan
7 Department of Psychiatry, Kaohsiung Medical University Hospital, Kaohsiung 80708, Taiwan
* Correspondence: kunhualee627@gmail.com (K.-H.L.); chfaye@cc.kmu.edu.tw (C.-F.Y.)

Abstract: Internet addiction (IA) has become a major public health problem among college students. The aim of this study was to examine the relationship between self-identity confusion and IA and the mediating effects of psychological inflexibility and experiential avoidance (PI/EA) indicators in college students. A total of 500 college students (262 women and 238 men) were recruited. Their levels of self-identity were evaluated using the Self-Concept and Identity Measure. Their levels of PI/EA were examined using the Acceptance and Action Questionnaire-II. The severity of IA was assessed using the Chen Internet Addiction Scale. The relationships among self- identity, PI/EA, and IA were examined using structural equation modeling. The severity of self-identity confusion was positively associated with both the severity of PI/EA and the severity of IA. In addition, the severity of PI/EA indicators was positively associated with the severity of IA. These results demonstrated that the severity of self-identity confusion was related to the severity of IA, either directly or indirectly. The indirect relationship was mediated by the severity of PI/EA. Self-identity confusion and PI/EA should be taken into consideration by the community of professionals working on IA. Early detection and intervention of self-identity confusion and PI/EA should be the objectives for programs aiming to lower the risk of IA.

Keywords: internet addiction; PI; EA; self-identity

---

1. Introduction

1.1. Internet Addiction in College Students

Internet addiction (IA) has become a major global public health problem. Several studies have proposed diagnostic criteria for IA based on various concepts originally adopted from formal psychiatric disorders such as substance dependence [1] and pathological gambling [2] on the *Diagnostic and Statistical Manual of Mental Disorders, Fourth Edition (DSM-IV)* and impulse control disorder in the

DSM-IV Text Revision [3]. Although IA has not been recognized as a disorder by the DSM-5 or the World Health Organization, the related diagnosis of internet gaming disorder and gaming disorder have been included in the Conditions for Further Study section of the DSM-5 [4] and the International Classification of Diseases, respectively. The common concepts of IA in previous studies include poorly controlled preoccupations, urges, withdrawal, tolerance, or behaviors associated with Internet use which lead to psychosocial distress and significant impairment at home, school, and work, as well as in health or interpersonal relationships [5–7]. The measures developed based on these concepts of IA can be used to evaluate the individuals' severity of IA on the evidence base.

IA is predominant among young people, especially college students. College students normally have free and unlimited access to the Internet, flexible schedules, and are free from their parents' interference. They use the Internet for studying, gaming, social networking, gambling, chatting, shopping, and watching pornographic videos [8,9]. Previous epidemiological studies revealed that the prevalence of IA in college students varied by country. Specifically, IA prevalence ranged from 3.7% in Japan [10] to 13.6% in China [11] and 15.3% in Taiwan [12]. Such deviation has been attributed to differences in study design, sampling, assessment tools, diagnostic criteria, and cultural backgrounds. IA has been associated with sleep disturbance [13], poor physical health [14], low self-esteem [15], poor academic performance [16], and mental health problems [17]. Therefore, IA is a crucial problem among college students and requires investigation.

Investigating the factors related to IA is the first step toward preventing its incidence and providing early treatment to improve mental health. IA is the result of interaction between individuals and their environment [18,19]. Several individual factors have been discovered as being related to IA. Research has demonstrated that depression and anxiety [20,21], a decreased sense of meaning in life [22], personality traits such as psychosis and bizarre mentation [23], low self-esteem [24,25], cognitive distortion [26], high impulsivity [27], and poor emotional regulation [28] are all associated with IA.

1.2. *Self-Identify Confusion and IA*

Self-concept formation, also termed personal identity formation, as a main developmental task in adolescence, includes the acceptance of physical changes and the development of social and emotional competencies and self-efficacy [29]. Previous studies have indicated significant deficits in self-concept formation among individuals with IA compared with those without [30,31]. Deficits in self-concept are characterized by low self-esteem; indecisiveness; inability to concentrate on required or suggested tasks; uncertainty regarding future objectives; an unclear description of self; problems in engaging in intimate relationships; and difficulties in social roles, values, and selections [29]. The Internet provides individuals with deficits in self-concept with a tempting environment to socially interact with others anonymously and to obtain success through Internet gaming or other such activities. These characteristics of the Internet increase the risk of IA in individuals with deficits in self-concept [32,33]. However, a lack of performance-related positive experiences on the Internet might also further deteriorate a self-concept deficit [31]. Therefore, investigating the relationship between self-identify confusion and IA is crucial to understand the mechanism of developing IA.

1.3. *Psychological Inflexibility and Experiential Avoidance and IA*

Psychological inflexibility and experiential avoidance (PI/EA) are defined as rigid strategies guided by psychological reactions and an unwillingness to experience unpleasant events or privations [34]. PI/EA contributes to the development, maintenance, and exacerbation of problematic behaviors [35], problematic substance use [36,37], and addictive behaviors [38]. PI/EA was reported as being positively associated with IA in one cross-sectional study [39].

1.4. *Self-Identify Confusion and PI/EA*

Research has determined three common types of self-identity confusion: Disturbed identity (a strong tendency to acquire the thoughts, feelings, beliefs, and problems of others in adulthood) [40], unconsolidated identity (failure to take on self-defining roles and demonstrate stable beliefs, attitudes, and values) [41], and lack of identity (sudden and dramatic shifts in self-image with respect to goals, values, vocational aspirations, sexual identity, and types of friends) [4]. People with self-identity confusion may experience difficulties accepting themselves and defusing cognitive stockades, and therefore, tend to develop PI/EA [42]. Some studies have revealed the therapeutic importance of cultivating psychological flexibility in the face of a self-identity crisis resulting from physical illness [43,44]. Throughout the process of accepting one's current self, psychological flexibility is essential for reconstructing one's self-concept, such that behaviors can be changed or redirected according to personal long-term values [44]. Although it is also possible that PI/EA may predate the maturity of self-concept, the present study focused on the influence of self-identity confusion on PI/EA and examined the mediating effects of PI/EA on the relationship between self-identity confusion and IA [45].

1.5. *Aims of This Study*

No study has examined the relationship between self-identify confusion, PI/EA, and IA. This study investigated the mediating effects of PI/EA on the relationship between self-identity confusion and IA among college students. We hypothesized that self-identity confusion is positively associated with IA and that PI/EA mediate the relationship between self-identity confusion and IA.

2. Materials and Methods

2.1. *Participants*

Participants were recruited using an advertisement posted for college students aged between 20 and 30 years. Five hundred and three college students responded to the advertisement. Of them, three were excluded due to difficulties in understanding the meaning of research questionnaires. In total, 238 male and 262 female college students coming from 70 colleges located across Taiwan participated in this study. Their mean age was 22.1 years, with a standard deviation of 1.8 years. Written informed consent was obtained from all the participants prior to the assessment. The study was approved by the Institutional Review Board of Kaohsiung Medical University Hospital.

2.2. *Measures*

Self-Concept and Identity Measure. We used the Self-Concept and Identity Measure (SCIM) to assess the level of self-identity confusion [46]. The 27-item SCIM contains three subscales: Disturbed identity, unconsolidated identity, and lack of identity. Exploratory factor analysis revealed a three-factor structure of the SCIM in the college students. Confirmatory factor analysis validated the three-factor structure in the community sample. The correlations between the three subscales ranged from 0.32 to 0.53 [46]. Each item was rated using a seven-point Likert scale ranging from 1 (strongly disagree) to 7 (strongly agree). High total scores on the three subscales indicated tendencies for disturbed identity, unconsolidated identity, and lack of identity. The Cronbach's α of the subscales in the present study ranged from 0.74 to 0.82.

Chen Internet Addiction Scale. We used the self-administered Chen Internet Addiction Scale (CIAS) to evaluate the participants' severity of IA in the month preceding the study. The CIAS contains 26 items that are rated using a four-point Likert-type scale, with the total score ranging from 26 to 104 [47]. A higher total score indicated a more severe level of IA. The CIAS contains five subscales, including symptoms of compulsive use, withdrawal, tolerance, and problems in interpersonal relationships and health/time management. The Cronbach's α of the five subscales of the CIAS in the present study ranged from 0.78 to 0.90. The 67/68 cutoff point of the CIAS is the optimal diagnostic cutoff point for Internet addiction in college students [48].

The Acceptance and Action Questionnaire-II. The Acceptance and Action Questionnaire-II (AAQ-II) [49] was revised from the original AAQ [50]. The AAQ-II consists of seven statements that represent various aspects of PI (e.g., "My painful experiences and memories make it difficult for me to live a life that I would value") and EA (e.g., "I am afraid of my feelings"). The participants were asked to rate each of these statements on a scale of 1 (never true) to 7 (always true) based on their current experiences. A higher total score indicated a higher level of PI/EA. A study reported that the AAQ-II has adequate internal consistency and convergent and divergent validity [49]. The Cronbach's α of the AAQ-II in the present study was 0.88.

2.3. Procedure and Statistical Analysis

Research assistants explained the procedures and methods for completing the research questionnaires to the participants individually. The participants were allowed to ask questions if they encountered problems while completing the questionnaires, and the research assistants helped them to resolve their problems.

The hypothesized model for the relationships among self-identity confusion, PI/EA, and IA is presented in Figure 1. Structural equation modeling (SEM) was used to estimate the parameters, test the model adequacy, and evaluate the extent of agreement between the observed data and the covariance matrix estimated from the model [51]. Amos version 18.0 software (IBM SPSS) was used to examine the goodness-of-fit index (GFI). The maximum likelihood method was used to analyze the data. In addition, the GFI, non-normed fit index (NFI), incremental fit index (IFI), comparative fit index (CFI), root mean square error of approximation (RMSEA), and standardized root mean square residual (SRMR) were used to evaluate the goodness of fit of the model [52]. On the basis of the goodness-of-fit requirement, the NFI, GFI, IFI, and CFI should be higher than 0.9; values of the RMSEA and SRMR lower than 0.05 are good; and values ranging between 0.05 and 0.09 are acceptable [52]. The Sobel test was applied to examine the mediating effect of PI/EA on the relationship between self-identity confusion and IA. A two-tailed p value of <0.05 was considered statistically significant.

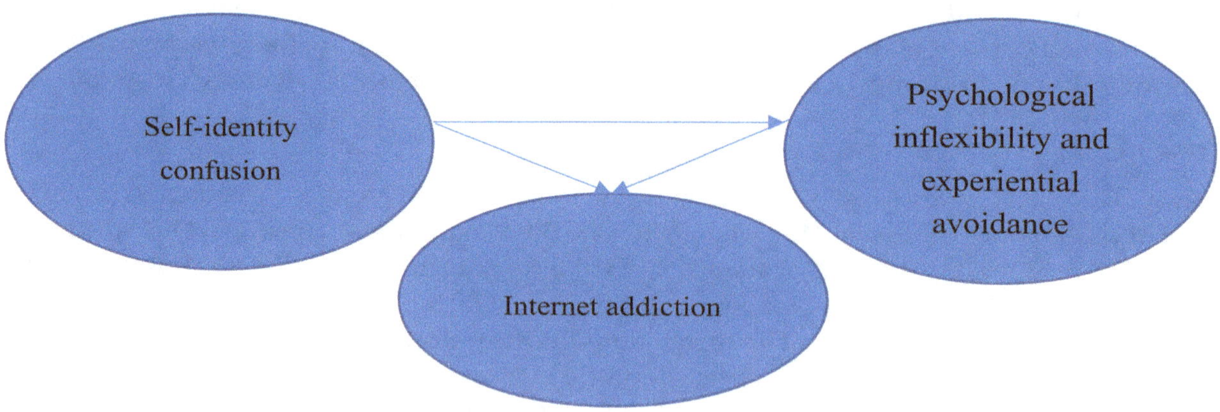

Figure 1. Hypothesized model of the associations among self-identity confusion, Internet addiction, and psychological inflexibility and experiential avoidance (PI/EA).

2.4. Ethics

The study procedures were carried out in accordance with the Declaration of Helsinki. The Institutional Review Boards of Kaohsiung Medical University Hospital approved the study (ethical approval code number: KMUH-IRB-20120249; date of ethical approval: 30 August 2012). All participants were informed about the study and provided written informed consent.

3. Results

In total, 85 (17%) participants were identified as having Internet addiction. The means, standard deviations, and correlation matrices of the measured variables are shown in Table 1. The results revealed significant correlations among the measured variables.

Table 1. The correlation matric of measured variables.

	Mean (SD)	1	2	3	4	5	6	7	8	9	10
1. Tolerance	8.9 (2.5)	1	0.66 *	0.67 *	0.57 *	0.70 *	0.26 *	0.28 *	0.26 *	0.24 *	0.30 *
2. Withdrawal	11.4 (3.3)		1	0.77 *	0.52 *	0.58 *	0.30 *	0.31 *	0.28 *	0.24 *	0.31 *
3. Compulsion	10.6 (3.1)			1	0.58 *	0.69 *	0.28 *	0.32 *	0.30 *	0.27 *	0.37 *
4. Time manage	10.5 (3.4)				1	0.68 *	0.20 *	0.27 *	0.23 *	0.21 *	0.29 *
5. Interpersonal	14.2 (4.2)					1	0.25 *	0.36 *	0.28 *	0.27 *	0.37 *
6. Psychological inflexibility	7.4 (3.3)						1	0.63 *	0.29 *	0.36 *	0.47 *
7. Experiential avoidance	9.8 (3.8)							1	0.35 *	0.39 *	0.52 *
8. Disturbed identity	33.7 (8.6)								1	0.24 *	0.56 *
9. Unconsolidated identity	18.4 (8.7)									1	0.52 *
10. Lack of identity	24.8 (8.4)										1

* $p < 0.001$.

The goodness-of-fit indices of SEM for the hypothesized model on the relationships among self-identity confusion, PI/EA, and IA are listed in Table 2. The estimated coefficients of paths in the hypothesized model are presented in Figure 2. The results found that all NFI, GFI, IFI, and CFI values were higher than 0.9 and the SRMR value was lower than 0.05, which indicated the goodness of fit of the model was good. According to Hu and Bentler [52], the value of the RMSEA (0.085) was at the acceptable level. The result of the Sobel test confirmed the mediating effect of PI/EA on the relationship between self-identity confusion and IA ($Z = 5.135$, $p < 0.05$).

Moreover, all paths in the hypothesized model were significant. The severity of self-identity confusion was positively associated with the severity of IA and PI/EA. In addition, the severity of PI/EA was positively associated with the severity of IA. The severity of self-identity confusion was directly related to the severity of IA and indirectly related to the severity of IA through the increasing severity of PI/EA.

Table 2. The goodness-of-fit index of structural equation modeling for the hypothesized model.

Type	Goodness of Fit Index	The Full Model
Absolute fit indices	χ^2	4.620
	df	32
	RMSEA	0.085 ($p < 0.09$)
	GFI	0.940 ($p > 0.09$)
Relative fit indices	NFI	0.941 ($p > 0.09$)
	IFI	0.953 ($p > 0.09$)
	CFI	0.953 ($p > 0.09$)
	SRMR	0.036 ($p < 0.05$)

χ^2: chi-square; RMSEA: Root Mean Square Error of Approximation; GFI: Goodness-of-Fit Index; NFI: Non-normed-Fit Index; IFI: Incremental Fit Index; CFI: Comparative Fit Index; SRMR: Standardized Root Mean Square Residual.

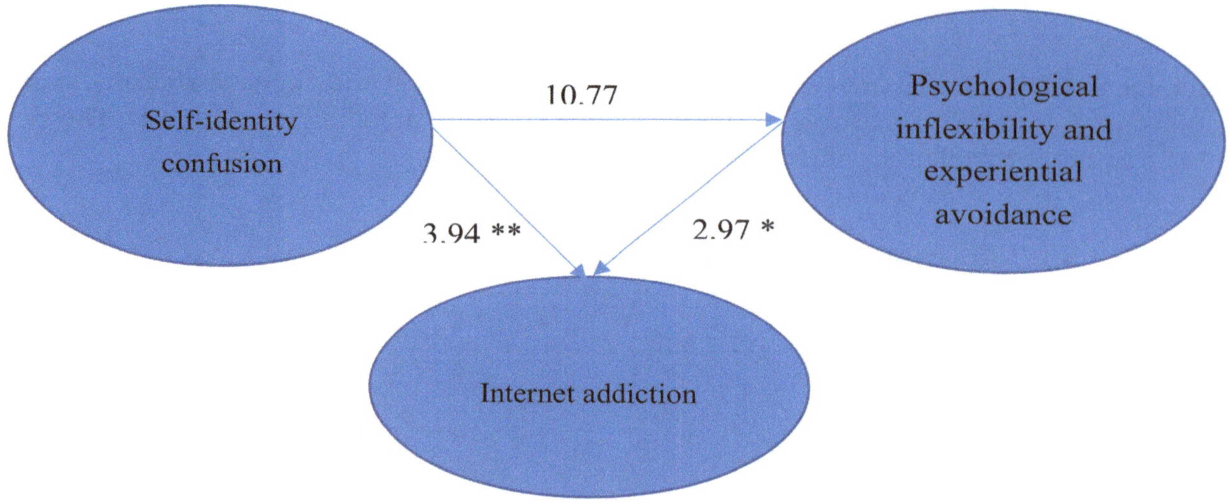

Figure 2. The estimated coefficients of the paths in the hypothesized model for the relationships among self-identity confusion, Internet addiction, and PI/EA. (* $p < 0.05$; ** $p < 0.01$).

4. Discussion

This was the first study to examine the association between self-identity confusion, PI/EA, and IA. The results of this study revealed that self-identity confusion was directly related to IA and indirectly related to IA by the mediation of PI/EA. The results of previous studies on the relationship between self-identity styles and IA have been mixed. Some studies have demonstrated that normative styles of self-identity are protective factors of IA, whereas diffuse-avoidant styles are the risk factors of IA [53,54]. Several possible etiologies may account for the positive association between self-identity confusion and IA. First, the Internet provides college students who have self-identity confusion with an environment to explore their personal values, beliefs, and goals, and college students may use the Internet to escape the daily problems that they encounter which result from self-identity confusion. Second, according to the self-concept fragmentation hypothesis, college students with self-identity confusion may use their own different personalities to interact with others in online environments and feel more at ease within these various online environments than in the real world [55–58]. Third, young adults with self-identity confusion may seek peer advice from others online on issues related to developing self-identity during adolescence [59]. Although college students may use the Internet as a tool to develop their self-identity, IA may limit real-world interaction and therefore slow the development of self-identity [56]. In addition, exposure to different identities in online activities may exacerbate their self-identity confusion [60]. Therefore, college students require help with self-identity confusion to develop adaptive ways to interact with others and develop interpersonal relationships in order to improve their self-identity and consequently reduce their dependence on the Internet. Positive self-identity development could be promoted using Borba's Esteem Builders Curriculum, which is one of the most comprehensive and widely used skills-based curricula [61]. Based on Marcia's identity status theory [62], providing clarity of identity through fostering exploration creates the platform for identity commitment [63] and helps individuals become mature and competent during life transitions [64].

The present study discovered that PI/EA were significantly associated with IA in college students. The relationship between PI and IA has also been supported by the results of an imaging study that suggested that people with IA had difficulties in executive control and attention when switching tasks [65]. People with PI may experience psychosocial maladjustment, and stressful events [66] may cause them to use the Internet to avoid real-world stressors.

In this study, we found that PI/EA mediated the relationship between self-identify confusion and IA. A few possible mechanisms may account for the result. First, an unsuccessful formation of self-concept may lead individuals to experience self-identity diffusion, thereby increasing the risk of mental disorders, such as personality, depressive, and addictive disorders. These disorders usually persist into adulthood if they are not treated appropriately [29,63] and can compromise an individual's self-concept. Persistent self-identity confusion may result in PI/EA [43,44] and result in psychological maladjustment [66]. The Internet may provide individuals with an opportunity to compensate for their self-directed negative feelings by providing opportunities for anonymous social interaction.

Second, people may experience various social-cognitive processes to construct and maintain their self-identity. Beronsky (1992) proposed three processing orientations that contribute to form and maintain a sense of self-identity: A procrastinating, diffuse-avoidant style; an open, informational style; and a conforming, normative style [67]. The individuals with a diffuse-avoidant identity style may tend to use the defense mechanism of avoidance, denial, suppression, and immaturity for masking painful inner conflicts [68,69]. Moreover, the individuals with the normative style may tend to use the defense mechanism of distorting, repressing, or denying reality that may limit self-awareness [70,71]. Therefore, the individuals with diffuse-avoidant or normative identity styles may develop PI/EA and are more likely to use the Internet than those with an informational identity style.

On the basis of our study results, we suggest that school counselors and mental health professionals routinely evaluate whether college students with IA have self-identity confusion and high PI/EA. For self-identity confusion, interventions that provide relational safety and support self-validity and self-exploration may be helpful in reducing the risk of IA [72].

The development of IA should be considered on the basis of ecological systems concepts [73]. Self-identity confusion is an individual factor related to IA. However, self-identity confusion may be influenced by sociocultural factors. Taiwanese culture based on Confucianism is more collectivistic-orientated than Western culture [74], and the difference in value orientation may make college students in Taiwan place greater importance on social relationships than those in Western societies. Whether the collectivistic-orientated culture may influence the development of self-identity and its relationship with IA warrants further study. It is also necessary to replicate the results of the present study in the individualistic-orientated societies.

Our study had a number of limitations. First, the cross-sectional research design limited our ability to draw conclusions regarding the causal relationship among self-identity confusion, PI/EA, and IA. Second, the study data were exclusively self-reported and may have therefore suffered from shared-method variance. Third, the participants in this study were college students who responded to the recruitment advertisement. Therefore, the results of this study might not be generalized to college students who did not participate in this study. Fourth, the present study used the AAQ-II to measure PI/EA. Although research determined that AAQ-II has adequate internal consistency and convergent and divergent validity [49], the items from the AAQ-II were found to be highly correlate with depression, anxiety, and stress, and therefore decreased its discriminant validity [75]. It is suggested that other measures, for example, the CompACT [76], might be needed in combination with the AAQ-II in assessing PI/EA.

Despite these limitations, this study contributes to the literature, as it is the first study to examine the relationship between self-identity confusion and IA and the mediating effects of PI/EA. Further research replicating this SEM model across different samples is suggested.

5. Conclusions

On the basis of our study, we found that self-identity confusion was directly related to IA and indirectly related to IA by the mediation of PI/EA. Therefore, self-identity confusion and PI/EA should be taken into consideration by the professionals working on prevention of IA. Moreover, we proposed that early detection and intervention for self-identity confusion may help college students to develop and consolidate self-identity, reduce PI/EA, and lower the risk of IA.

Author Contributions: Conceptualization, K.-Y.H., R.C.H., K.-H.L. and C.-F.Y.; methodology, C.-F.Y. and K.-H.L.; software, Y.-H.Y.; formal analysis, K.-Y.H., Y.-H.Y., K.-H.L. and C.-F.Y.; writing—original draft preparation, K.-Y.H.; writing—review and editing, K.-Y.H. and C.-F.Y.; supervision, R.C.H., K.-H.L. and C.-F.Y.; funding acquisition, R.C.H., K.-H.L. and C.-F.Y.

References

1. Anderson, K.J. Internet use among college students: An exploratory study. *J. Am. Coll. Health* **2001**, *50*, 21–26. [CrossRef] [PubMed]
2. Young, K.S. Internet addiction: The emergence of a new clinical disorder. *CyberPsychol. Behav.* **1998**, *1*, 237–244. [CrossRef]
3. Shapira, N.A.; Goldsmith, T.D.; Keck, P.E., Jr.; Khosla, U.M.; McElroy, S.L. Psychiatric features of individuals with problematic internet use. *J. Affect. Disord.* **2000**, *57*, 267–272. [CrossRef]
4. American Psychiatric Association. *Diagnostic and Statistical Manual of Mental Disorders*, 5th ed.; American Psychiatric Association: Washington, DC, USA, 2013; ISBN 9780890425558.
5. Weinstein, A.; Lejoyeux, M. Internet addiction or excessive internet use. *Am. J. Drug Alcohol Abuse* **2010**, *36*, 277–283. [CrossRef] [PubMed]
6. Widyanto, L.; Griffiths, M. 'Internet addiction': A critical review. *Int. J. Ment. Health Addict.* **2006**, *4*, 31–51. [CrossRef]
7. Young, K.S. Internet Addiction: A new clinical phenomenon and its consequences. *Am. Behav. Sci.* **2004**, *48*, 402–415. [CrossRef]
8. Kuss, D.J.; Griffiths, M.D. Online social networking and addiction—A review of the psychological literature. *Int. J. Environ. Res. Public Health* **2011**, *8*, 3528–3552. [CrossRef] [PubMed]
9. Kuss, D.J.; Griffiths, M.D.; Binder, J.F. Internet addiction in students: Prevalence and risk factors. *Comput. Hum. Behav.* **2013**, *29*, 959–966. [CrossRef]
10. Tateno, M.; Teo, A.R.; Shirasaka, T.; Tayama, M.; Watabe, M.; Kato, T.A. Internet addiction and self-evaluated attention-deficit hyperactivity disorder traits among Japanese college students. *Psychiatry Clin. Neurosci.* **2016**, *70*, 567–572. [CrossRef]
11. Yang, T.; Yu, L.; Oliffe, J.L.; Jiang, S.; Si, Q. Regional contextual determinants of internet addiction among college students: A representative nationwide study of China. *Eur. J. Public Health* **2017**, *27*, 1032–1037. [CrossRef]
12. Lin, M.P.; Ko, H.C.; Wu, J.Y. Prevalence and psychosocial risk factors associated with internet addiction in a nationally representative sample of college students in Taiwan. *Cyberpsychol. Behav. Soc. Netw.* **2011**, *14*, 741–746. [CrossRef] [PubMed]
13. Abolghasem, P.; Eftekhari, M.; Rezania, S.; Jafarisani, M.; Soleimani, R.; Khalafi, A. Studying the relationship between quality of sleep and addiction to internet among students. *Nova J. Med. Biol. Sci.* **2016**, *5*, 1–7. [CrossRef]
14. Güzel, N.; Kahveci, I.; Solak, N.; Cömert, M.; Turan, F. Internet addiction and its impact on physical health. *Turk. Med. Stud. J.* **2018**, *5*, 32–36. [CrossRef]
15. Budak, E.; Taymur, I.; Askin, R.; Belkiz Gungor, B.; Demirci, H.; Ikra Akgul, A.; Anil Sahin, Z. Relationship between internet addiction, psychopathology and self-esteem among university students. *Eur. Res. J.* **2015**, *1*, 128–135. [CrossRef]
16. Fragkos, C.C.; Fragkos, C.C.; Kiohos, A.P. Internet addiction among Greek university students: Demographic associations with the phenomenon, using the Greek version of young's internet addiction test. *Int. J. Econ. Sci. Appl. Res.* **2010**, *3*, 49–74.
17. Gupta, A.; Khan, A.M.; Rajoura, O.P.; Srivastava, S. Internet addiction and its mental health correlates among undergraduate college students of a university in north India. *J. Family Med. Prim. Care* **2018**, *7*, 721–727. [CrossRef] [PubMed]
18. Li, C.; Dang, J.; Zhang, X.; Zhang, Q.; Guo, J. Internet addiction among Chinese adolescents: The effect of parental behavior and self-control. *Comput. Hum. Behav.* **2014**, *41*, 1–7. [CrossRef]

19. Hyun, G.J.; Han, D.H.; Lee, Y.S.; Kang, K.D.; Yoo, S.K.; Chung, U.-S.; Renshaw, P.F. Risk factors associated with online game addiction: A hierarchical model. *Comput. Hum. Behav.* **2015**, *48*, 706–713. [CrossRef]
20. Bonnaire, C.; Baptista, D. Internet gaming disorder in male and female young adults: The role of alexithymia, depression, anxiety and gaming type. *Psychiatry Res.* **2018**, *272*, 521–530. [CrossRef]
21. Li, G.; Hou, G.; Yang, D.; Jian, H.; Wang, W. Relationship between anxiety, depression, sex, obesity, and internet addiction in Chinese adolescents: A short-term longitudinal study. *Addict. Behav.* **2019**, *90*, 421–427. [CrossRef]
22. Laudet, A.B.; Morgen, K.; White, W.L. The role of social supports, spirituality, religiousness, life meaning and affiliation with 12-step fellowships in quality of life satisfaction among individuals in recovery from alcohol and drug problems. *Alcohol Treat. Q.* **2006**, *24*, 33–73. [CrossRef]
23. Munno, D.; Cappellin, F.; Saroldi, M.; Bechon, E.; Guglielmucci, F.; Passera, R.; Zullo, G. Internet addiction disorder: Personality characteristics and risk of pathological overuse in adolescents. *Psychiatry Res.* **2017**, *248*, 1–5. [CrossRef]
24. Steinfield, C.; Ellison, N.B.; Lampe, C. Social capital, self-esteem, and use of online social network sites: A longitudinal analysis. *J. Appl. Dev. Psychol.* **2008**, *29*, 434–445. [CrossRef]
25. Steinfield, C.; Lampe, C.; Ellison, N.B. The benefits of Facebook "friends": Social capital and college students' use of online social network sites. *J. Comput. Mediat. Commun.* **2007**, *12*, 1143–1168. [CrossRef]
26. Lu, X.; Yeo, K.J. Pathological internet use among Malaysia university students: Risk factors and the role of cognitive distortion. *Comput. Hum. Behav.* **2015**, *45*, 235–242. [CrossRef]
27. Reed, P.A.; Osborne, L.; Romano, M.; Truzoli, R. Higher impulsivity after exposure to the internet for individuals with high but not low levels of self-reported problematic internet behaviours. *Comput. Hum. Behav.* **2015**, *49*, 512–516. [CrossRef]
28. Hormes, J.M.; Kearns, B.; Timko, C.A. Craving Facebook? Behavioral addiction to online social networking and its association with emotion regulation deficits. *Addiction* **2014**, *109*, 2079–2088. [CrossRef]
29. Erikson, E. *Identity: Youth and Crisis*; W. W. Norton & Company: New York, NY, USA, 1968.
30. Lemenager, T.; Dieter, J.; Hill, H.; Hoffmann, S.; Reinhard, I.; Beutel, M.; Vollstadt-Klein, S.; Kiefer, F.; Mann, K. Exploring the neural basis of avatar identification in pathological internet gamers and of self-reflection in pathological social network users. *J. Behav. Addict.* **2016**, *5*, 485–499. [CrossRef]
31. Lemenager, T.; Hoffmann, S.; Dieter, J.; Reinhard, I.; Mann, K.; Kiefer, F. The links between healthy, problematic, and addicted Internet use regarding comorbidities and self-concept-related characteristics. *J. Behav. Addict.* **2018**, *7*, 31–43. [CrossRef]
32. Brand, M.; Young, K.S.; Laier, C.; Wolfling, K.; Potenza, M.N. Integrating psychological and neurobiological considerations regarding the development and maintenance of specific Internet-use disorders: An interaction of person-affect-cognition-execution (I-PACE) model. *Neurosci. Biobehav. Rev.* **2016**, *71*, 252–266. [CrossRef]
33. Tavolacci, M.P.; Ladner, J.; Grigioni, S.; Richard, L.; Villet, H.; Dechelotte, P. Prevalence and association of perceived stress, substance use and behavioral addictions: A cross-sectional study among university students in France, 2009–2011. *BMC Public Health* **2013**, *13*, 724. [CrossRef]
34. Bond, F.W.; Hayes, S.; Barnes-Homes, D. Psychological flexibility, act, and organizational behavior. *J. Organ. Behav. Manag.* **2006**, *26*, 25–54. [CrossRef]
35. Hayes, S.C.; Wilson, K.G.; Gifford, E.V.; Follette, V.M.; Strosahl, K. Experimental avoidance and behavioral disorders: A functional dimensional approach to diagnosis and treatment. *J. Consult. Clin. Psychol.* **1996**, *64*, 1152–1168. [CrossRef]
36. Bricker, J.B.; Schiff, L.; Comstock, B.A. Does avoidant coping influence young adults' smoking? A ten-year longitudinal study. *Nicotine Tob. Res.* **2011**, *13*, 998–1002. [CrossRef]
37. Levin, M.E.; Lillis, J.; Seeley, J.; Hayes, S.C.; Pistorello, J.; Biglan, A. Exploring the relationship between experiential avoidance, alcohol use disorders, and alcohol-related problems among first-year college students. *J. Am. Coll. Health* **2012**, *60*, 443–448. [CrossRef]
38. Kingston, J.; Clarke, S.; Remington, B. Experiential avoidance and problem behavior: A mediational analysis. *Behav. Modif.* **2010**, *34*, 145–163. [CrossRef]
39. Chou, W.P.; Lee, K.H.; Ko, C.H.; Liu, T.L.; Hsiao, R.C.; Lin, H.F.; Yen, C.F. Relationship between PI/EA and internet addiction: Mediating effects of mental health problems. *Psychiatry Res.* **2017**, *257*, 40–44. [CrossRef]

40. Westen, D.; Heim, A.K. Disturbances of self and identity in personality disorders. In *Handbook of Self and Identity*; Leary, M.R., Tangney, J.P., Eds.; Guilford Press: New York, NY, USA, 2003; pp. 643–664. ISBN 978-1593852375.
41. Kroger, J.; Marcia, J.E. The identity statuses: Origins, meanings, and interpretations. In *Handbook of Identity Theory and Research*; Schwartz, S.J., Luyckx, K., Vignoles, V.L., Eds.; Springer: New York, NY, USA, 2011; pp. 31–53. ISBN 978-1-4419-7988-9.
42. Hayes, S.C.; Strosahl, K.; Wilson, K.G. *Acceptance and Commitment Therapy: An Experiential Approach to Behavior Change*; Guilford Press: New York, NY, USA, 1999; ISBN 978-1572304819.
43. Lundgren, T.; Dahl, J.; Hayes, S.C. Evaluation of mediators of change in the treatment of epilepsy with acceptance and commitment therapy. *J. Behav. Med.* **2008**, *31*, 225–235. [CrossRef]
44. Whiting, D.L.; Deane, F.P.; Ciarrochi, J.; McLeod, H.J.; Simpson, G.K. Validating measures of psychological flexibility in a population with acquired brain injury. *Psychol. Assess.* **2015**, *27*, 415–423. [CrossRef]
45. Kwok, S.S.W.; Chan, E.C.C.; Chen, P.P.; Lo, B.C.Y. The "self" in pain: The role of PI in chronic pain adjustment. *J. Behav. Med.* **2016**, *39*, 908–915. [CrossRef]
46. Kaufman, E.A.; Cundiff, J.M.; Crowell, S.E. The development, factor structure, and validation of the self-concept and identity measure (SCIM): A self-report assessment of clinical identity disturbance. *J. Psychopathol. Behav. Assess.* **2015**, *37*, 122–133. [CrossRef]
47. Chen, S.; Weng, L.; Su, Y.; Wu, H.; Yang, P. Development of a Chinese internet addiction scale and its psychometric study. *Chin. J. Psychol.* **2003**, *45*, 279. [CrossRef]
48. Ko, C.H.; Yen, J.Y.; Chen, S.H.; Yang, M.J.; Lin, H.C.; Yen, C.F. Proposed diagnostic criteria and the screening and diagnosing tool of Internet addiction in college students. *Compr. Psychiatry* **2009**, *50*, 378–384. [CrossRef]
49. Bond, F.W.; Hayes, S.C.; Baer, R.A.; Carpenter, K.M.; Guenole, N.; Orcutt, H.K.; Waltz, T.; Zettle, R.D. Preliminary psychometric properties of the acceptance and action questionnaire–II: A revised measure of PI/EA. *Behav. Ther.* **2011**, *42*, 676–688. [CrossRef]
50. McCurry, S.M.; Hayes, S.C.; Strosahl, K.; Wilson, K.G.; Bissett, R.T.; Pistorello, J.; Toarmino, D.; Polusny, M.A.; Dykstra, T.A.; Batten, S.V. Measuring EA: A preliminary test of a working model. *Psychol. Rec.* **2004**, *54*, 553–578. [CrossRef]
51. Jöreskog, K.G.; Sörbom, D. *LISREL 8: Structural Equation Modeling with the SIMPLIS Command Language*; Scientific Software International: Chicago, IL, USA, 1993; ISBN 978-0894980336.
52. Hu, L.-T.; Bentler, P.M. Fit indices in covariance structure modeling: Sensitivity to underparameterized model misspecification. *Psychol. Methods* **1998**, *3*, 424. [CrossRef]
53. Tabaraei, N.; Nikoogoftar, M.; Minoosepehr, S. Determination of problematic internet use: Identity styles and social skills. *IAU Int. J. Soc. Sci.* **2014**, *4*, 27–34.
54. Sinatra, M.; de Palo, V.; Contini, P.; Volpicella, V. Identity styles and internet-related addictive behaviors in adolescents. *Turk. Online J. Educ. Technol.* **2016**, *2016*, 1161–1165.
55. Matsuba, M.K. Searching for self and relationships online. *Cyberpsychol. Behav.* **2006**, *9*, 275–284. [CrossRef]
56. Mazalin, D.; Moore, S. Internet use, identity development and social anxiety among young adults. *Behav. Chang.* **2004**, *21*, 90–102. [CrossRef]
57. Israelashvili, M.; Kim, T.; Bukobza, G. Adolescents' over-use of the cyber world—Internet addiction or identity exploration? *J. Adolesc.* **2012**, *35*, 417–424. [CrossRef]
58. Lee, C.; Aiken, K.D.; Hung, H.C. Effects of college students' video gaming behavior on self-concept clarity and flow. *Soc. Behav. Personal. Int. J.* **2012**, *40*, 673–679. [CrossRef]
59. Allen, K.A.; Ryan, T.; Gray, D.L.; McInerney, D.M.; Waters, L. Social media use and social connectedness in adolescents: The positives and the potential pitfalls. *Aust. Educ. Dev. Psychol.* **2014**, *31*, 18–31. [CrossRef]
60. Sharif, S.P.; Khanekharab, J. Identity confusion and materialism mediate the relationship between excessive social network site usage and online compulsive buying. *Cyberpsychol. Behav. Soc. Netw.* **2017**, *20*, 494–500. [CrossRef]
61. Michele Borba, E.D.; Craig Borba, E.D.; Robert, R. A Research Summary: Effectiveness of Implementing the Esteem Builders Program School-Wide on Elementary Students' Behavior and Academic Self-Concept. 1999. Available online: http://www.micheleborba.com/Pages/PilotStudy.htm (accessed on 30 June 2019).
62. Marcia, J.E. Development and validation of ego-identity status. *J. Personal. Soc. Psychol.* **1966**, *3*, 551–558. [CrossRef]

63. Zaff, J.F.; Hair, E.C. In Well-being: Positive development across the life course. In *Positive Development of the Self: Self-Concept, Self-Esteem, and Identity*; Lawrence Erlbaum Associates Publishers: Mahwah, NJ, USA, 2003; pp. 235–251.
64. Finkenauer, C.; Engels, R.C.M.E.; Meeus, W.H.J.; Oosterwegel, A. Self and identity in early adolescence: The pains and gains of knowing who and what you are. In *Understanding Early Adolescent Self and Identity*; Brinthaupt, T.M., Lipka, R.P., Eds.; State University of New York Press: Albany, NY, USA, 2002; pp. 25–56.
65. Dong, G.; Lin, X.; Zhou, H.; Lu, Q. Cognitive flexibility in internet addicts: fMRI evidence from difficult-to-easy and easy-to-difficult switching situations. *Addict. Behav.* **2014**, *39*, 677–683. [CrossRef]
66. Cheng, C.; Sun, P.; Mak, K.K. Internet addiction and psychosocial maladjustment: Avoidant coping and coping inflexibility as psychological mechanisms. *Cyberpsychol. Behav. Soc. Netw.* **2015**, *18*, 539–546. [CrossRef]
67. Berzonsky, M.D. Identity style and coping strategies. *J. Personal.* **1992**, *60*, 771–788. [CrossRef]
68. Luyckx, K. Identity styles, self-reflective cognition, and identity processes: A study of adaptive and maladaptive dimensions of self-analysis au—Berzonsky, Michael, D. *Identity* **2008**, *8*, 205–219. [CrossRef]
69. Beaumont, S.L. Identity processing styles and defense styles during emerging adulthood: Implications for life distress AU—Seaton, Cherisse, L. *Identity* **2011**, *11*, 1–24. [CrossRef]
70. Berzonsky, M.; Kinney, A. Identity processing style and defense mechanisms. *Pol. Psychol. Bull.* **2008**, *39*, 111–117. [CrossRef]
71. Soenens, B.; Duriez, B.; Goossens, L. Social–psychological profiles of identity styles: Attitudinal and social-cognitive correlates in late adolescence. *J. Adolesc.* **2005**, *28*, 107–125. [CrossRef]
72. Gonzalez-Bueso, V.; Santamaria, J.J.; Fernandez, D.; Merino, L.; Montero, E.; Jimenez-Murcia, S.; Del Pino-Gutierrez, A.; Ribas, J. Internet gaming disorder in adolescents: Personality, psychopathology and evaluation of a psychological intervention combined with parent psychoeducation. *Front. Psychol.* **2018**, *9*, 787. [CrossRef]
73. Bronfenbrenner, U. *The Ecology of Human Development*; Harvard University Press: Cambridge, MA, USA, 1979; ISBN 9780674224575.
74. Triandis, H.C. Individualism-collectivism and personality. *J. Personal.* **2001**, *69*, 907–924. [CrossRef]
75. Tyndall, I.; Waldeck, D.; Pancani, L.; Whelan, R.; Roche, B.; Dawson, D. The Acceptance and Action Questionnaire-II (AAQ-II) as a Measure of EA: Concerns over Discriminant Validity. *J. Contextual Behav. Sci.* **2019**, *12*, 278–284. [CrossRef]
76. Frances, A.W.; Dawson, D.L.; Golijani-Moghaddam, N.G. The development and validation of the comprehensive assessment of Acceptance and Commitment Therapy processes (CompACT). *J. Contextual Behav. Sci.* **2016**, *5*, 134–145. [CrossRef]

5

Internet Addiction in the Web of Science Database

Antonio-José Moreno-Guerrero, Gerardo Gómez-García, Jesús López-Belmonte and Carmen Rodríguez-Jiménez *

Department of Didactics and School Organization, University of Granada, 18071 Granada, Spain; ajmoreno@ugr.es (A.-J.M.-G.); gomezgarcia@ugr.es (G.G.-G.); jesuslopez@ugr.es (J.L.-B.)
* Correspondence: carmenrj@ugr.es

Abstract: Information and communication technologies (ICT) is a major element of today's society with great potential that can offer both advantages and disadvantages. Addiction to the Internet and social networks is a growing problem in all age groups. Education is the context in which to work and train in the correct use of these media. The objective of the study focuses on knowing the scientific production and the performance of the concepts "addiction" and "internet" (ADIN). A bibliometric methodology complemented with the scientific mapping technique was followed. Different processes related to the quantification, analysis, evaluation, and estimation of scientific documents were carried out. The literature was analyzed by specific programs such as SciMAT, Analyze Results, and Creation Citation Report. The unit of analysis was specified in 5644 scientific publications extracted from Web of Science (WoS), belonging to the period of years between 1996 and 2019. The results showed that the evolution in the study of the addiction to the Internet is constant and continuous, with articles in English being the most used means to present the information on the part of the investigators. In addition, the subject of study was based on time, given that the coincidence of key words between the periods analyzed was high. In conclusion, the importance of promoting healthy living habits that include responsible use of the Internet are discussed.

Keywords: scientific production; bibliometric analysis; scientific mapping; addiction; internet; Web of Science

---

1. Introduction

Today's society is increasingly focused on technology and therefore people are progressively more dependent on it, particularly with regards to the Internet [1,2]. Mobile phones and different technological devices have made the world of video games and online shopping more accessible to everyone, making markets even more desirable and broad than before [3].

The Internet and the different social networks have become popular instruments that are currently used to communicate and exchange information, among the most outstanding actions [4]. The way in which people interact with each other, entertain themselves, and consume through the media has been modified through the Internet [5]. However, as more people connect to multimedia devices to share information and make use of the possibilities they are offered, cases of media addiction are growing at a dangerous pace [6,7]. These addictions have grown significantly over the last decade [8], surpassing other types of addictions.

There is a great deal of scientific evidence showing how there is a serious risk associated with excessive use of the Internet and everything that derives from it [9], where, in addition, personal characteristics, gender, socio-cultural differences [10], and biological factors could play an important role in the appearance of an addiction to these media. The literature reveals an association between the Internet and social networks and an increase in so-called techno-stress [11–13].

The constant use of the Internet and social networks leads to an addiction and obsession, which results in negative behavior [14]. The consequences of these habits regarding the excessive use of different smart devices and the Internet can affect both the physical and mental health of users [15]. Issues such as anxiety, depression, impulsiveness, and aggressive behavior can also result or be increased from uncontrolled use [16]. Those with internet addiction have higher levels of depression, anxiety, and impulsivity than those without such an addiction [9].

Numerous studies address internet and smartphone addiction, regardless of the age of those suffering from it [17] or even the field in which they are trained or work [18]. In addition, the literature contains relevant research that addresses this type of addiction and its relationship to the educational setting [8,19]. Technology, the Internet, and the impact of the digital world have a great influence on the student body and the development of their personality [20] and health [21].

At present, students, regardless of their educational stage, are one of the groups most closely related to everything related to ICT and its use for different purposes, such as socialization or proper academic development [22]. Experts on the field state that those students who use the Internet for purposes that go beyond simple socialization through the different social networks and video games have a better level with regard to problems related to the use of this technology [23]. The exclusive use of these media for playful or socializing purposes without an educational perspective or previous training in the correct use and handling can lead to problems such as sexting [24], cyberbullying [25], or video game addiction [26]. The consequences derived from these phenomena can affect the academic, social, and emotional spheres.

In this respect, from the educational field, mechanisms of prevention and action should be established in the face of these new existing trends. Therefore, it is necessary to educate in terms of the correct handling of the devices at a technical level, but also at a regulatory level, where the self-regulation of certain behaviors towards these devices is promoted, always extracting the maximum potential for all the areas of the life of the students, including their academic life [27]. The objective from the educational point of view should be to form digitally competent citizens who have positively developed their ethical, literacy, participatory, and critical aspects towards technology and the use of the Internet [28,29].

In recent times, there have been constant publications that analyze ICT, as well as the Internet and its relationship with education [30,31], as the tendency of these topics is to increase and acquire more relevance in terms of research. On the other hand, studies approached from bibliometrics, such as the one presented in this paper, are in recent times a constant that addresses a multitude of topics of incidence, such as medical research [32], virtual reality [33,34], or the area of sports [35].

2. Justification of Study

In the research presented, the concepts "addiction" and "internet" (ADIN) are analyzed in the impact scientific literature collected from the Web of Science (WoS) database. Web of Science is an online platform containing databases of bibliographic information and information analysis resources that allow the evaluation and analysis of research performance, especially in the field of social sciences. In addition, it presents a series of analysis tools that allow specific and concrete searches to be carried out [36]. This study acquires a bibliometric nature with the purpose of analyzing the publications by means of a scientific mapping developed as a result of various bibliometric indicators and a dynamic and structural evolution of the aforementioned terms.

To carry out and follow a study model validated by experts in this field of research, other impact investigations taken from the Journal Citation Reports were taken as a reference (JCR) [36,37].

This study focused on the evaluation of the trajectory and evolution of the mentioned concepts of the main WoS collection. Initially, a search was carried out in such a database to know the status of the terms issue and, in addition, to check if there were any studies of similar characteristics to the one presented in this work. After the search phase, no publication was found that analyzed both terms with a scientific mapping, and thus this study acquired an exploratory nuance about the state of the art in impact literature. Therefore, this study helps to increase the findings and reduce the gap found in the literature concerning the relationship between "addiction" and "internet". Therefore, the results obtained will acquire a relevant value as they will contribute to the advancement of science, in addition to serving as a basis for successive research.

3. Materials and Methods

3.1. Research Objectives

The general objective of this study was to analyze the scientific literature on ADIN indexed in the WoS database. This general objective is articulated in the following specific objectives:

- To determine the performance of publications on ADIN in WoS.
- To decree the scientific evolution of ADIN in WoS.
- To find out the most incident issues about ADIN in WoS.
- To identify the most influential authors in ADIN in WoS.

The research questions posed are

- RQ1: What is the performance of ADIN publications in WoS?
- RQ2: What is the scientific evolution of ADIN in WoS?
- RQ3: What are the most frequent problems of ADIN in WoS?
- Q4: Who are the most influential authors of ADIN in WoS?

3.2. Research Design

The research methodology adopted in this study to achieve the proposed objectives was bibliometry. This choice is justified in the scientometric potentialities linked to the actions of searching, recording, analyzing, and predicting scientific literature [38]. Similarly, the guidance and considerations of experts in this type of study were followed [39].

Specifically, this work was based on the analysis of co-words [40] and various bibliometric indicators such as the h-index, taken as a reference, in addition to other indices (g, hg, q2) [41]. This gave rise to the creation of node maps whose interpretation determined the performance and position of conceptual subdomains alluding to ADIN. In addition, the analytical treatment delimited the thematic development of these concepts in WoS [42]. From this database, we used the complete record in order to obtain as much information as possible, in order to have the most relevant data to perform the co-word analysis [43].

3.3. Procedure and Data Analysis

This investigation was carried out following various actions that specified the following procedures: (a) selection of the database (WoS), (b) determination of the keywords ("addiction" and "internet") after consultation in specialized thesauri (ERIC and UNESCO) and in the information provided in the Special Issue of the *International Journal of Environmental Research and Public Health*, and (c) construction of a precise search equation to obtain significant results ("addiction*" [TOPIC] AND "internet" [TOPIC]) and report documents containing both terms in different metadata (title, abstract, and keywords).

The first search action compiled a scientific volume of 5776 publications. In addition, the entire report was analyzed to eliminate repeated documents, those belonging to the year 2020 and the poorly indexed ones. After this, an analysis unit of 5644 publications remained, as a result of the configuration of various production indicators with their respective inclusion criteria (Table 1).

Table 1. Production indicators and inclusion criteria.

Indicators	Criteria
Year of publication	All production except 2020
Language	x ≥ 50
Publication area	x ≥ 300
Type of documents	x ≥ 300
Organizations	x ≥ 70
Authors	x ≥ 60
Sources of origin	x ≥ 100
Countries	x ≥ 400
Citation	The four most cited documents

To improve the understanding and visualization of the different actions carried out, the following flow chart was established following the protocols of the PRISMA-P matrix (Figure 1).

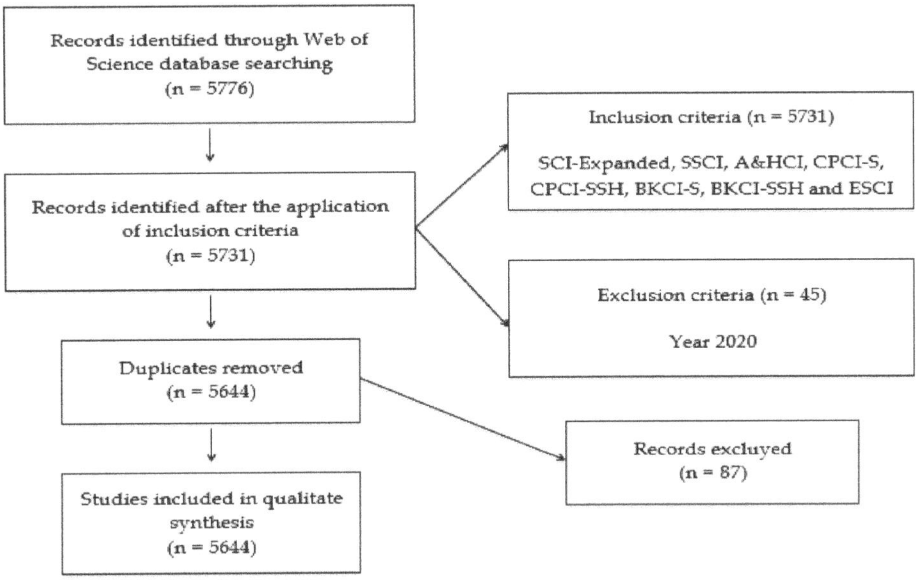

Figure 1. Flowchart according to the PRISMA Declaration.

The documents obtained were analyzed with various programs (Analyze Results, Creation Citation Report, and SciMAT). The first two tools are provided by WoS and were used to obtain data concerning the year, authorship, country, type of document, institution, language, means of publication, and most cited documents. For the structural and dynamic development of a longitudinal nature of the scientific volume, SciMAT was used, under the considerations of the experts [44].

With SciMAT, a co-word analysis of the topics was carried out through the following processes:

- Recognition: In this process, various actions were carried out. The keywords of the literature obtained were analyzed (n = 10,555). A map of co-occurrence nodes was generated. A standardized network of co-words was developed. The most significant keywords were detected (n = 9842), and the themes and concepts with greater predominance were represented with a clustering algorithm.
- Reproduction: In this process, a strategic diagram and a thematic network based on the principles of centrality and density were prepared. In the generated graphs, four regions can be seen: (1) top right (motor themes and highlights), (2) upper left (rooted and isolated themes); (3) lower left (themes to disappear or project), and (4) lower right (underdeveloped and transversal themes).
- Determination: In this process, the evolution of the nodes in certain periods or intervals of time was analyzed. In particular, four periods were defined (P_1 = 1996-2010; P_2 = 2011-2014; P_3 = 2015-2017; P_4 = 2018-2019), except in the authorship that one that covered the entire documentary volume

was established (P_X = 1996-2019). The number of matching keywords determined the strength of association between the configured periods.

- Performance: In this process, a set of production indicators associated with inclusion criteria that determine the scientific works that become part of the study were delimited (Table 2).

Table 2. Production indicators and inclusion criteria.

Configuration	Values
Analysis unit	Keywords authors, keywords WoS
Frequency threshold	Keywords: P_1 = (5), P_2 = (7), P_3 = (7), P_4 = (7) Authors: P_X = (10)
Network type	Co-occurrence
Co-occurrence union value threshold	Keywords: P_1 = (2), P_2 = (4), P_3 = (5), P_4 = (5) Authors: P_X = (6)
Normalization measure	Equivalence index
Clustering algorithm	Maximum size: 9; minimum size: 3
Evolutionary measure	Jaccard index
Overlapping measure	Inclusion rate

4. Results

4.1. Performance and Scientific Production

The evolution of the 5644 documents in the scientific production on ADIN has been constant and continuous over time, showing an exponential growth from its beginnings until the year 2019 (Figure 2). In this sense, and according to the Price law about growth of scientific information, visualization of the distribution of publications on internet addiction doubled in its development 10 years after its first publication. At present, productivity on the subject is in a phase of linear growth.

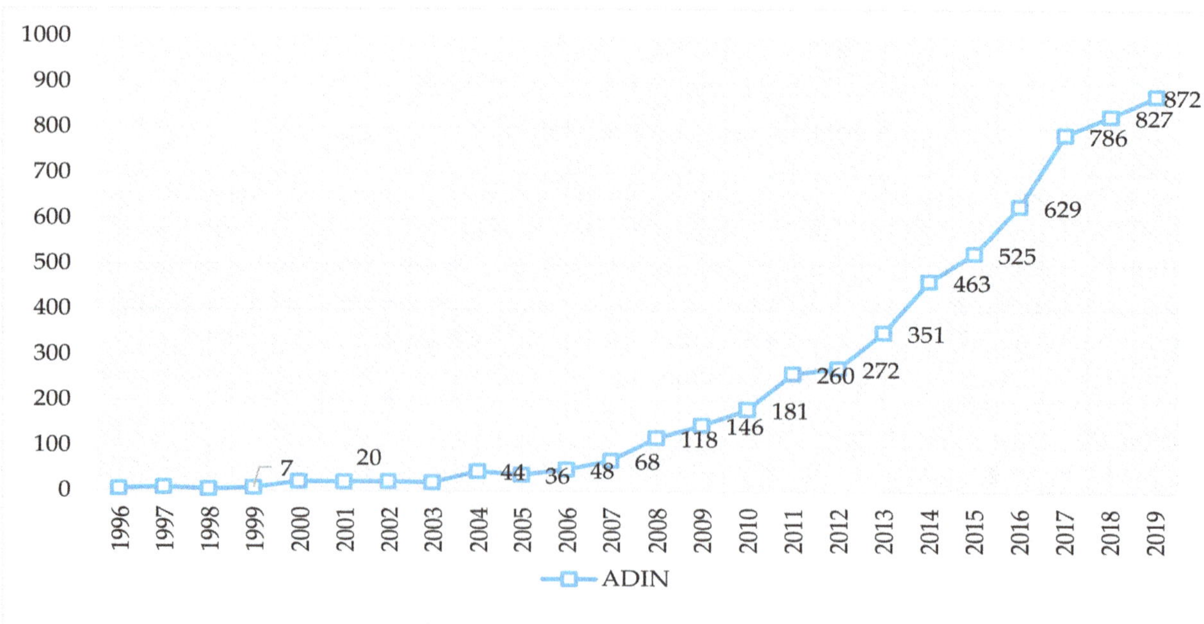

Figure 2. Evolution of scientific production of the keywords "addiction" and "internet" (ADIN) in the Web of Science (WoS).

The language chosen by the various authors for the presentation of the academic results was English (Table 3).

Table 3. Scientific language used in ADIN.

Language	*n*
English	5265
Spanish	119
German	95
French	56
Russian	53

The main area of knowledge in ADIN studies is psychiatry, distanced considerably from other areas of knowledge (Table 4).

Table 4. Research areas.

Research Area	*n*
Psychiatry	1649
Psychology (multidisciplinary)	801
Substance abuse	678
Psychology (clinical)	522
Psychology (experimental)	374
Education educational research	313

The type of document mainly used by the various scientists are articles (Table 5).

Table 5. Document types.

Document Types	*n*
Article	4467
Meeting abstract	383
Proceedings paper	347
Review	320

Nottingham Trent University is the leading organization in ADIN studies (Table 6).

Table 6. Institutions.

Institution	*n*
Nottingham Trent University	242
Seoul National University (SNU)	107
Catholic University of Korea	105
Yale University	98
Kaohsiung Medical University	87
Chung Ho Memorial Hospital	76
Johannes Gutenberg Univesrity of Mainz	72

The most prolific author is Griffinths, M.D., with considerable scientific output on ADIN (Table 7).

Table 7. Authors.

Authors	*n*
Griffinths, M.D.	183
Kim, D.J.	72
Ko, C.H.	67
Yen, C.F.	66

Table 7. *Cont.*

Authors	*n*
Potenza, M.N.	65
Billieux, J.	63
Brand, M.	60
Wolfling, K.	60

The main source of presentation of studies on ADIN are, with similar productions, *Computers in Human Behavior* and the *Journal of Behavioral Addictions* (Table 8).

Table 8. Source titles.

Source Titles	*n*
Computers in Human Behavior	356
Journal of Behavioral Addictions	331
Cyberpsychology Behavior and Social Networking	168
Addictive Behaviors	105
International Journal of Mental Health Addiction	105

The country with the greatest interest in production on ADIN is the United States (Table 9).

Table 9. Countries.

Country	*n*
United States	1263
China	773
England	511
South Korea	469
Turkey	406
Germany	405

The reference author for the scientific community in relation to the subject of ADIN, in terms of number of citations, is Davis (2001), followed at a short distance by Morahan-Martin and Schumacher (2000) and Block (2008) (Table 10).

Table 10. Most cited articles and main conclusions.

Reference	Citations	Main Conclusion
[45]	881	The model implies a more important role of cognitions in pathological internet use (PIU), and describes the means by which PIU is both developed and maintained. Furthermore, it provides a framework for the development of cognitive-behavioral interventions for PIU.
[46]	593	Pathological users, for pathological internet use (PIU), scored significantly higher on the UCLA Loneliness Scale, and were socially disinhibited online.
[47]	579	This document refers to how the DSM-IV considers internet addiction.
[48]	535	Among the findings are the urgent need to develop research on best practices for treating pain in adolescents, as well as the development of prevention strategies to reduce diversion and abuse.

4.2. *Structural and Thematic Development*

The evolution of keywords shows information about the number of keywords in each of the established time intervals, the number of matching keywords between the periods, and the number of keywords leaving and entering a certain period with respect to another. The studies on ADIN, taking into account the evolution of keywords in scientific production, mark a settled and consolidated line of research, given that the level of coincidence between periods was between 40% and 50% (Figure 3).

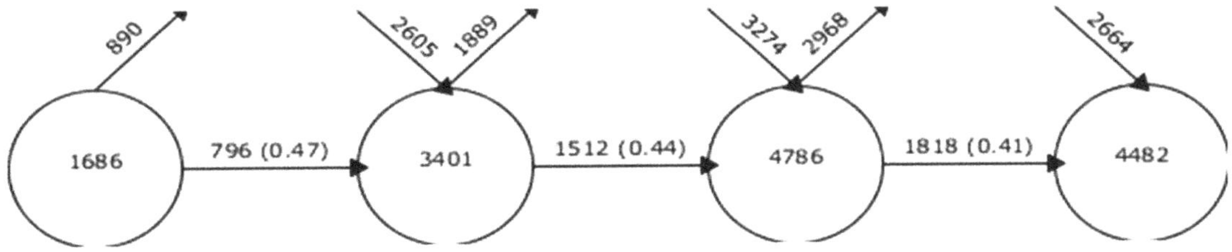

Figure 3. Continuity of keywords between contiguous intervals.

The academic performance in the established periods offers the subjects with the greatest bibliometric indicators, using the h-index as the main reference, and completing this information with the g-index, hg-index and q2-index, in addition to the number of citations. On the subject of ADIN, the subjects with the highest bibliometric indicators varied between periods. In the first time period (1996–2010), the topic with the highest bibliometric indicator was "addiction"; in the second time period (2011–2014) it was "prevalence"; in the third time period (2015–2017) it was "depression" and "addiction"; and in the last time period (2018–2019) it was "adolescents". This shows changes in the interests of researchers in this field of study. We also observed the changes between periods of the topics of greatest interest to researchers, showing the main lines of research in each of the established time intervals (Table 11).

Table 11. Thematic performance.

			Interval 1996–2010			
Denomination	**Works**	**Index h**	**Index g**	**Index hg**	**Index q^2**	**Citations**
Health-care	12	8	10	8.94	13.86	210
Addiction	238	76	130	99.4	108.19	18,177
Impulse-control-disorder	13	11	12	11.46	25.48	1203
Prevalence	62	37	61	47.51	65.8	5423
Symptoms	20	15	20	17.32	48.68	2216
Computer-games	13	11	11	11	29.1	1328
Sensation-seeking	15	14	14	14	31.3	1547
Technology	22	12	20	15.49	35.16	2060
Online	42	26	38	31.43	43.86	3061
Students	17	13	17	14.87	24.45	848
Intervention	11	8	10	8.94	22.09	523
Scale	21	17	19	17.97	31.4	1488
Alcohol-use	5	5	5	5	10.72	491
Video-games	6	6	6	6	21.77	489
Support	6	6	6	6	21.21	591
Model	5	4	5	4.47	25.14	611
Risk	4	4	4	4	21.82	466
			Interval 2011–2014			
Denomination	**Works**	**Index h**	**Index g**	**Index hg**	**Index q^2**	**Citations**
Prevalence	519	69	105	85.12	83.89	19,238
College-students	95	39	71	52.62	54.44	5256
Children	44	23	37	29.17	33.57	1384
Behavior	115	38	61	48.15	54.79	4168
Loneliness	81	30	56	40.99	46.8	3339
Alcohol	30	17	30	22.58	28.57	1026
Motivations	28	20	27	23.24	36.06	2048
Gender	27	13	23	17.29	19.42	596

Table 11. *Cont.*

Interval 2011–2014						
Denomination	**Works**	**Index h**	**Index g**	**Index hg**	**Index q^2**	**Citations**
FMRI	15	13	14	13.49	28.62	870
Treatment	26	17	25	20.62	29.15	1038
Validation	16	13	16	14.42	22.8	681
Health	15	10	15	12.25	15.81	228
Pornography	12	10	12	10.95	17.03	406
TDAH	8	7	8	7.48	12.69	481
DSM-5	18	11	17	13.67	26.12	759
Play	10	8	9	8.49	14.7	296
Computer-use	20	15	19	16.88	24.49	724
Anterior-cingulate-cortex	5	5	5	5	16.28	414
Aggression	7	7	7	7	20.32	579
Interval 2015–2017						
Denomination	**Works**	**Index h**	**Index g**	**Index hg**	**Index q^2**	**Citations**
Funcional-connectivity	54	21	29	24.68	25.51	998
Depression	571	42	63	51.44	51.44	8642
Addiction	680	42	63	51.44	51.03	9259
Self-esteem	108	22	33	26.94	27.75	1492
Decision-making	35	17	29	22.2	22.58	866
DSM-5	73	21	38	28.25	29.7	1627
Smartphone-addiction	44	17	26	24.74	29.44	1314
Validation	85	16	25	20	21.54	937
Substance-use	52	15	26	19.75	21.21	821
Children	53	15	24	18.97	18.57	763
Facebook	44	11	15	12.85	12.85	331
Students	45	15	22	18.17	18.97	596
Model	47	13	23	17.29	18.73	605
Internet-pornography	43	13	26	18.38	17.66	736
Play	19	11	16	13.27	16.58	361
Smoking	15	6	13	8.83	12.73	179
Technology	10	8	10	8.94	13.56	244
Computer-games	12	6	9	7.35	11.22	126
Substance-use-disorders	8	6	7	6.48	10.39	207
Gaming-disorder	9	5	7	5.92	7.07	68
Interval 2018–2019						
Denomination	**Works**	**Index h**	**Index g**	**Index hg**	**Index q^2**	**Citations**
Adolescents	860	17	22	19.34	19.34	2433
Internet-pornography	48	8	13	10.2	11.66	231
Mobile-phone	66	8	14	10.58	12.33	262
Self-esteem	138	11	17	13.97	15.56	544
Facebook	73	7	8	7.48	7.94	200
Impulsivity	68	9	11	9.95	9.95	229
Video-games	82	6	10	7.75	8.49	180
Validation	74	7	9	7.94	7.94	177
Children	112	8	10	8.94	9.8	263
Problematic-internet-use	119	10	13	11.4	11.83	399
University-students	45	8	13	10.2	10.95	222
Prefrontal-cortex	20	5	7	5.92	6.71	60
Internet-use	25	5	7	5.92	7.42	83
Life	16	4	7	5.29	6.93	55
Cue-reactivity	7	3	4	3.46	3.46	20
International-consensus	12	5	7	5.92	6.71	59
Stress	12	3	5	3.87	3.46	33
Risk	16	3	4	3.46	4.58	29

The diagrams of the intervals developed show data on the importance of each of the themes in the different periods. For this purpose, a grouping process was developed, according to Callon's indicators, which assesses the degree of interaction of a network with respect to other networks, from two axes: centrality, which analyses the strength of the relationship of external links with other topics, where it shows the importance of the development of a topic in a field of research; and density, which assesses the internal strength of the network, analyzing the internal links between the key words that are grouped around a specific topic, giving information on the degree of development of a field of study. In the first period (1996–2010), the driving themes were "addiction", "prevalence", "symptoms", "health-care", and "sensation-seeking". In the second period (2011–2014), the themes were "prevalence", "children", "computer-use", and "loneliness". In the third period (2015–2017), themes were "depression", "addiction", "DSM-5", "functional-connectivity", "self-esteem", "children", and "validation". In the last period (2018–2019), themes were "adolescents", "self-esteem", "impulsivity", "children", and "video-games". From this last period, we should also highlight the themes "international-consensus", "stress", "risk", "life", and "internet-use", given that their location in the diagram makes them unknown themes, as they may be the next references in the next few years in this field of study, or they may disappear. Generally speaking, the interests of ADIN researchers are focused on aspects related to adolescents, children, frequency, and addiction, as these are the issues that most appear in the motor themes of the diagram (Figure 4).

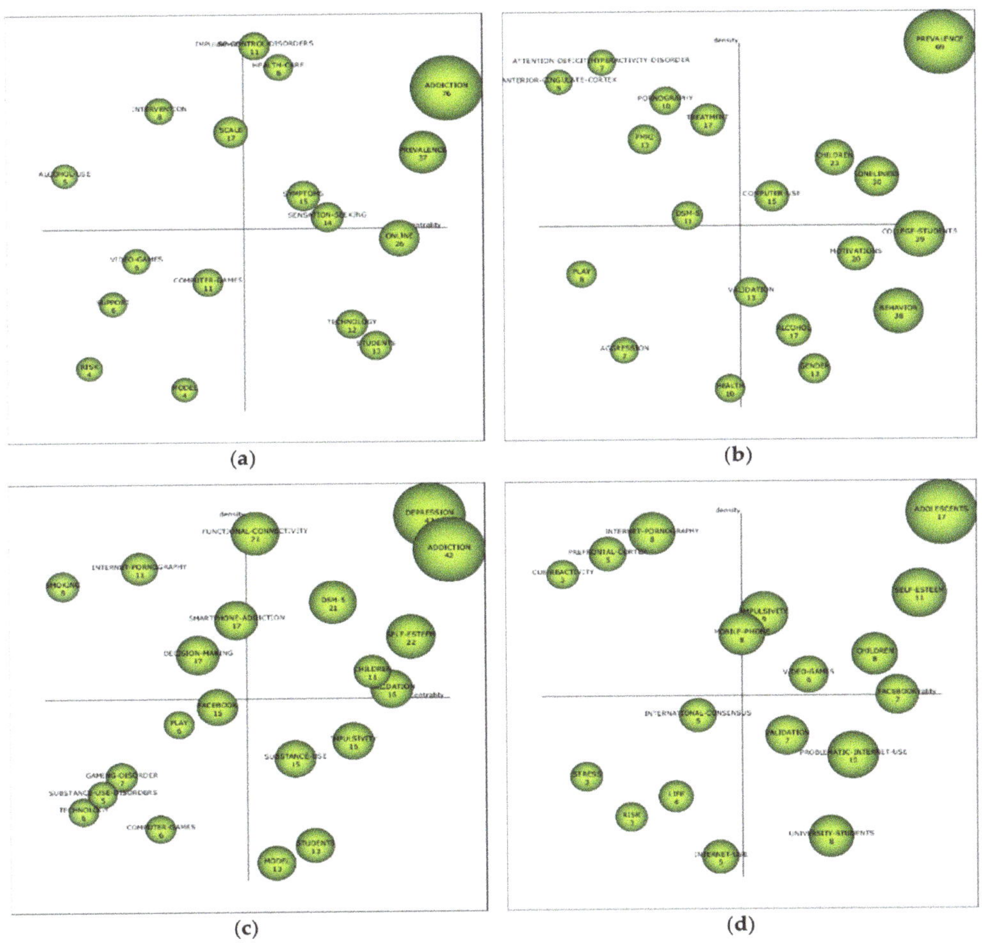

Figure 4. ADIN's strategic diagram by h-index. Note: (**a**) interval 1996–2010; (**b**) interval 2011–2014; (**c**) interval 2015–2017; (**d**) interval 2018–2019.

4.3. Thematic Evolution of the Terms

The thematic evolution offers the strength of the relationship maintained between the themes of the various intervals generated according to the Jaccard index. The development is generated if a theme of a particular interval shares keywords or themes with the subsequent or previous periods. The greater the number of keywords between the two themes of consecutive intervals, the more solid its evolution will be. The possible connections are continuous line, where its connection is thematic, and discontinuous line, whose connection is by keywords. The thickness of the lines shows the strength of the relationship between the themes. The data showed a conceptual gap in the thematic evolution in the ADIN study, as there was no keyword that was repeated in all the established periods. Even so, there were themes that were repeated in at least two or more periods. The timeline with the greatest connecting force was the one established between "prevalence-prevalence-depression-adolescent", being the basis of the studies on the research topic. There were other strong connections, such as those established between "play-play", from the second and third period, and "impulsivity-impulsivity" or "self-esteem" from the third and fourth period. In addition, Figure 5 shows that there were an even number of thematic connections and keyword connections. The studies on ADIN had an established basis, focusing mainly on people under 18 years of age and the different pathologies caused by internet use addiction.

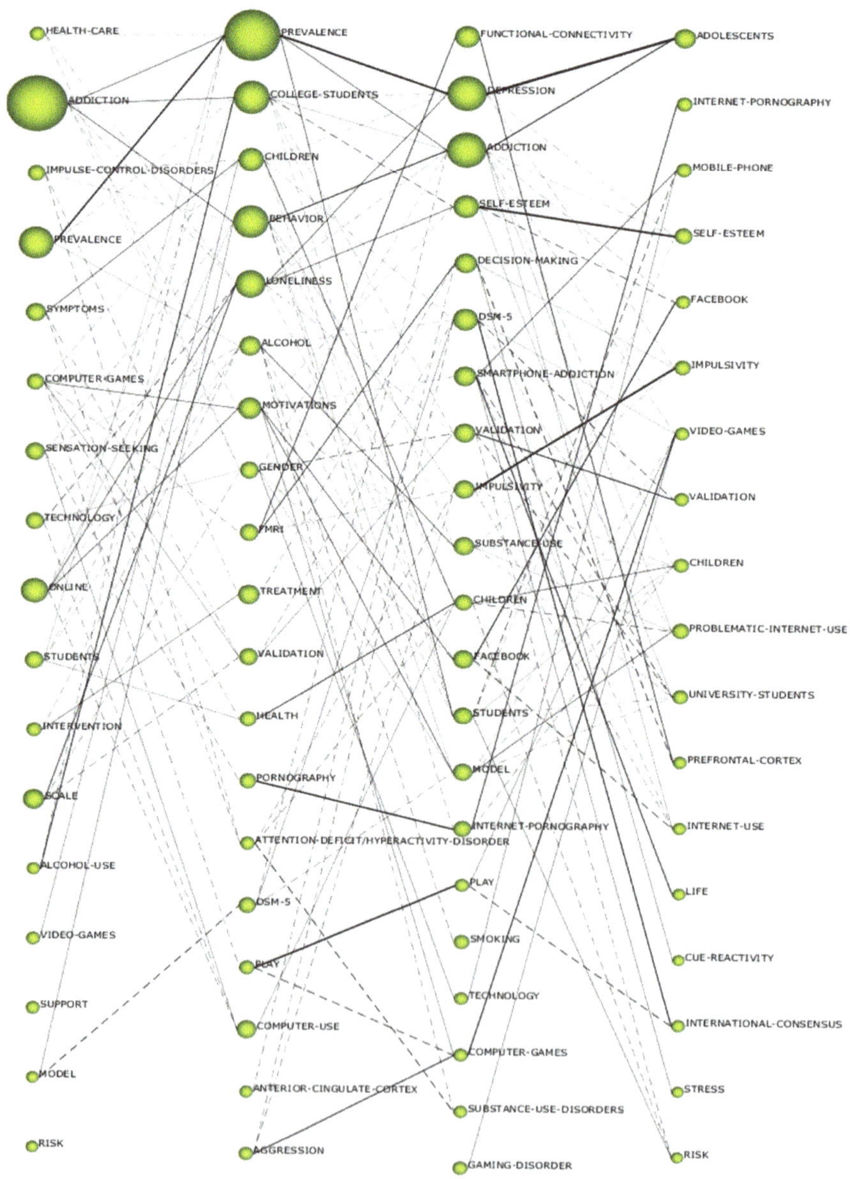

Figure 5. Thematic evolution by h-index.

4.4. Authors with a Higher Relevance Index

The driving authors on the field of study of ADIN are Mihara, S.; Marino, C.; and Levine, S. In addition, the author that have a great relevance for the scientific community, bearing in mind their h-index, are Yen, J.Y., and Griffiths, M.D., although their location in the diagram placed them as isolated or cross-sectional authors. For the next few years, we should bear in mind the authors Brand, M.; Dong, G.H.; and Montag, C., because their location in the diagram placed them as unknown authors, and they may disappear or be the reference authors in this field of study (Figure 6).

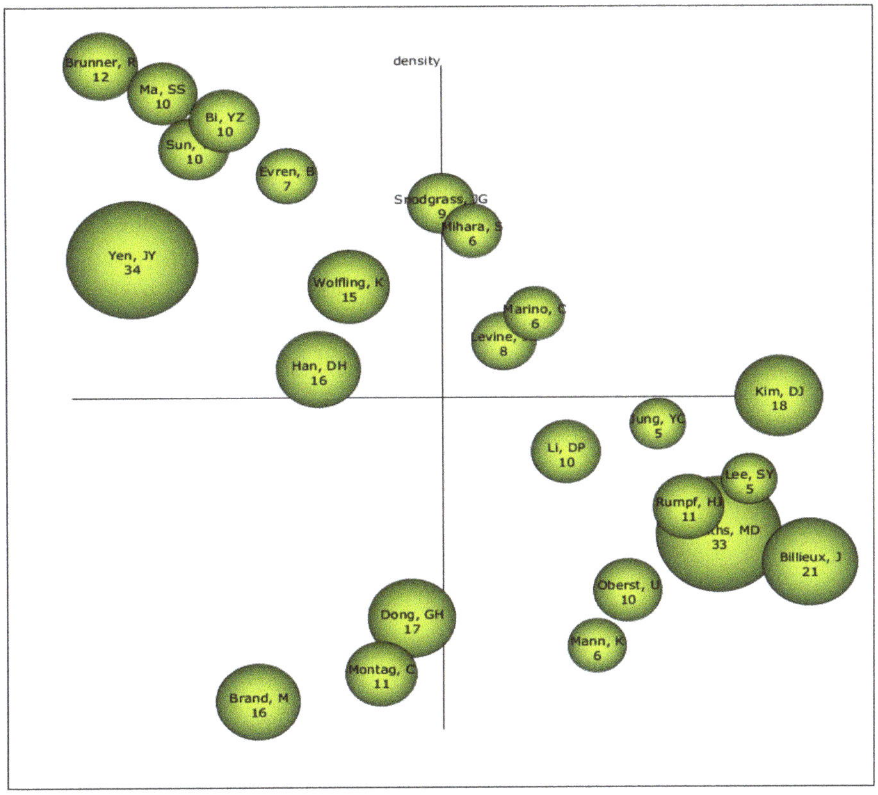

Figure 6. Strategic authoring diagram.

5. Discussion

ADIN has become one of the most frequented topics in the scientific panorama over the last years. The arrival of the Internet in people's lives has brought many benefits, but also risks that citizens must be aware of in order to take preventive measures [9].

The present work aimed to establish a state of the art study on scientific productivity on ADIN in one of the most prestigious databases at present (WoS). The analysis of the data allowed the elucidation of the exponential growth in which the discipline of knowledge finds itself at present, doubling in 10 years from its origin the number of publications and being nowadays in a phase of linear growth [44]. The large percentage of manuscripts found belonged mainly to the psychiatric and psychological area, linked to the treatment of addictions, drugs, and harmful substances, which denotes that this is a global concern that particularly affects the compendium of the health discipline [32]. However, there is also an emerging amount of research concerning the educational branch, which allows us to see that ADIN is beginning to be a concern for experts in the field of education, in order to promote a practice of a prophylactic nature [33].

Likewise, the analysis on the most prolific institutions and authors in the area allowed us to know that the research on ADIN is an object of study by multiple researchers from different parts of the world, with numerous countries being among the biggest producers of scientific works on the subject, and therefore configuring one of the most important risks that reside in the society [1].

In this sense, the co-word analysis provided an understanding of which of the descriptors had the highest academic performance over the years about ADIN, in addition to being able to visualize its evolution over the years. By way of this, it was possible to distinguish how there was an evolution in this issue, from the origin of ADIN to the present, starting with descriptors such as "sensation-seeking" or "symptoms", to "loneliness", "depression", "self-esteem", "stress", "video-games", or "impulsivity". Undoubtedly, a negative progression is visualized that began with descriptors that alluded to minor symptoms and disorders, and ended with descriptors referring to risks related to serious disorders or diseases such as depression, social isolation, or serious self-esteem problems. This indicates that there has been an increase in ADIN in society and, therefore, there are publications that refer to this phenomenon associated with this type of disease [9,16].

In sum, the results indicated that, to a greater extent, risks associated with the Internet, such as the consumption of pornography and young people's addiction to video games and the behavioral disorders associated with them, obtained a considerable density of publication, and therefore these are risks that affect society today [23,24]. In a similar vein, the analysis of the relationship between issues through the Jaccard index allowed us to discern relevant connections between issues, as was the case with the one maintained between "prevalence-prevalence-depression-adolescent", "addiction-behavior-addiction-adolescent", or "online-loneliness-self-esteem". These links allowed us to corroborate the interest of the research community in the risks associated with ADIN over the years, an idea similar to those expressed in previous research [7,17,33,34]. Specifically, the main population under study, according to the works analyzed, are young people, especially adolescents.

Finally, the scientific mapping of authors with a higher index of relevance allowed us to know a considerable compendium of experts in the present on ADIN, which indicates the importance that this topic is gaining within the current scientific panorama, as well as the need for its study and deepening by the research community.

6. Conclusions

ADIN is among the most threatening risks to society today and in the future, especially among the younger population, who live more with technological devices continuously, which can lead to severe consequences associated with serious behavioral disorders and psychological diseases.

Through this work, we intended to establish a general state on the productivity and scientific performance of the subject, trying to contribute interesting ideas about the evolution of the subject and about which are the most frequent aspects to be developed by the researchers, who focus their attention on the study of ADIN. All of this information can be used in order to be able to elucidate the working path in the near future.

Among the limitations that comprise this work is the debugging of the data presented in WoS, where in some cases some repeated or unrelated documents are presented. This was also the case in the establishment of the intervals, this being a question of equity, given that the researchers tried to maintain a similar density of manuscripts in each of them. This study focused solely on the WoS database to show the scientific community the state of the art research on the existing literature on the subject. This may also be a limitation of the study. Therefore, as a future line of research, it is proposed that the analysis be replicated in other impact databases such as Scopus. On the other hand, as future lines of research, it is recommended that future authors investigate the search for new risks associated with the excessive use of the Internet, as well as the establishment of effective educational research to help combat and prevent this dangerous phenomenon for present and future generations.

In conclusion, the idea of continuing on the path of promoting healthy living habits with respect to digital health, especially among the youngest people, through a responsible practice to promote a healthy society that avoids coming into contact with the risks associated with the digital world, is stressed.

Author Contributions: Conceptualization, C.R.-J. and A.-J.M.-G.; methodology, A.-J.M.-G. and J.L.-B.; software, A.-J.M.-G.; validation, J.L.-B. and G.G.-G.; formal analysis, J.L.-B.; investigation, A.-J.M.-G.; resources, G.G.-G.;

data curation, A.-J.M.-G.; writing—original draft preparation, C.R.-J.; writing—review and editing, C.R.-J. and G.G.-G.; visualization, C.R.-J. and G.G.-G.; supervision, A.-J.M.-G. and J.L.-B. All authors have read and agreed to the published version of the manuscript.

Acknowledgments: To the researchers of the research group Análisis de la Realidad Educativa (AREA) (HUM-672). Research group by belonging to the Ministry of Education and Science of the Junta de Andalucía and based in the Department of Didactics and School Organization of the Faculty of Education Sciences of the University of Granada.

References

1. Brooks, S.; Wang, X.; Schneider, C. Technology Addictions and Technostress: An Examination of the US and China. *J. Organ. End User Comput. (JOEUC)* **2020**, *32*, 1–19. [CrossRef]
2. Sahu, M.; Gandhi, S.; Sharma, M.K. Mobile Phone Addiction Among Children and Adolescents: A Systematic Review. *J. Addictions Nurs.* **2019**, *30*, 261–268. [CrossRef] [PubMed]
3. San-Martín, S.; Jimenez, N.; Camarero, C.; San-José, R. The Path between Personality, Self-Efficacy, and Shopping Regarding Games Apps. *J. Theor. Appl. Electron. Commer. Res.* **2020**, *15*, 59–75. [CrossRef]
4. Aparicio-Martínez, P.; Ruiz-Rubio, M.; Perea-Moreno, A.J.; Martínez-Jiménez, M.P.; Pagliari, C.; Redel-Macías, M.D.; Vaquero-Abellán, M. Gender differences in the addiction to social networks in the Southern Spanish university students. *Telemat. Inform.* **2020**, *46*, 1–12. [CrossRef]
5. Firth, J.; Torous, J.; Stubbs, B.; Firth, J.A.; Steiner, G.Z.; Smith, L.; Álvarez-Jiménez, M.; Gleeson, J.; Vancampfort, D.; Armitage, C.J.; et al. The "online brain": How the Internet may be changing our cognition. *World Psychiatry* **2019**, *18*, 119–129. [CrossRef]
6. Molavi, P.; Mikaeili, N.; Ghaseminejad, M.A.; Kazemi, Z.; Pourdonya, M. Social Anxiety and Benign and Toxic Online Self-Disclosures: An Investigation into the Role of Rejection Sensitivity, Self-Regulation, and Internet Addiction in College Students. *J. Nerv. Ment. Dis.* **2018**, *206*, 598–605. [CrossRef]
7. Rodríguez-García, A.M.; Moreno-Guerrero, A.J.; López Belmonte, J. Nomophobia: An Individual's Growing Fear of Being without a Smartphone—A Systematic Literature Review. *Int. J. Environ. Res. Public Health* **2020**, *17*, 580. [CrossRef]
8. Carbonell, X.; Chamarro, A.; Oberst, U.; Rodrigo, B.; Prades, M. Problematic use of the internet and smartphones in university students: 2006–2017. *Int. J. Environ. Res. Public Health* **2018**, *15*, 475. [CrossRef] [PubMed]
9. Bisen, S.S.; Deshpande, Y.M. Prevalence, predictors, psychological correlates of internet addiction among college students in India: A comprehensive study. *Anatol. J. Psychiatry.* **2020**, *21*, 117–123. [CrossRef]
10. Urbanova, L.B.; Holubcikova, J.; Madarasova Geckova, A.; Reijneveld, S.A.; van Dijk, J.P. Does Life Satisfaction Mediate the Association between Socioeconomic Status and Excessive Internet Use? *Int. J. Environ. Res. Public Health* **2019**, *16*, 3914. [CrossRef] [PubMed]
11. Cuervo-Carabel, T.; Orviz-Martínez, N.; Arce-García, S.; Fernández-Suárez, I. Tecnoestrés en la Sociedad de la Tecnología y la Comunicación: Revisión bibliográfica a partir de la Web of Science. *Arch. Prevención Riesgos Labor.* **2018**, *21*, 18–25. [CrossRef]
12. Kim, Y.J.; Jang, H.M.; Lee, Y.; Lee, D.; Kim, D.J. Effects of internet and smartphone addictions on depression and anxiety based on propensity score matching analysis. *Int. J. Environ. Res. Public Health* **2018**, *15*, 859. [CrossRef] [PubMed]
13. Xie, J.Q.; Zimmerman, M.A.; Rost, D.H.; Yin, X.Q.; Wang, J.L. Stressful life events and problematic smartphone usage among Chinese boarding-school adolescents: A moderated mediation model of peer support and depressive symptoms. *Addict. Res. Theory* **2019**, 1–8. [CrossRef]
14. Masi, L.; Herba, C.; Garel, P. Projet pilote: Exploration de l'utilisation d'Internet et des médias sociaux chez un groupe d'adolescents ayant participé à Espace Transition. *Ann. Médico-Psychologiques Rev. Psychiatr.* **2019**, *177*, 319–326. [CrossRef]
15. Savolainen, I.; Oksanen, A.; Kaakinen, M.; Sirola, A.; Paek, H.J. The Role of Perceived Loneliness in Youth Addictive Behaviors: Cross-National Survey Study. *JMIR Men. Health* **2020**, *7*, e14035. [CrossRef]

16. Obeid, S.; Saade, S.; Haddad, C.; Sacre, H.; Khansa, W.; Al Hajj, R.; Kheir, N.; Hallit, S. Internet addiction among Lebanese adolescents: The role of self-esteem, anger, depression, anxiety, social anxiety and fear, impulsivity, and aggression—A cross-sectional study. *J. Nerv. Ment. Dis.* **2019**, *207*, 838–846. [CrossRef]
17. Lyvers, M.; Cutinho, D.; Thorberg, F.A. Alexithymia, impulsivity, disordered social media use, mood and alcohol use in relation to facebook self-disclosure. *Comput. Hum. Behav.* **2020**, *103*, 174–180. [CrossRef]
18. Rafiee, F.; Ghamari Zare, Z.; Adib-Hajbaghery, M.; Bakhtiari Zade, S. Internet addiction and psychological strain in nursing and midwifery students. *Nurs. Midwifery Stud.* **2020**, *9*, 36–42. [CrossRef]
19. Bhatt, S.; Gaur, A. Psychological risk factors associated with internet and smartphone addiction among students of an Indian dental institute. *Indian J. Public Health* **2019**, *63*, 313–317. [CrossRef]
20. Al Majali, S.A. The Digital World for Children and its Relationship with Personality Disorders: Exploring Emerging Technologies. *Int. J. Emerg. Technol. Learn. (iJET)* **2020**, *15*, 213–221. [CrossRef]
21. Lai, H.Y.; Cheah, W.L. Stress and its association with sociodemographic characteristics, coping and internet use among late adolescent university students in East Malaysia. *J. Indian Assoc. Child. Adolesc. Ment. Health* **2020**, *16*, 13–32.
22. Ergun-Basak, B.; Aydin, M. Problematic Internet Use in Terms of the Purposes of Internet Use, Irrational Beliefs, Feelings of Inferiority, and Gender. *Addicta: The Turkish J. Addict.* **2019**, *6*, 469–494. [CrossRef]
23. Truzoli, R.; Viganò, C.; Galmozzi, P.G.; Reed, P. Problematic internet use and study motivation in higher education. *J. Comput. Assist. Learn.* **2019**, 1–7. [CrossRef]
24. Cooper, K.; Quayle, E.; Jonsson, L.; Svedin, C.G. Adolescents and self-taken sexual images: A review of the literature. *Comput. Hum. Behav.* **2016**, *55*, 706–716. [CrossRef]
25. Cardozo, G.; Dubini, P.; Lorenzino, L. Bullying y ciberbullying: Un estudio comparativo con adolescentes escolarizados. *Rev. Mex. Psicol.* **2017**, *34*, 101–109.
26. Griffiths, M.D.; Nuyens, F. An Overview of Structural Characteristics in Problematic Video Game Playing. *Curr. Addict. Rep.* **2017**, *4*, 272–283. [CrossRef]
27. Caro-Amada, C.; Plaza, J. Intervención educativa familiar y terapia sistémica en la adicción adolescente a internet: Fundamentación teórica. *Rev. Española Orientac. Psicopedag. (REOP)* **2016**, *27*, 99–113. [CrossRef]
28. Choi, M. A concept analysis of digital citizenship for democratic citizenship education in the internet age. *Theory Res. Soc. Educ.* **2016**, *44*, 565–607. [CrossRef]
29. Hartley, J. *The Uses of Digital Literacy*; Routledge: New York, NY, USA, 2017.
30. Van Laar, E.; Van Deursen, A.J.; Van Dijk, J.A.; De Haan, J. The relation between 21st-century skills and digital skills: A systematic literature review. *Comput. Hum. Behav.* **2017**, *72*, 577–588. [CrossRef]
31. Rodríguez-Jiménez, C.; Gómez-García, G.; Romero-Rodríguez, J.M. Los retos tecnológicos del docente del siglo XXI/Technological challenges of the 21st century teacher. *Educ. Soc.* **2019**, *17*, 44–56.
32. Liao, H.; Tang, M.; Luo, L.; Li, C.; Chiclana, F.; Zeng, X.J. A bibliometric analysis and visualization of medical big data research. *Sustainability* **2018**, *10*, 166. [CrossRef]
33. Aznar, I.; Trujillo, J.M.; Romero-Rodríguez, J.M. Estudio bibliométrico sobre la realidad virtual aplicada a la neurorrehabilitación y su influencia en la literatura científica. *Rev. Cuba. Inf. Cienc. Salud* **2018**, *29*, 1–10.
34. Salmeron-Manzano, E.; Manzano-Agugliaro, F. The Higher Education Sustainability through Virtual Laboratories: The Spanish University as Case of Study. *Sustainability* **2018**, *10*, 4040. [CrossRef]
35. Sánchez-Santos, J.M.; Castellanos-García, P.A. Bibliometric analysis of sports economics research. *Int. J. Sport Financ.* **2011**, *6*, 222–244.
36. López, J.; Moreno-Guerrero, A.J.; López, J.A.; Pozo, S. Analysis of the Productive, Structural, and Dynamic Development of Augmented Reality in Higher Education Research on the Web of Science. *Appl. Sci.* **2019**, *9*, 1–21.
37. Rodríguez-García, A.M.; López, J.; Agreda, M.; Moreno-Guerrero, A.J. Productive, Structural and Dynamic Study of the Concept of Sustainability in the Educational Field. *Sustainability* **2019**, *11*, 5613. [CrossRef]
38. Martínez, M.A.; Cobo, M.J.; Herrera, M.; Herrera, E. Analyzing the scientific evolution of social work using science mapping. *Res. Soc. Work Pract.* **2015**, *25*, 257–277. [CrossRef]
39. Moral-Muñoz, J.A.; Herrera-Viedma, E.; Santisteban-Espejo, A.; Cobo, M.J. Software tools for conducting bibliometric analysis in science: An up-to-date review. *Prof. Inf.* **2020**, *29*, 1–20. [CrossRef]
40. Hirsch, J.E. An index to quantify an individual´s scientific research output. *Proc. Natl. Acad. Sci. USA* **2005**, *102*, 16569–16572. [CrossRef]

41. Cobo, M.J.; López, A.G.; Herrera, E.; Herrera, F. Science mapping software tools: Review, analysis, and cooperative study among tools. *J. Am. Soc. Inf. Sci. Technol.* **2011**, *62*, 1382–1402. [CrossRef]
42. López-Robles, J.R.; Otegi-Olaso, J.R.; Porto, I.; Cobo, M.J. 30 years of intelligence models in management and business: A bibliometric review. *Int. J. Inf. Manag.* **2019**, *48*, 22–38. [CrossRef]
43. Belli, S.; Baltá, J. Stocktaking scientific publication on bi-regional collaboration between Europe 28 and Latin America and the Caribbean. *Scientometrics* **2019**, *121*, 1447–1480. [CrossRef]
44. Montero-Díaz, J.; Cobo, M.J.; Gutiérrez-Salcedo, M.; Segado-Boj, F.; Herrera-Viedma, E. Mapeo científico de la Categoría «Comunicación» en WoS (1980–2013). *Comunicar* **2018**, *26*, 81–91. [CrossRef]
45. Davis, R.A. A cognitive-behavioral model of pathological Internet use. *Comput. Hum. Behav.* **2001**, *17*, 187–195. [CrossRef]
46. Morahan-Martin, J.; Schumacher, P. Incidence and correlates of pathological Internet use among college students. *Comput. Hum. Behav.* **2000**, *16*, 13–29. [CrossRef]
47. Block, J.J. Issues for DSM-V: Internet addiction. *Am. J. Psychiatry* **2008**, *165*, 306–307. [CrossRef]
48. Compton, W.M.; Volkow, N.D. Major increases in opioid analgesic abuse in the United States: Concerns and strategies. *Drug Alcohol Depend.* **2006**, *81*, 103–107. [CrossRef]

6

Gaming Device Usage Patterns Predict Internet Gaming Disorder: Comparison across Different Gaming Device Usage Patterns

Soo-Hyun Paik, Hyun Cho, Ji-Won Chun, Jo-Eun Jeong and Dai-Jin Kim *

Department of Psychiatry, Seoul St. Mary's Hospital, The Catholic University of Korea, Seoul 06591, Korea; suehime@gmail.com (S.-H.P.); sonap1@hanmail.net (H.C.); cuneus@naver.com (J.-W.C.); goodi11@hanmail.net (J.-E.J.)

* Correspondence: kdj922@catholic.ac.kr

Abstract: Gaming behaviors have been significantly influenced by smartphones. This study was designed to explore gaming behaviors and clinical characteristics across different gaming device usage patterns and the role of the patterns on Internet gaming disorder (IGD). Responders of an online survey regarding smartphone and online game usage were classified by different gaming device usage patterns: (1) individuals who played only computer games; (2) individuals who played computer games more than smartphone games; (3) individuals who played computer and smartphone games evenly; (4) individuals who played smartphone games more than computer games; (5) individuals who played only smartphone games. Data on demographics, gaming-related behaviors, and scales for Internet and smartphone addiction, depression, anxiety disorder, and substance use were collected. Combined users, especially those who played computer and smartphone games evenly, had higher prevalence of IGD, depression, anxiety disorder, and substance use disorder. These subjects were more prone to develop IGD than reference group (computer only gamers) (B = 0.457, odds ratio = 1.579). Smartphone only gamers had the lowest prevalence of IGD, spent the least time and money on gaming, and showed lowest scores of Internet and smartphone addiction. Our findings suggest that gaming device usage patterns may be associated with the occurrence, course, and prognosis of IGD.

Keywords: Internet gaming disorder; game device usage pattern; smartphone; comorbidity

1. Introduction

Playing online games is one of the most popular recreational activities. According to a Korean national survey conducted in 2016, 67.9% of the general population aged from 10 to 65 years old played online games [1]. Though gaming is a pleasurable and stimulatory activity, the dark side of excessive gaming is evident as well. Excessive use and loss of control over gaming has brought about various mental health and social concerns [2]. As numerous psychological and neurobiological correlates of excessive Internet gaming have been elucidated, such as impulsivity, reward sensitivity, and altered brain structure and function [3,4], the revised version of the Diagnostic and Statistical Manual of Mental Disorder, fifth edition (DSM-5) has listed the phenomenon of Internet gaming disorder (IGD) as a condition for further research [5].

To date, studies on IGD have mainly focused on personal computer (PC) games, especially massive multiplayer online role-playing games (MMORPGs) [3], and consistently reported that IGD was highly prevalent among male adolescents [6]. However, the spread of smartphones has explosively increased the number of gamers in female and in all age groups and subsequently changed the demographics and characteristics of online gamers. According to a Korean national survey conducted in 2015, among Korean smartphone users, 86.5% of the forties, 85.4% of the fifties, and 88.8% of females reported they had experiences of playing online games [7]. In addition, recent advances in smartphone game platforms have increased accessibility to various game genres including real-time strategy, MMORPG, or shooting games. Accordingly, the number of gamers who played with both devices has rapidly grown as well: 56.9% of the responders played smartphone games only while 20% played PC games only, and the remaining played both PC and smartphone games [7].

Given that each device has unique interface features and characteristics, gaming device usage patterns, such as single or combined use or time dedicated to each device, may play an important role on gaming behaviors and clinical characteristics and the occurrence of IGD. However, only a few studies have investigated the role of gaming device usage patterns on gaming-related attitudes or comorbid psychopathology. This study was designed to explore gaming behaviors and clinical characteristics across different gaming device usage patterns and their role on IGD.

2. Materials and Methods

2.1. Participants and Procedures

Data was collected from a large online survey conducted between April and September 2016 on online gaming and smartphone usage behaviors. Participants aged from 14 to 39 years were recruited from a pool of panelists registered for online panels at Panel Marketing Interactive (PMI), a research company that provides survey-related technology and data collection. The participants were given tokens that could be used as cybermoney as an incentive for their participation. In total, 9474 people were contacted and ultimately 7200 people (76% of those contacted) participated in our online survey. From the total 7200 responders, adults aged from 20 to 39 who both played online games and owned smartphones were included in this study (n = 3470). Since adolescents are considered to be more vulnerable to addictive disorders due to high novelty seeking and risk-taking temperament during adolescent period and immature cortical growth, which plays a critical role in cognitive control [8,9], we decided that the adult sample should be analyzed separately from adolescents. Though about 80% of smartphone users aged over 40 years had experiences of playing online games, the number of PC-based online gamers in this age are much lower than younger adults [1]. Thus, we set the upper age limit as 40 years old. We excluded responders who used game consoles (n = 412, 11.8% of total responders) for two reasons: (1) most of them also played PC and smartphone games (397, 96.3%), and (2) the aim of this study was to investigate the gaming characteristics among PC and smartphone gamers. Finally, 3058 subjects were selected (1548 males and 1510 females). The mean age was 26.95 years (standard deviation (SD) = 5.859 years).

All study procedures were performed in accordance with the guidelines of the Declaration of Helsinki. The Institutional Review Boards of Seoul St. Mary's Hospital approved the study protocol (KC15EISI0103). All subjects were informed about the study and all provided informed consent.

2.2. Measures

2.2.1. Demographic and Gaming Characteristics

Demographic information on education levels and occupation status was asked. Education levels were classified into two categories: (1) up to 12 years (up to high school graduates), and (2) more than 13 years (currently in university/college or higher education). Occupational status was classified into three categories: (1) current students; (2) individuals currently with full-time jobs, and (3) individuals currently without full-time jobs.

All participants were asked to answer dichotomously (1: Yes, 2: No) to nine diagnostic criteria questions for IGD according to the DSM-5. Participants who answered "yes" to five or more criteria for questions pertaining to the previous 12 months were defined as the IGD group in line with previous studies [10–12], and those with four or less affirmative answers were defined as the non-IGD group. Gaming device usage patterns were determined by reports from the responders on the time proportion dedicated to either PC or smartphone (SM) and were classified into five groups: (1) PC only group: individuals who played only PC games, 100% dedicated to PC games ($n = 720$); (2) PC > SM group: individuals who played more PC games than SM games, 60% to 99% dedicated to PC games and 1% to 40% to SM ($n = 580$); (3) PC = SM group: individuals who played PC and SM games evenly, 41% to 59% dedicated to both PC and SM games ($n = 326$); (4) PC < SM group: individuals who played SM games more than PC games, 60% to 99% dedicated to SM games and 1% to 40% to PC ($n = 735$), and (5) SM only group: individuals who played only SM games, 100% to SM games ($n = 697$). Additionally, time (minutes) and money (by Korean currency, KRW, per month) spent on gaming, whether they owned game community memberships, and whether they have any experience of attending offline meetings were asked. The most preferred game was asked and classified into five genres according to the White Paper on Korean Games [13]: (1) simulation and real-time strategy (i.e., League of Legends, StarCraft, and the Sims); (2) role-playing game (RPG) (i.e., World of Warcraft and Lineage); (3) sports and racing (i.e., FIFA, Winning Eleven, Need for Speed, and Tales Runner); (4) shooting and action (i.e., Sudden Attack, Counter Strike, and Virtual Fighter) and (5) puzzle, arcade, and board games (i.e., Candy Crush Saga, Monopoly, and rhythm games). The main motive for gaming was selected from the following categories: (1) for fun; (2) for killing time; (3) for relieving stress; (4) for need (i.e., to maintain interpersonal relationship), and (5) for sense of achievement.

2.2.2. Clinical Characteristics

Participants were asked to answer the following questionnaires in order to determine clinical characteristics: Young's Internet Addiction Test (YIAT), Smartphone Addiction Scale-Short Version (SAS-SV), Brief Self-Control Scale (BSCS), Patient Health Questionnaire-9 (PHQ-9), Generalized Anxiety Disorder-7 (GAD-7), Alcohol Use Disorder Identification Test (AUDIT), and Fagerstrom Test for Nicotine Dependence (FTND).

YIAT, a 20-item scale which is rated by a five-point Likert scale (1: Not at all, 5: Almost always) [14], was used to assess the severity of Internet addiction [15]. In South Korea, YIAT had acceptable internal consistency and reliability (Cronbach's alpha = 0.921) [16] and Cronbach's alpha for YIAT was 0.956 in this sample.

SAS-SV, a 10-item scale which is rated by a six-point Likert scale (1: Strongly disagree, 6: Strongly agree), was used to assess the severity of smartphone addiction [17]. SAS-SV has excellent concurrent validity and highly correlated with the original version (Cronbach's alpha = 0.958, $p < 0.001$). SAS-SV has been used in adult sample to assess the degree of smartphone addiction across various countries; a higher score indicated a higher degree of smartphone addiction [18,19]. Cronbach's alpha was 0.773 in this study.

BSCS, a 13-item questionnaire with a five-point Likert scale (1: Strongly disagree, 5: Strongly agree), was used to measure self-control ability. BSCS measures the ability to override or change one's inner response as well as to interrupt undesired behavioral tendencies and refrain from acting on them, with higher scores indicating lower self-control ability. BSCS had good internal consistency (Cronbach's alpha = 0.85) in the original study [20]. Cronbach's alpha was 0.757 in this study.

PHQ-9 is a nine-item depression rating scale which corresponds to the major depressive episode criteria of the DSM-IV with a four-point Likert scale (0: Not at all, 3: Almost every day) [19]. We defined individuals with scores of 10 or more as having depression according to Manea and colleagues [21]. The Korean version of PHQ-9 has proven to have excellent validity and reliability in primary care patients for detecting major depressive disorder (Cronbach's alpha = 0.852) [22]. Cronbach's alpha was 0.893 in this study.

GAD-7, a seven-item scale with a four-point Likert scale (0: Not at all, 3: Nearly every day), was used to screen generalized anxiety disorder (GAD) [23]. GAD-7 is particularly useful in assessing symptom severity. We defined individuals with scores of 10 or greater as having GAD according to Plummer and colleagues [24]. GAD-7 had excellent internal consistency (Cronbach's alpha = 0.92) [23]. Cronbach's alpha was 0.908 in this study.

AUDIT, developed by the World Health Organization, is a 10-item scale to identify alcohol-related problems [25]. Total scores range from 0 to 40 and the optimal cut-off point to identify at-risk alcohol users is 10 for males and 6 for females in South Korea [26]. In this study, alcohol use disorder (AUD) was defined for males as a score of 10 or more and for females as a score of 6 or more. AUDIT had good internal consistency (Cronbach's alpha = 0.80–0.93) and Cronbach's alpha was 0.859 in this study.

FTND is a six-item scale which is most widely used to measure nicotine dependence [27]. Total scores range from 0 to 10 and individuals with scores of four or more were determined to have nicotine dependence [28]. The Korean version of FTND was standardized and Cronbach's alpha was 0.6913, which was similar in this study, 0.636.

2.3. Statistical Analysis

The quantitative variables are presented as means ± SD and the qualitative data are presented as absolute numbers (N) and percentages (%). To compare differences between IGD and non-IGD groups, and across different gaming device usage pattern groups, non-parametric Mann-Whitney U tests and Kruskal-Wallis H tests were used, respectively. Additional post-hoc tests were done by the Mann-Whitney U tests. To examine the predictive values of each variable for IGD, binary logistic regression analysis was performed and the results are shown by odds ratios (ORs) and 95% confidential intervals (CIs). All statistical works were performed by using SPSS version 24.0 (SPSS Inc., Chicago, IL, USA).

3. Results

3.1. Comparison between the IGD and Control Groups

Table 1 shows differences in gaming behaviors and clinical characteristics between IGD and non-IGD subjects. From the total 3058 participants, 396 (12.9%) were classified as having IGD. IGD subjects had higher mean age, were more likely to be males, had lower prevalence of participants with higher education or who currently had full-time jobs, spent more time and money on gaming, and had more game community membership and experience of offline meeting attendance than non-IGD subjects. IGD was more prevalent in combined user groups (PC > SM, PC = SM, and PC < SM groups) than in the single user groups (PC and SM only groups) (66.4% vs. 51.7%, respectively). Preferred game genres were different; IGD subjects preferred simulation/strategy (28.5%) and RPG (27.3%) genres while non-IGD subjects did puzzle, arcade, and board games (31.0%). The main motives for gaming were different as well; the proportions of gamers who played for fun and for killing time were higher in non-IGD subjects (43.5% vs. 37.4%, 25.2% vs. 16.4%, respectively) while the proportion of gamers who played for relieving stress and for the sense of achievement was higher in IGD subjects (25.5% vs. 20.1%, and 15.2% vs. 8.2%, respectively). Scores of YIAT, SAS-SV, and BSCS and the prevalence of depression, GAD, AUD, and nicotine dependence were significantly higher among IGD subjects.

We performed two additional subgroup analyses to explore the gender role in IGD. First, we compared between IGD and non-IGD subjects for males and females separately (see Table S1 in the Supplementary Materials), and then between males and females in the IGD group (see Table S2 in the Supplementary Materials). The difference of education levels and occupational status between IGD and non-IGD groups was not observed in females, whereas that of preferred game genre was not found in males. Other findings were comparable to the findings of the whole sample. When compared between the male IGD group and female IGD group, the male IGD group had a higher proportion of individuals who currently had full-time jobs, game community membership, and nicotine dependence, and spent more money on gaming, while the female IGD group had higher scores for SAS-SV and BSCS, indicating lower self-control ability, and higher prevalence of AUD than the male IGD group. Gaming device usage patterns differed between genders. PC > SM (448, 28.9%) and PC only (431, 27.8%) patterns were more prevalent in males, and these patterns persisted in the male IGD group. Females had a higher proportion of PC < SM (417, 27.6%) and SM only (505, 33.4%) patterns, while the female IGD group showed higher PC < SM and PC = SM patterns.

Table 1. Comparison between the IGD and non-IGD groups.

Variables	IGD	Non-IGD	X^2/U	*p*
N (%)	396 (12.9%)	2662 (87.1%)		
Age	27.63 ± 5.797	26.85 ± 5.862	572,613.000	0.005 *
Male (%)	220 (55.6%)	1328 (49.9%)	4.431	0.035 *
Education levels				
Up to 12 years (high school)	63 (15.9%)	276 (10.4%)	10.731	0.001 **
More than 13 years	333 (84.1%)	2386 (89.6%)		
Occupational status				
Student	123 (31.1%)	1029 (38.7%)	8.472	0.014 *
Current full-time job	213 (53.8%)	1227 (48.0%)		
No currently full-time job	60 (15.2%)	356 (13.4%)		
Time spent on gaming				
Weekday (min)	167.79 ± 124.190	107.63 ± 96.227	722,949.000	0.000 **
Weekend (min)	253.76 ± 152.207	169.02 ± 131.868	729,658.000	0.000 **
Money spent on gaming (KRW)	32,270.45 ± 48,491.203	11,599.61 ± 27,190.750	752,279.500	0.000 **
Game community membership	253 (63.9%)	818 (30.7%)	166.566	0.000 **
Ever attended offline meeting	179 (45.2%)	352 (13.2%)	59.393	0.000 **
Gaming device usage pattern				
PC only	87 (22.0%)	633 (23.8%)	51.909	0.000 **
PC > SM	90 (22.7%)	490 (18.4%)		
PC = SM	71 (17.9%)	255 (9.6%)		
PC < SM	102 (25.8%)	633 (23.8%)		
SM only	46 (11.6%)	651 (24.5%)		
Preferred game genre				
Simulation/strategy	113 (28.5%)	708 (26.6%)	23.102	0.000 **
RPG	108 (27.3%)	521 (19.6%)		
Sports/racing	60 (15.2%)	413 (15.5%)		
Shooting/action	33 (8.3%)	196 (7.4%)		
Puzzle/arcade/board game	82 (20.7%)	824 (31.0%)		
Reason for gaming				
For fun	148 (37.4%)	1159 (43.5%)	44.352	0.000 **
For killing time	65 (16.4%)	671 (25.2%)		
For relieving stress	101 (25.5%)	535 (20.1%)		
For need	22 (5.6%)	80 (3.0%)		
For achievement	60 (15.2%)	217 (8.2%)		
YIAT	53.98 ± 26.267	36.80 ± 18.800	788,470.500	0.000 **
SAS-SV	39.97 ± 9.015	28.75 ± 10.114	838,582.000	0.000 **
BSCS	53.98 ± 26.267	36.80 ± 18.800	775,457.500	0.000 **
Depression (%)	252 (63.6%)	631 (23.7%)	267.652	0.000 **
Generalized anxiety disorder (%)	179 (45.2%)	383 (14.4%)	218.205	0.000 **
Alcohol use disorder (%)	139 (35.1%)	446 (16.8%)	75.003	0.000 **
Nicotine dependence (%)	55 (59.8%)	133 (31.7%)	25.675	0.000 **

Abbreviations: IGD: Internet Gaming Disorder; KRW: Korean Won; PC: Personal computer; SM: Smartphone; RPG: Role-playing game; YIAT: Young's Internet Addiction Test; SAS-SV: Smartphone Addiction Scale-Short Form; BSCS: Brief Self-Control Scale. * $p < 0.05$, ** $p < 0.005$.

3.2. Comparison across Different Gaming Device Usage Patterns

Table 2 shows the results of a comparison analysis across the five different gaming device usage groups. The mean age was highest in the SM only group and males were most prevalent in the PC only and PC > SM groups. PC only and PC = SM groups had higher prevalence of individuals with lower education. The PC only and PC > SM groups had higher proportions of students whereas the SM only and PC = SM groups had higher proportions of individuals who currently had full-time jobs. IGD was most prevalent in the PC = SM group (21.8%), followed by the PC > SM (15.5%) and PC < SM (13.9%) groups, and least prevalent in the SM only (6.6%) group. Time and money spent on gaming was highest in the PC > SM group and lowest in the SM only group. The PC > SM and PC = SM groups had the highest prevalence of game community membership and experience of offline meeting attendance.

Preferred game genres and motives for gaming were different across groups. The SM only group preferred puzzle, arcade, and board games while the other groups preferred simulation/strategy and RPG games. PC predominant groups (PC only, PC > SM, PC = SM groups) mainly played games "for fun" and "for relieving stress" while SM predominant groups (PC < SM and SM only groups) chose to play games more "for killing time". The SM only group had the lowest scores on YIAT, SAS-SV, and BSCS and proportions of depression, GAD, AUD, and nicotine dependence and PC = SM had the highest scores and proportions of comorbid psychopathology.

3.3. *Predictive Value of the Gaming Device Usage Patterns*

Table 3 shows the results of a binary logistic regression analysis predicting IGD using age, gender, time and money spent on gaming game community membership, device usage patterns, the scores of SAS-SV and BSCS, and the presence of depression, GAD, AUD, and nicotine dependence as covariates. Since the ranges of time and money spent on gaming were too broad to calculate odds ratios, these variables were divided dichotomously according to the median value: time spent on gaming during weekday (0: Minimum to 90 min, 1: 91 min to maximum) and weekend (0: Minimum to 150 min, 1: 151 min to maximum), and money (0: Minimum to KRW2000 (approximately 1.84 USD (1 USD = KRW1088.00, December 2017), 1: KRW2001 to maximum). When analyzed in a single equation, the input variables accounted for 39.5% of the total variance (Nagelkerke R^2 = 0.395) and the prediction success was 89.1%.

Individuals with higher age (B = 0.032, OR = 1.033), who spent 150 min or more on gaming during the weekend (B = 0.542, OR = 1.720), who spent more than KRW2001 on gaming per month (B = 0.729, OR = 2.072) and who owned a game community membership (B = 0.851, OR = 2.341) were likely to become IGD. As for the gaming device usage patterns, the PC = SM pattern increased the probability of IGD in comparison to the reference (PC only) group (B = 0.457, OR = 1.579). Individuals with higher SAS-SV and BSCS scores and depression were more prone to become IGD (B = 0.090, 0.043, and 0.667, OR = 1.094, 1.044, and 1.949 for SAS-SV, BSCS, and depression, respectively).

Table 2. Differences across device usage patterns.

Variables	PC Only	PC > SM	PC = SM	PC < SM	SM Only	X^2/H	p	Post-Hoc
N (%)	720 (23.5%)	580 (19.0%)	326 (10.7%)	735 (24.0%)	697 (22.8%)			
Age	25.70 ± 5.306	25.74 ± 5.458	27.16 ± 5.800	27.11 ± 5.890	28.95 ± 6.142	140.747	0.000 **	e > a,b,c,d, a,b < c,d
Male (%)	448 (62.2%)	431 (74.3%)	159 (48.8%)	318 (43.3%)	192 (27.5%)	333.801	0.000 **	
Education levels								
Up to 12 years	95 (13.2%)	66 (11.4%)	46 (14.1%)	65 (8.8%)	67 (9.6%)	11.608	0.021 *	
More than 13 years	625 (86.8%)	514 (88.6%)	280 (85.9%)	670 (91.2%)	630 (90.4%)			
Occupational status								
Student	330 (45.8%)	292 (50.3%)	107 (32.8%)	254 (34.6%)	169 (24.2%)			
Current full-time job	281 (39.0%)	217 (37.4%)	180 (55.2%)	383 (42.1%)	429 (61.5%)	134.837	0.000 **	
No current full-time job	109 (15.1%)	71 (12.2%)	39 (12.0%)	98 (13.3%)	99 (14.2%)			
IGD (%)	87 (12.1%)	90 (15.5%)	71 (21.8%)	102 (13.9%)	46 (6.6%)	51.909	0.000 **	
Time spent on gaming								
Weekday (min)	111.65 ± 103.703	139.56 ± 105.489	120.45 ± 112.919	110.11 ± 87.180	96.75 ± 103.262	122.254	0.000 **	e < a,b,c,d, b > a,c,d
Weekend (min)	194.60 ± 148.341	220.82 ± 134.656	180.53 ± 124.000	172.78 ± 123.798	137.61 ± 135.296	226.227	0.000 **	e < a,b,c,d, b > a,c,d
Money spent on gaming (KRW)	17,298.34 ± 37,995.779	24,993.36 ± 36,335.539	19,647.24 ± 34,119.854	11,973.13 ± 29,297.559	2082.50 ± 7421.816	577.364	0.000 **	e < a,b,c,d, b > a,c,d d < a,c
Game community membership	220 (30.6%)	304 (52.4%)	153 (46.9%)	273 (37.7%)	117 (16.8%)	207.871	0.000 **	
Ever attended offline meeting	101 (45.9%)	172 (56.6%)	88 (57.5%)	128 (46.2%)	42 (35.9%)	21.019	0.000 **	
Preferred game genre								
Simulation/strategy	255 (35.4%)	230 (39.7%)	77 (23.6%)	152 (20.7%)	107 (15.4%)			
RPG	183 (25.4%)	132 (22.8%)	79 (24.2%)	157 (21.4%)	78 (11.2%)			
Sports/racing	119 (16.5%)	89 (15.3%)	69 (21.2%)	123 (16.7%)	73 (10.5%)	591.480	0.000 **	
Shooting/action	88 (12.2%)	59 (10.2%)	21 (6.4%)	40 (5.4%)	12 (3.0%)			
Puzzle/arcade/board game	75 (10.4%)	70 (12.1%)	80 (24.5%)	263 (29.0%)	418 (60.0%)			
Reason for gaming								
For fun	237 (45.4%)	267 (46.0%)	147 (45.1%)	318 (43.3%)	248 (35.6%)			
For killing time	120 (16.7%)	88 (15.2%)	66 (20.2%)	181 (24.6%)	281 (38.2%)			
For relieving stress	178 (24.7%)	134 (23.1%)	69 (21.2%)	153 (20.8%)	102 (14.6%)	164.244	0.000 **	
For need	34 (4.7%)	24 (4.1%)	13 (4.0%)	21 (2.9%)	10 (1.4%)			
For achievement	61 (8.5%)	67 (11.6%)	31 (9.5%)	62 (8.4%)	56 (8.0%)			
YIAT	38.65 ± 20.899	43.56 ± 18.530	44.08 ± 21.511	40.73 ± 20.591	31.36 ± 19.930	145.760	0.000 **	e < a,b,c,d, a < b,c
SAS-SV	29.50 ± 10.646	30.19 ± 11.029	31.58 ± 11.149	31.60 ± 10.392	28.76 ± 10.657	31.614	0.000 **	e < c,d, a < c,d
BSCS	36.51 ± 6.663	36.17 ± 6.959	36.73 ± 6.920	36.49 ± 6.742	35.33 ± 6.795	17.479	0.002 **	e < a,c,d
Depression (%)	218 (30.3%)	156 (26.9%)	116 (35.6%)	233 (31.7%)	160 (23.0%)	23.687	0.000 **	
Generalized anxiety disorder (%)	141 (19.6%)	101 (17.4%)	74 (22.7%)	144 (19.6%)	102 (14.6%)	12.350	0.015 *	
Alcohol use disorder (%)	141 (31.6%)	84 (22.0%)	82 (36.4%)	160 (31.3%)	118 (26.3%)	19.325	0.001 **	
Nicotine dependence (%)	35 (31.0%)	50 (38.8%)	23 (44.2%)	60 (43.2%)	20 (25.3%)	10.006	0.040 *	

Abbreviations: PC: Personal computer; SM: Smartphone; IGD: Internet Gaming Disorder; KRW: Korean Won; RPG: Role-playing game; YIAT: Young's Internet Addiction Test; SAS-SV: Smartphone Addiction Scale Short Form; BSCS: Brief Self-Control Scale. * $p < 0.05$, ** $p < 0.005$.

Table 3. Logistic regression results predicting Internet gaming disorder.

Variables	B (s.e.)	OR	95% CI	*p*
Age	0.032 (0.011)	1.033	1.010–1.056	0.005 *
Gender (male)	0.260 (0.144)	1.296	0.977–1.719	0.072
Weekday gaming hour (>90 min)	0.262 (0.144)	1.300	0.931–1.816	0.124
Weekend gaming hour (>150 min)	0.542 (0.170)	1.720	1.232–2.399	0.001 **
Money spent on gaming (>KRW2000)	0.729 (0.144)	2.072	1.562–2.749	0.000 **
Game community membership	0.851 (0.137)	2.341	1.791–3.061	0.000 **
Gaming device usage pattern				
PC only		Reference		0.000 **
PC > SM	−0.085 (0.196)	0.919	0.626–1.349	0.666
PC = SM	0.457 (0.213)	1.579	1.040–2.397	0.032 *
PC < SM	0.019 (0.189)	1.019	0.703–1.476	0.921
SM only	−0.144 (0.229)	0.866	0.552–1.357	0.529
SAS-SV	0.090 (0.008)	1.094	1.076–1.112	0.000 **
BSCS	0.043 (0.013)	1.044	1.018–1.070	0.001 **
Depression	0.667 (0.168)	1.949	1.403–2.708	0.000 **
Generalized anxiety disorder	0.132 (0.173)	1.141	0.812–1.603	0.447
Alcohol use disorder	0.254 (0.150)	1.2899	0.961–1.728	0.090
Nicotine dependence	0.384 (0.223)	1.468	0.949–2.271	0.085

Abbreviations: s.e.: standard error; KRW: Korean Won; PC: Personal computer; SM: Smartphone; SAS-SV: Smartphone Addiction Scale Short Form; BSCS: Brief Self-Control Scale; OR: odds ratio; CI: confidence interval.
* $p < 0.05$, ** $p < 0.005$.

4. Discussion

4.1. Characteristics of IGD in Smartphone Era

Overall, the prevalence of IGD was 12.9% in this study. The prevalence of IGD ranged from 0.6% to 46% depending on the sample and methods [29]. According to a Korean national survey conducted in 2015, the prevalence of Internet addiction was 5.8% in an adult population with ages ranging from 20 to 59 years old [7], which was lower than our results. Given that our sample was recruited from online survey responders who played online games and included those age ranged from 20 to 39, it seems reasonable that the prevalence of IGD is higher in our sample, though a direct comparison is impossible due to the differences in the sample collecting methods and applied diagnostic criteria. Rather, this result was in line with a previous study reporting that 38.7% of adult MMORPG players were IGD [30], since 20.5% of the responders played RPGs, most of which were MMORPGs. The prevalence of IGD is higher in Korea than in the other countries. The prevalence of IGD has been considered to be high in East Asian countries [31]. Cultural differences, such as Internet accessibility (speed of Internet access, availability of Wi-Fi, the cost paid for using Internet, or accessibility of Internet cafes), social norms for Internet gaming and device usage patterns, and government regulations for Internet gaming, as well as the sample recruitment and applied measurements may account for the different prevalence across different countries. Considering that IGD subjects in this study showed comparable clinical characteristics to previous studies, such that they owned game community memberships and attended offline meetings more frequently, spent more time and money on gaming, showed more preference for the simulation/strategy and RPG genres, were motivated to play games more to relieve stress, manifested higher degrees of smartphone addiction and lower levels of self-control, and had higher prevalence of depression, GAD, AUD, and nicotine dependence than non-IGD individuals [3,6,32–36], our sample may represent the general IGD population. In contrast to prior findings that IGD was frequently observed in male adolescents [37,38], the proportion of females in the IGD group was 44.4% and the mean age was higher among those with IGD. Given that our sample only included an adult population, this would be a unique feature of adult IGD, distinct from adolescent IGD. The spread of smartphone games, which provide easier accessibility and portability than PC games, may increase the number of female and middle-aged adult gamers.

Some gaming-related and clinical characteristics were significantly different between male and female participants. Preferred game genre and reason for gaming were different between genders, in line with previous findings [39–41]. Males displaying IGD spent more money on gaming and had more game community memberships, both classical features of IGD, while females displaying IGD had higher smartphone addiction severity and lower self-control ability, which may indicate the role of problematic smartphone use on IGD in females [42,43]. The proportion of nicotine dependence was higher among males with IGD, while that of AUD was higher among females with IGD. This may be due to an increased risk of AUD in the presence of comorbid psychiatric condition in females [44]. Gaming device usage patterns were significantly different between genders as well; males had a tendency to play PC games more than SM games while females seemed to play more SM games. The features of each device, which are described below, differences in time spent on gaming, preference of specific game genres that were more suitable for PC interface, and social expectation toward gaming behavior between genders may account for the results [41].

4.2. *Characteristics across Different Gaming Device Usage Patterns*

When comparing across different gaming device usage patterns, several intriguing findings were observed. First, IGD was more prevalent in combined user groups (PC > SM, PC = SM, and PC < SM groups), especially in the PC = SM group, than the single user groups (PC and SM only). IGD is a behavioral addiction that psychologically and neurobiologically resembles substance addiction [3]. As substance abusers frequently co-administer multiple substances simultaneously [45], IGD subjects may need multiple methods of playing games. In particular, the PC = SM group had the highest prevalence of IGD, possibly due to the differences in motivational background and gaming interface of each device. Though both PC and SM games provide a sense of reward and relatedness as well as escape from negative emotions [46,47], each device may satisfy different needs. Since PC games usually provide high quality sound and visual effects and necessitate substantial duration for playing, they may have the potential to provide a sense of immersion, achievement, and competitiveness [47]. Meanwhile, SM games may increase a sense of social relatedness and attenuate loneliness and negative emotion [48], since SM games are easily played in association with social networking service (SNS) applications. In this study, motives for gaming were significantly different across groups; PC predominant gamers played games "for fun", "for relieving stress", and "for achievement", while SM predominant gamers played games "for killing time", "for fun", and "for relieving stress". Considering that the PC = SM group manifested more comorbid psychopathology, which can be taken as being more defective in self-soothing ability, they may need both devices to satisfy different needs and become more indulged in gaming than the other groups.

Second, each combined user group (PC > SM, PC = SM, and PC < SM groups) had unique clinical characteristics that may modify the course and prognosis of IGD. Individuals in the PC > SM group showed typical behavioral manifestations of IGD [32]. They were younger, had a higher male proportion, spent more time and money on gaming, and had more game community memberships, but had less prevalence of comorbid psychopathology than other combined user groups. Meanwhile, the PC = SM group showed the highest prevalence of comorbid psychopathology, implying that they may be suffering from more difficulty in academic or occupational adaptation and impelled to continuously play games to soothe their negative emotions or to alleviate substance craving. The PC < SM group manifested similar gaming behaviors to the SM only group while comorbidity patterns were comparable to the PC = SM group. These findings suggest an important clinical implication that detailed investigations of the gaming device usage patterns may provide precise estimation of current status and prediction of prognosis.

Third, the PC only group spent less time and money on gaming and showed lower scores on YIAT and SAS-SV than the combined user groups. PC games usually need special environmental requisites, such as fast online connection speeds, high-resolution large screens, and charged memberships, which may paradoxically keep the PC gamers away from playing anytime and anywhere. In addition, since PC games offer excellent visual and sound effects and sophisticated game platforms, PC gamers may not be satisfied with SM games. Another interesting finding was that PC only gamers manifested as high prevalence of depression, GAD, and AUD as the PC < SM group. Considering that PC games had more addictive potential than SM games [49,50], PC only gamers may have difficulty in functioning as is the case for the combined users despite less behavioral disturbances.

Fourth, the SM only group had a higher mean age and proportion of females, spent less time and money on gaming, and had lower severity of Internet and smartphone addiction and prevalence of IGD, depression, GAD, AUD, and nicotine dependence and higher self-control ability than the other groups. Explanations can be drawn from the unique characteristics of SM game interfaces and smartphones themselves. First is the structural characteristic of smartphone games. Despite substantial technical advances that enable sophisticated games to be played on smartphone platforms, simpler games such as puzzle, arcade, or board games are still more suitable and preferred for the SM gamers, possibly due to unchangeable structures such as small screens and viewing angles, which interfere with the sense of immersion [51]. Secondly, the emergence of the social networking games (SNGs), a hybrid game genre that connects games with SNSs, should be considered. SNG players can play games and interact with online friends simultaneously within existing SNS applications. Many responders in the SM only group answered that they preferred to play SNGs, such as "Farmville" or "I Love Coffee", to mention but a few. Considering that getting something useful out of playing, such as the improvement of relationships, was the major motive to play SNGs [52], SM gamers, especially SNG players, may prefer to play games to get something that classical PC games cannot provide, such as enhancement of social relatedness and the alleviation of feelings of loneliness. Third, the unique properties of smartphones themselves can be considered. In addition to the portability and availability for easy and frequent access that leads to habitual checking behavior [53], the multi-tasking function enables SM users to play games while they are doing other things, such as searching on websites or sending messages. Though SM gamers may not spend as much time and money on gaming and feel as much immersion in games as PC gamers do, they may use games to "kill time" between tasks or during "empty" hours of waiting.

4.3. The Role of Gaming Device Usage Patterns on IGD

Logistic regression analysis revealed that the PC = SM pattern was a predictor of IGD, along with time and money spent on gaming, game community membership, the severity of smartphone addiction, self-control ability, and the presence of depression. As mentioned above, individuals in the PC = SM group had the highest prevalence of comorbidity and thus they may feel that it is difficult to quit games probably due to lack of tolerability for withdrawal symptoms or negative emotions. Another possibility lays in that the PC = SM pattern may have an intrinsic risk potential for IGD since no multicollinearity was observed among variables. Further studies are necessary to elucidate the neurobiology that underlies this distinct device usage pattern. An important finding that higher financial investment was associated with increased risk of IGD should be marked. This was in line with previous findings demonstrating that higher money spent on gaming was associated with IGD in adolescents and had a predictive value of IGD in adults [32,54]. Most online games are freemium services, which are free for download, but require payment for additional features or virtual goods [55]. Even though the amount is small, as much as $2, it could cause a big financial problem if accumulated, as is the case of gambling disorder, and could induce more commitment toward the games. Increased risk of IGD with individuals who spent more than 2000 won (approximately $1.84) for gaming per month would support the danger of accumulated micropayments.

There are some limitations that should be noted. First, the causality of IGD and the device usage patterns were not elucidated due to the cross-sectional nature of this study. Second, the distinction between the game genres may not be mutually exclusive because of the fast evolution of hybrid game genres. For example, Cookie Run is a hybrid form of running and action games. Likewise, the distinction between the games and other smartphone applications were not exclusive, such as with SNGs. Further research studies need to investigate the role of hybrid games or applications on IGD or other technological addiction. Third, IGD was determined by self-reports of endorsement to five or more DSM-5 IGD criteria, which was originally developed for professional usage. However, Lemmens and colleagues have demonstrated solid psychometric property and high practicality of The Short, Nine-Item IGD Scale, which assessed IGD using the self-reporting of nine items of DSM-5 IGD criteria with a dichotomous scale [12]. Despite deviation from original professional purposes, the self-rating IGD would be a valid tool for identifying IGD, especially in a large sample. Fourth, since comorbid psychopathology and gaming device usage patterns were assessed via self-report, over- or under-estimation of psychopathology and a recall bias may be present. Overestimation of IGD should be considered when determining IGD by the self-report as well. As mentioned above, the prevalence of IGD was higher in this study than in the national survey. Further research studies may need to validate the findings using diagnostic interviews and machinery collecting methods. Lastly, we did not include console users. In contrast to the United States of America and European countries, only a small number of gamers used video and portable consoles for gaming [1]. Console games had different features than PC and SM games, such as the need for buying consoles and software, and may manifest unique gaming-relate behaviors and characteristics. Further studies are necessary to investigate the characteristics of console gamers, especially in comparison with PC and SM gamers. Alternatively, was this meant to be "the United States of America"? If so, please specify to avoid potential ambiguity with the continents.

5. Conclusions

In this study, we investigated how gaming device usage patterns influenced gaming behaviors and clinical characteristics. To the best of our knowledge, this is the first study to elucidate the differences in gaming behavior and comorbid psychopathology across gaming device usage patterns and the role of specific usage patterns on IGD. Despite limitations, this study is notable for having been conducted using a large sample and having covered a diverse range of gaming behaviors and clinical characteristics, and thus contributes to deepening our understanding of IGD in the smartphone era. Our findings suggest that gaming device usage patterns may be associated with the occurrence, course, and prognosis of IGD. An important clinical implication can be drawn that the evaluation of gaming device usage patterns would help to determine the risk, predict outcome, and offer optimized treatment options for IGD.

Acknowledgments: This work was supported by a grant from the Brain Research Program through the National Research Foundation of Korea (NRF) funded by the Ministry of Science, ICT & Future Planning (NRF-2014M3C7A1062893).

Author Contributions: All the authors contributed to the design and study planning and advised the course of study. S.-H.P. conducted the literature search, provided summaries of previous research studies, conducted the statistical analysis, and wrote the first draft of the manuscript. All authors contributed to the development of the manuscript, revised it critically, and approved the final manuscript.

References

1. Game Users Survey Report 2016. Available online: http://www.kocca.kr/cop/bbs/view/B0000147/1831102.do?menuNo=200904 (accessed on 18 July 2017).
2. Ferguson, C.J.; Coulson, M.; Barnett, J. A meta-analysis of pathological gaming prevalence and comorbidity with mental health, academic and social problems. *J. Psychiatr. Res.* **2011**, *45*, 1573–1578. [CrossRef] [PubMed]

3. Kuss, D.J.; Griffiths, M.D. Internet gaming addiction: A systematic review of empirical research. *Int. J. Ment. Health Addict.* **2012**, *10*, 278–296. [CrossRef]
4. Fauth-Bühler, M.; Mann, K. Neurobiological correlates of internet gaming disorder: Similarities to pathological gambling. *Addict. Behav.* **2017**, *64*, 349–356. [CrossRef] [PubMed]
5. American Psychiatric Association. *Diagnostic and Statistical Manual of Mental Disorders (DSM-5®)*; American Psychiatric Pub.: Arlington, VA, USA, 2013.
6. Ho, R.C.; Zhang, M.W.; Tsang, T.Y.; Toh, A.H.; Pan, F.; Lu, Y.; Cheng, C.; Yip, P.S.; Lam, L.T.; Lai, C.-M. The association between internet addiction and psychiatric co-morbidity: A meta-analysis. *BMC Psychiatr.* **2014**, *14*, 183. [CrossRef] [PubMed]
7. Survey on Internet Overdependence 2015. Available online: http://www.nia.or.kr/site/nia_kor/ex/bbs/View.do?cbIdx=65914&bcIdx=17132&parentSeq=17132 (accessed on 21 June 2016).
8. Kelley, A.E.; Schochet, T.; Landry, C.F. Risk taking and novelty seeking in adolescence: Introduction to part I. *Ann. N. Y. Acad. Sci.* **2004**, *1021*, 27–32. [CrossRef] [PubMed]
9. Crews, F.; He, J.; Hodge, C. Adolescent cortical development: A critical period of vulnerability for addiction. *Pharmacol. Biochem. Behav.* **2007**, *86*, 189–199. [CrossRef] [PubMed]
10. Kim, N.R.; Hwang, S.S.-H.; Choi, J.-S.; Kim, D.-J.; Demetrovics, Z.; Király, O.; Nagygyörgy, K.; Griffiths, M.; Hyun, S.Y.; Youn, H.C. Characteristics and psychiatric symptoms of internet gaming disorder among adults using self-reported DSM-5 criteria. *Psychiatr. Investig.* **2016**, *13*, 58–66. [CrossRef] [PubMed]
11. Wang, H.R.; Cho, H.; Dai-Jin, K. Prevalence and correlates of comorbid depression in a nonclinical online sample with DSM-5 internet gaming disorder. *J. Affect. Disord.* **2018**, *226*, 1–5. [CrossRef] [PubMed]
12. Lemmens, J.S.; Valkenburg, P.M.; Gentile, D.A. The Internet Gaming Disorder Scale. *Psychol. Assess.* **2015**, *27*, 567. [CrossRef] [PubMed]
13. Korean Creative Content Agency. *White Paper on Korean Games*; Korea Creative Content Agency: Seoul, Korea, 2013.
14. Young, K.S.; De Abreu, C.N. *Internet Addiction: A Handbook and Guide to Evaluation and Treatment*; John Wiley & Sons: Hoboken, NJ, USA, 2010.
15. Widyanto, L.; McMurran, M. The psychometric properties of the internet addiction test. *Cyberpsychol. Behav.* **2004**, *7*, 443–450. [CrossRef] [PubMed]
16. Gyeong, H.; Lee, H.-K.; Lee, K. Factor analysis of the Young's internet addiction test: In Korean College Students Group. *J. Korean Neuropsychiatr. Assoc.* **2012**, *51*, 45–51. [CrossRef]
17. Kwon, M.; Kim, D.-J.; Cho, H.; Yang, S. The smartphone addiction scale: Development and validation of a short version for adolescents. *PLoS ONE* **2013**, *8*, e83558. [CrossRef] [PubMed]
18. Hawi, N.S.; Samaha, M. To excel or not to excel: Strong evidence on the adverse effect of smartphone addiction on academic performance. *Comput. Educ.* **2016**, *98*, 81–89. [CrossRef]
19. Haug, S.; Castro, R.P.; Kwon, M.; Filler, A.; Kowatsch, T.; Schaub, M.P. Smartphone use and smartphone addiction among young people in Switzerland. *J. Behav. Addict.* **2015**, *4*, 299–307. [CrossRef] [PubMed]
20. Tangney, J.P.; Baumeister, R.F.; Boone, A.L. High self-control predicts good adjustment, less pathology, better grades, and interpersonal success. *J. Personal.* **2004**, *72*, 271–324. [CrossRef]
21. Manea, L.; Gilbody, S.; McMillan, D. Optimal cut-off score for diagnosing depression with the Patient Health Questionnaire (PHQ-9): A meta-analysis. *Can. Med. Assoc. J.* **2012**, *184*, E191–E196. [CrossRef] [PubMed]
22. Choi, H.S.; Choi, J.H.; Park, K.H.; Joo, K.J.; Ga, H.; Ko, H.J.; Kim, S.R. Standardization of the Korean version of Patient Health Questionnaire-9 as a screening instrument for major depressive disorder. *J. Korean Acad. Fam. Med.* **2007**, *28*, 114–119.
23. Spitzer, R.L.; Kroenke, K.; Williams, J.B.; Löwe, B. A brief measure for assessing generalized anxiety disorder: The GAD-7. *Arch. Intern. Med.* **2006**, *166*, 1092–1097. [CrossRef] [PubMed]
24. Plummer, F.; Manea, L.; Trepel, D.; McMillan, D. Screening for anxiety disorders with the GAD-7 and GAD-2: A systematic review and diagnostic metaanalysis. *Gen. Hosp. Psychiatry* **2016**, *39*, 24–31. [CrossRef] [PubMed]
25. Saunders, J.B.; Aasland, O.G.; Babor, T.F.; De la Fuente, J.R.; Grant, M. Development of the alcohol use disorders identification test (AUDIT): WHO collaborative project on early detection of persons with harmful alcohol consumption-II. *Addiction* **1993**, *88*, 791–804. [CrossRef] [PubMed]
26. Joe, K.H.; Chai, S.H.; Park, A.; Lee, H.K.; Shin, I.H.; Min, S.H. Optimum Cut-Off Score for Screening of Hazardous Drinking Using the Korean Version of Alcohol Use Disorder Identification Test(AUDIT-K). *J. Korean Addict. Psychiatry* **2009**, *13*, 34–40.

27. Heatherton, T.F.; Kozlowski, L.T.; Frecker, R.C.; Fagerstrom, K.O. The Fagerström test for nicotine dependence: A revision of the Fagerstrom Tolerance Questionnaire. *Addiction* **1991**, *86*, 1119–1127. [CrossRef]
28. Ahn, H.K.; Lee, H.J.; Jung, D.S.; Lee, S.Y.; Kim, S.W.; Kang, J.H. The reliability and validity of Korean version of questionnaire for nicotine dependence. *J. Korean Acad. Fam. Med.* **2002**, *23*, 999–1008.
29. Festl, R.; Scharkow, M.; Quandt, T. Problematic computer game use among adolescents, younger and older adults. *Addiction* **2013**, *108*, 592–599. [CrossRef] [PubMed]
30. Charlton, J.P.; Danforth, I.D. Distinguishing addiction and high engagement in the context of online game playing. *Comput. Hum. Behav.* **2007**, *23*, 1531–1548. [CrossRef]
31. Rho, M.J.; Jeong, J.-E.; Chun, J.-W.; Cho, H.; Jung, D.J.; Choi, I.Y.; Kim, D.-J. Predictors and patterns of problematic Internet game use using a decision tree model. *J. Behav. Addict.* **2016**, *5*, 500–509. [CrossRef] [PubMed]
32. Lemmens, J.S.; Hendriks, S.J. Addictive online games: Examining the relationship between game genres and internet gaming disorder. *Cyberpsychol. Behav. Soc. Netw.* **2016**, *19*, 270–276. [CrossRef] [PubMed]
33. Choi, S.-W.; Kim, D.-J.; Choi, J.-S.; Ahn, H.; Choi, E.-J.; Song, W.-Y.; Kim, S.; Youn, H. Comparison of risk and protective factors associated with smartphone addiction and Internet addiction. *J. Behav. Addict.* **2015**, *4*, 308–314. [CrossRef] [PubMed]
34. Yen, J.Y.; Ko, C.H.; Yen, C.F.; Chen, C.S.; Chen, C.C. The association between harmful alcohol use and Internet addiction among college students: Comparison of personality. *Psychiatry. Clin. Neurosci.* **2009**, *63*, 218–224. [CrossRef] [PubMed]
35. Kim, E.J.; Namkoong, K.; Ku, T.; Kim, S.J. The relationship between online game addiction and aggression, self-control and narcissistic personality traits. *Eur. Psychiatr.* **2008**, *23*, 212–218. [CrossRef] [PubMed]
36. Rehbein, F.; Kliem, S.; Baier, D.; Mößle, T.; Petry, N.M. Prevalence of internet gaming disorder in German adolescents: Diagnostic contribution of the nine DSM-5 criteria in a state-wide representative sample. *Addiction* **2015**, *110*, 842–851. [CrossRef] [PubMed]
37. Kuss, D.J. Internet gaming addiction: Current perspectives. *Psychol. Res. Behav. Manag.* **2013**, *6*, 125. [CrossRef] [PubMed]
38. Ko, C.-H.; Yen, J.-Y.; Chen, C.-C.; Chen, S.-H.; Yen, C.-F. Gender differences and related factors affecting online gaming addiction among Taiwanese adolescents. *J. Nerv. Ment. Dis.* **2005**, *193*, 273–277. [CrossRef] [PubMed]
39. Weiser, E.B. Gender differences in Internet use patterns and Internet application preferences: A two-sample comparison. *Cyberpsychol. Behav.* **2000**, *3*, 167–178. [CrossRef]
40. Winn, J.; Heeter, C. Gaming, gender, and time: Who makes time to play? *Sex Roles* **2009**, *61*, 1–13. [CrossRef]
41. Mok, J.-Y.; Choi, S.-W.; Kim, D.-J.; Choi, J.-S.; Lee, J.; Ahn, H.; Choi, E.-J.; Song, W.-Y. Latent class analysis on internet and smartphone addiction in college students. *Neuropsychiatr. Dis. Treat.* **2014**, *10*, 817. [PubMed]
42. Kim, Y.; Jeong, J.-E.; Cho, H.; Jung, D.-J.; Kwak, M.; Rho, M.J.; Yu, H.; Kim, D.-J.; Choi, I.Y. Personality factors predicting smartphone addiction predisposition: Behavioral inhibition and activation systems, impulsivity, and self-control. *PLoS ONE* **2016**, *11*, e0159788. [CrossRef] [PubMed]
43. Burns, L.; Teesson, M. Alcohol use disorders comorbid with anxiety, depression and drug use disorders: Findings from the Australian National Survey of Mental Health and Well Being. *Drug Alcohol Depend.* **2002**, *68*, 299–307. [CrossRef]
44. Barrett, S.P.; Darredeau, C.; Pihl, R.O. Patterns of simultaneous polysubstance use in drug using university students. *Hum. Psychopharmacol.* **2006**, *21*, 255–263. [CrossRef] [PubMed]
45. Demetrovics, Z.; Urbán, R.; Nagygyörgy, K.; Farkas, J.; Zilahy, D.; Mervó, B.; Reindl, A.; Ágoston, C.; Kertész, A.; Harmath, E. Why do you play? The development of the motives for online gaming questionnaire (MOGQ). *Behav. Res. Methods* **2011**, *43*, 814–825. [CrossRef] [PubMed]
46. Kuss, D.J.; Louws, J.; Wiers, R.W. Online gaming addiction? Motives predict addictive play behavior in massively multiplayer online role-playing games. *Cyberpsychol. Behav. Soc. Netw.* **2012**, *15*, 480–485. [CrossRef] [PubMed]
47. Park, N.; Lee, H. Social implications of smartphone use: Korean college students' smartphone use and psychological well-being. *Cyberpsychol. Behav. Soc. Netw.* **2012**, *15*, 491–497. [CrossRef] [PubMed]
48. Lee, C.; Kim, O. Predictors of online game addiction among Korean adolescents. *Addict. Res. Theory* **2017**, *25*, 58–66. [CrossRef]

49. Jeong, S.-H.; Kim, H.; Yum, J.-Y.; Hwang, Y. What type of content are smartphone users addicted to? SNS vs. games. *Comput. Hum. Behav.* **2016**, *54*, 10–17. [CrossRef]
50. Hou, J.; Nam, Y.; Peng, W.; Lee, K.M. Effects of screen size, viewing angle, and players' immersion tendencies on game experience. *Comput. Hum. Behav.* **2012**, *28*, 617–623. [CrossRef]
51. Park, E.; Baek, S.; Ohm, J.; Chang, H.J. Determinants of player acceptance of mobile social network games: An application of extended technology acceptance model. *Telemat. Inform.* **2014**, *31*, 3–15. [CrossRef]
52. Liu, C.-H.; Lin, S.-H.; Pan, Y.-C.; Lin, Y.-H. Smartphone gaming and frequent use pattern associated with smartphone addiction. *Medicine* **2016**, *95*, e4068. [CrossRef] [PubMed]
53. Dreier, M.; Wölfling, K.; Duven, E.; Giralt, S.; Beutel, M.; Müller, K. Free-to-play: About addicted Whales, at risk Dolphins and healthy Minnows. Monetarization design and internet gaming disorder. *Addict. Behav.* **2017**, *64*, 328–333. [CrossRef] [PubMed]
54. Evans, E. The economics of free: Freemium games, branding and the impatience economy. *Convergence* **2016**, *22*, 563–580. [CrossRef]
55. Kwon, M.; Nam, K.; Seo, B. *A Survey on Internet Overdependence, 2015*; Ministry of Science, ICT, and Future Planning: Seoul, Korea, 2016.

7

Relationships between Severity of Internet Gaming Disorder, Severity of Problematic Social Media Use, Sleep Quality and Psychological Distress

Hiu Yan Wong [1], Hoi Yi Mo [1], Marc N. Potenza [2,3,4], Mung Ni Monica Chan [1], Wai Man Lau [1], Tsz Kwan Chui [1], Amir H. Pakpour [5,6,*] and Chung-Ying Lin [1,*]

1 Department of Rehabilitation Sciences, The Hong Kong Polytechnic University, Hung Hom, Hong Kong; anniehiuyan@gmail.com (H.Y.W.); elainemohoiyi@gmail.com (H.Y.M.); monicachan0710@gmail.com (M.N.M.C.); sunny313971048@gmail.com (W.M.L.); chuitszkwan1996@gmail.com (T.K.C.)

2 Departments of Psychiatry and Neuroscience and the Child Study Center, School of Medicine, Yale University, New Haven, CT 06511, USA; marc.potenza@yale.edu

3 Connecticut Council on Problem Gambling, Wethersfield, CT 06109, USA

4 Connecticut Mental Health Center, New Haven, CT 06519, USA

5 Social Determinants of Health Research Center, Research Institute for Prevention of Non-Communicable Diseases, Qazvin University of Medical Sciences, Qazvin 3419759811, Iran

6 Department of Nursing, School of Health and Welfare, Jönköping University, 55511 Jönköping, Sweden

* Correspondence: pakpour_amir@yahoo.com (A.H.P.); cylin36933@gmail.com (C.-Y.L.)

Abstract: Internet gaming and social media use are prevalent and integral to many people's lives. However, excessive engagement in either could lead to negative health impacts. This study aimed to investigate relationships between severities of internet gaming disorder (IGD) and problematic social media use (operationalized as social media addiction; SMA) with sleep quality and psychological distress among young adults. A cross-sectional study with snowball sampling was conducted among Hong Kong university students in 2019. All participants (n = 300; mean (SD) age = 20.89 (1.48); 122 males (40.67%)) responded to an online survey that included Chinese versions of the Internet Gaming Disorder Scale-Short Form (IGDS9-SF), Bergen Social Media Addiction Scale (BSMAS), Pittsburgh Sleep Quality Index (PSQI), and Depression Anxiety Stress Scales (DASS-21). Multiple linear regressions demonstrated that IGDS-SF9 scores demonstrated associations with psychological distress measures (standardized coefficient (β) = 0.295 for depression, 0.325 for anxiety, 0.339 for stress, all $p < 0.001$). BSMAS scores showed similar albeit numerically less robust associations ($\beta = 0.235$ for depression, $p < 0.001$; 0.219 for anxiety, $p = 0.001$; 0.262 for stress, $p < 0.001$). BSMAS scores demonstrated associations with poorer sleep quality ($\beta = 0.292$; $p < 0.001$) and IGDS9-SF scores ($\beta = 0.157$; $p = 0.024$) showed a significantly less robust association ($p = 0.01$ for comparing the two βs). These findings suggest that both severities of IGD and SMA associate with more psychological distress and poorer sleep quality, although the strengths of associations may differ.

Keywords: gaming; social media; behavior addiction; sleep quality; psychological distress

---

1. Introduction

Serious health concerns have been linked to specific types and patterns of engagement in internet usage, leading to the concept of "internet addiction" [1,2]. The availability, accessibility and affordability of internet usage worldwide may lead to worsening health problems. According to the International Telecommunication Union (ITU) [3], global internet usage increased from 1990 million in 2010 to 3385 million in 2016. In Hong Kong and Macau, it is estimated that 23.3% of young adults aged 18 to 30 years experience problems with online gaming [4]. Therefore, problematic gaming is a significant concern for young adults in these Asian jurisdictions, and findings suggest similar concerns in other (American, European) countries. In addition to online gaming, internet-based social media platforms (e.g., YouTube, Snapchat, and Instagram) are frequently used, with nearly three fourths (71%) of young adults aged 18–24 years in the US using these media platforms doing so multiple times per day [5]. As such, many young adults may be vulnerable to experiencing Internet gaming and/or social media addictions.

Definitions for addictions have changed over time. Recently, the American Society of Addiction Medicine defined addiction as, "a treatable, chronic medical disease involving complex interactions among brain circuits, genetics, the environment, and an individual's life experiences. People with addiction use substances or engage in behaviors that become compulsive and often continue despite harmful consequences" [6]. Indeed, *behavioral addictions* have been included in the latest edition of the *Diagnostic and Statistical Manual of Mental Disorders (DSM-5)*, with gambling disorder and internet gaming disorder (IGD) defined, with the latter as a provisional diagnostic entity [7]. Recently, *gaming disorder* has been added to the *International Classification of Diseases 11th Revision (ICD-11)* as a disorder due to addictive behaviors [8]. With poor control over repetitive, persistent, and dysfunctional behaviors, behavioral addictions can result in negative health consequences, including social relationship problems, impairments in functional roles and activities, sleep problems, and mental disorders [9]. Therefore, assisting people, especially young adults, in tackling behavioral addictions is important for healthcare providers.

Debates have focused on whether generalized internet addiction or specific internet addictions are diagnosable entities, and if the latter, which disorders constitute specific internet addictions [10,11]. In the current study, we focused on gaming and social media addictions given their potential impacts. Both social media addiction (SMA) and IGD have been associated with sleep disturbances, including sleep quality deterioration and reductions in sleep duration [12,13]. A potential reason for both SMA and IGD leading to sleep disturbances involves portable smartphones and other portable digital devices that may be brought to bed [13].

With portable smartphones and Wi-Fi access, internet (including of social media) may constitute an unstructured activity, one not limited in time and one that can displace time [14]. As such, SMA may lead to lack of sleep. Delayed bedtimes and late waking times may further lead to the rhythm desynchronization and impact school performance [15]. Other potential mechanisms in disrupting sleep may include psychological stimulation (i.e., excited mood due to use of social media) [16], light-emitting screens (i.e., light may suppress sleep-promoting hormones like melatonin that are typically elevated before bedtime) [17], and shortened sleep duration [18]. Similar considerations exist for online gaming. Gamers from different time zones often participate in multiplayers games [12]. Therefore, some gamers may avoid logging off or may arise in the middle of the night to continue gaming [19], leading to irregular or disorganized sleep-wake patterns. Individuals may become sleep-deprived in order to engage in virtual activities. Consistently, playing online games has been associated with longer sleep latencies and shorter total rapid eye movement (REM) sleep [20].

Apart from negative effects on sleep, SMA and IGD may impact psychological well-being, with associations with depression, anxiety, and stress [2,21]. "Fear of missing out" may keep individuals on social media sites and lead to stress and burnout [4,21]. Internet addiction, as a general concept, may lead to poor sleep quality and psychological problems [2,22–24]. Both SMA [25–29] and IGD [30–32] have been associated with poor psychological health. However, differential associations of IGD and SMA with health outcomes have been rarely examined and compared in the same studies. To our best knowledge, only one study has examined relationships between IGD/SMA and symptoms of psychiatric disorders (i.e., attention-deficit/hyperactivity disorder, obsessive- compulsive disorder, anxiety, and depression) [33] and another has examined relationships between IGD/SMA and psychological distress (i.e., anxiety, stress, and depression) [32]. Therefore, more research is needed. Specifically, the activity demands and behavioral patterns of the two addictions are different. As internet gaming and use of social media may have different activity demands and behavioral patterns, with gaming typically requiring more rapid reactions and sustained attention over a continuous time period than using social media use, IGD and SMA may differentially impact sleep quality and psychological distress.

The current preliminary study was designed to explore how severities of IGD and SMA relate to sleep quality and emotional distress in a population at risk of internet addiction (i.e., young adults) [34] in order to complement prior studies of primary and secondary school students [1,35]. We hypothesized that both severities of IGD and SMA would relate to poorer sleep quality and more emotional distress.

2. Materials and Methods

A cross-sectional study using convenience and snowball sampling was conducted among university students aged 18–24 in Hong Kong in 2019.

2.1. Participants and Procedure

Data were collected from April to June 2019 using *Google Form*. The inclusion criteria were: (1) currently studying as an undergraduate or a postgraduate in a university or college in Hong Kong; (2) able to understand written Chinese in traditional characters and spoken Chinese in Cantonese; (3) currently possessing a smartphone with Internet access. The exclusion criterion was having a self-reported diagnosis of psychiatric problems or neurological disease. Finally, 306 participants agreed to participate in this study and data from 300 were analyzed after removing data from those who were not eligible (the six participants were removed because they were not university students or not studying in Hong Kong).

An invitation message with an online link to the survey was sent to the existing social network of the present study's Hong Kong researchers. The recipients were invited to complete an online survey and spread the message to their university peers. The message explained the present study's objectives and the estimated time for completing the survey. Before survey commencement, a project information sheet explaining the study aims, survey structure, and confidentiality assurance was provided to the participants. Participants could enter the survey only after they provided an online consent form that expressed their willingness to participate. The survey included a background information sheet and the Chinese versions of the following questionnaires: the Internet Gaming Disorder Scale-Short Form (IGDS9-SF), Bergen Social Media Addiction Scale (BSMAS), Pittsburgh Sleep Quality Index (PSQI) and Depression Anxiety Stress Scales (DASS-21). The background information sheet included questions relating to age, gender, education level, height, weight, smoking history, monthly income, time spent on smartphone per day in the past month, time spent on internet gaming per day in the past month, and time spent on social media per day in the past month. Five university students completed the survey to help ensure the survey readability before recruiting study participants. The study was approved by the Human Subjects Ethics Subcommittee of The Hong Kong Polytechnic University (Ref No. HSEARS20190130006).

2.2. Instruments

2.2.1. Internet Gaming Disorder Scale- Short Form (IGDS9-SF)

The 9-item IGDS9-SF assesses the severity of Internet Gaming Disorder (IGD) and its detrimental effects over a 12-month period [36–42]. The nine questions correspond to the nine DSM-5 criteria for IGD [7]. The items are rated using a 5-point Likert scale from 1 (*Never*) to 5 (*Very often*). A total score can be obtained by summing responses with a range from 9 to 45 points, with higher scores reflecting greater IGD severity. The cut-off score over 21 indicates problematic internet gaming [43]. A sample question is, "Do you feel the need to spend increasing amount of time engaged gaming in order to achieve satisfaction or pleasure?" The instrument has demonstrated validity and reliability for assessing IGD [36–42]. IGDS9-SF scores have been correlated with weekly time spent gaming

($r = 0.325$, $p < 0.0001$) and IGD-20 Test scores ($r = 0.842$, $p < 0.0001$), providing evidence for validity [44]. The IGDS9-SF has demonstrated high internal consistency ($\alpha = 0.87$) and low floor or ceiling effects [44]. The IGDS9-SF has also been validated among Hong Kong participants [45,46]. The internal consistency of the IGDS9-SF in the present study was 0.91.

2.2.2. The Bergen Social Media Addiction Scale (BSMAS)

The BSMAS is a self-report scale for assessing SMA severity [33,47–49]. It contains six items relating to six core addiction components (salience, mood modification, tolerance, withdrawal, conflict, and relapse) [50]. Each item examines the experience of using social media over the last year and is rated on a five-point Likert scale ranging from 1 (*very rarely*) to 5 (*very often*), producing a composite score ranging from 6 to 30. A sample question from the BSMAS is, "How often during the last year have you used social media so much that it has had a negative impact on your job/studies?" Higher BSMAS scores indicate greater SMA severity. A cut-off score over 19 indicates problematic social media use [51]. The BSMAS has satisfactory psychometric properties with high internal consistency ($\alpha = 0.819$) and low floor and ceiling effects [34]. BSMAS scores correlated with IGDS9-SF scores and assessments of anxiety and depression [34]. The BSMAS has been previously validated among Hong Kong participants [45,46]. The internal consistency of the BSMAS in the present study was 0.83.

2.2.3. Depression Anxiety Stress Scales (DASS-21)

The DASS-21 includes three self-reported subscales to measure negative emotional states, including depression, anxiety, and stress [52]. Each scale consists of seven items [52]. By using a four-point severity/ frequency scale, each participant is asked to rate the extent to the experiences relate to each negative emotion. The rating scale for each item is comprised of 0 (*did not apply to me at all*), 1 (applied *to me to some degree, or some of the time*), 2 (*applied to me to a considerable degree, or a good part of time*) and 3 (*applied to me very much, or most of the time*). A sample question from the DASS-21 depression subscale is, "I felt that I had nothing to look forward to." A sample question from the DASS-21 anxiety subscale is, "I was aware of dryness of my mouth." A sample question from the DASS-21 stress subscale is, "I found it hard to wind down." The scores for depression, anxiety, and stress are summed, respectively, to generate scores in each domain [52]. The high internal consistency ($\alpha = 0.94$, 0.88, and 0.93 for depression, anxiety, and stress, respectively) of the DASS-21 reflects its reliability [53]. The DASS-21 has been validated among Hong Kong participants [52]. The internal consistency of the DASS-21 in the present study was 0.88 (Depression domain), 0.83 (Anxiety domain), and 0.85 (Stress domain).

2.2.4. The Pittsburgh Sleep Quality Index (PSQI)

The PSQI assesses sleep quality in clinical populations using nineteen questions that can be classified into seven domains that include subjective sleep quality (Q6), sleep latency (Q2 and Q5a), sleep duration (Q4), habitual sleep efficiency (Q1, Q3 and Q4), sleep disturbances (Q5b-Q5j), use of sleeping medication (Q7), and daytime dysfunction (Q8 and Q9) [54]. The items examine sleep quality and disturbances over a 1-month period. A sample question from the PSQI is, "How often have you had trouble sleeping because you have bad dreams?" Scores for each question range from 0 (*no difficulty*) to 3 (*severe difficulty*). The summed component scores generate a global score ranging from 0 to 21, where higher scores represent poorer sleep quality. A cutoff score of 5 for sleep impairment has been proposed for distinguishing good sleep and poor sleep [54]. PSQI scores have correlated with severity of Internet addiction [55]. The PQSI has demonstrated high internal consistency ($\alpha = 0.83$). Both global scores (T1-T2 correlation coefficient = 0.85, $p < 0.001$) and component scores such as sleep latency (T1-T2 correlation coefficient = 0.84, $p < 0.001$) show high test-retest reliability [54]. The PSQI has suggested as a good screening test for insomnia in college students, with a recommended cut-off ≥ 6 due to its high diagnostic accuracy [56]. The Chinese PSQI has been validated among general and clinical populations in Hong Kong [57,58].

2.3. *Statistical Analysis*

Statistical analysis was performed using Statistical Package for the Social Sciences (SPSS) version 24.0 (IBM Inc., Armonk, NY, USA). Pearson's correlations were applied to examine the bivariate correlations between IGDS9-SF, BSMAS and PSQI scores and DASS-21 domains. Fisher's r-to-z transformation on dependent samples (http://quantpsy.org/corrtest/corrtest2.htm) was used to examine for significant differences in magnitudes of bivariate correlations. The associations of severities of IGD and SMA and health outcomes were further analyzed using regression models, which controlled for potential confounders. Specifically, DASS-21 domain scores (i.e., depression, anxiety, and stress domains) and PSQI score were entered as dependent variables; IGDS9-SF and BSMAS were used as independent variables; age, gender, time spent on smartphones, time spent on gaming on the internet, time spent on social media, and smoking history were treated as confounding variables. Further statistical testing on the differences of regression coefficients was conducted using a t-test statistic: dividing the difference between the two regression coefficients by the square root of their sum of the squared standard errors. All statistics were tested using two-tailed with significance level set at p-value < 0.05.

3. Results

Participants (N = 300) had a mean (SD) age of 20.89 (1.48) years. Less than half of the participants were male (40.67%), with small proportion of current smokers (0.36%). On average, participants spent 5.29 h (2.34) on smartphones, 3.09 h (1.80) on social networks and 1.19 h (1.53) gaming per day.

Participants had a mean (SD) score of 16.98 (6.48) on the IGDS9-SF, 15.37 (4.11) on the BSMAS, 5.16 (4.47) for Depression; 4.18 (3.83) for Anxiety; 6.72 (4.25) for Stress; and 6.63 (2.14) on the PSQI (Table 1). Additionally, all scores on the IGDS9-SF, BSMAS, DASS-21, and PSQI distributed normally or nearly normally as their skewness values were between 0.34 and 1.15 and kurtosis values were between −0.32 and 2.24. According to the cutoffs on the IGDS9-SF (score of 21 or above) and BSMAS (score of 19 or above), 77 (25.7%) of participants had IGD and 67 (22.3%) had SMA.

Table 1. Participant characteristics.

Characteristic	M ± SD or n (%)
Age (year)	20.89 ± 1.48
Gender (Male)	122 (40.67)
Height (cm)	165.57 ± 8.75
Weight (kg)	56.54 ± 10.24
Body mass index (kg/m^2)	20.52 ± 2.64
Smoke (No) [1]	279 (99.64)
Monthly income (HKD)	
≤ 1000	34 (12.27)
1001–2000	52 (18.77)
2001–3000	59 (21.30)
3001–5000	88 (31.77)
≥5001	44 (15.88)
Time on smartphones (hours/day)	5.29 ± 2.34
Time spent gaming on the internet (hours/day)	1.19 ± 1.53
Time spent on social media (hours/day)	3.09 ± 1.80
IGDS9-SF score (range: 9–45)	16.98 ± 6.45
BSMAS score (range: 6–30)	15.37 ± 4.11
Depression (range: 0–21)	5.16 ± 4.47
Anxiety (range: 0–21)	4.18 ± 3.83
Stress (range: 0–21)	6.72 ± 4.25
PSQI score (range: 0–21)	6.63 ± 2.14

[1] With 10 missing values. IGDS9-SF = Internet Gaming Disorder Scale-Short Form; BSMAS = Bergen Social Media Addiction Scale; DASS-21= Depression Anxiety Stress Scales; PSQI = Pittsburgh Sleep Quality Index; HKD = Hong Kong Dollar, 1 HKD ≈ 7.8 UDS. Depression, Anxiety, and Stress were subdomains of the DASS-21.

Table 2 shows that all the studied variables were significantly correlated ($p < 0.001$). More specifically, IGDS9-SF, BSMAS, depression, anxiety, stress, and PSQI scores were all positively correlated (r = 0.221 to 0.363). The magnitudes of correlations between DASS-21 subscales and IGDS9-SF (r = 0.331 to 0.363) were similar to those between DASS-21 subscales and BSMAS (r = 0.336 to 0.384). Indeed, the Fisher's r-to-z transformation on dependent samples showed non-significant findings (z = 0.227 to 0.807; p = 0.42 to 0.82). Although the correlation between BSMAS and PSQI scores (r = 0.351) showed a numerically larger magnitude than that between IGDS9-SF and PSQI (r = 0.249), the Fisher's r-to-z transformation on dependent samples showed no significant difference in the correlation comparison (z = 1.509; p = 0.13).

Table 2. Correlation matrix between IGDS9-SF, BSMAS, DASS-21, and PSQI scores.

	r					
	IGDS9-SF	**BSMAS**	**Depression**	**Anxiety**	**Stress**	**PSQI**
IGDS9-SF	–					
BSMAS	0.221	–				
Depression	0.351	0.336	–			
Anxiety	0.363	0.344	0.792	–		
Stress	0.331	0.384	0.792	0.815	–	
PSQI	0.249	0.351	0.351	0.411	0.386	–

IGDS9-SF = Internet Gaming Disorder Scale-Short Form; BSMAS = Bergen Social Media Addiction Scale; DASS-21 = Depression Anxiety Stress Scales; PSQI = Pittsburgh Sleep Quality Index. Depression, anxiety, and stress were subdomains of the DASS-21. All p-values < 0.001.

Multiple linear regressions in Table 3 (F-values ranged between 6.916 and 10.323; all $p < 0.001$) showed that both IGDS9-SF and BSMAS were associated with all outcome variables (i.e., depression, anxiety, stress, and sleep quality) after controlling for age, gender, time spent on smartphones, time spent on social media, and time spent gaming. As shown by the standardized coefficient (β), IGDS9-SF had a higher association with depression (β = 0.295), anxiety (β = 0.325), and stress (β = 0.339) as compared to BSMAS (β = 0.235 for depression; 0.219 for anxiety; 0.262 for stress) without significance (t = 0.116 to 0.577; p = 0.56 to 0.91). In contrast, BSMAS scores had a significantly higher association with poor sleep quality (β = 0.292) as compared to IGDS9-SF scores (β = 0.157; t = 2.436; p = 0.01).

Table 3. Regression models assessing associations between problematic use of Internet and health outcomes.

	Coefficient (SE)/Standardized Coefficient			
	Depression	**Anxiety**	**Stress**	**Sleep Quality**
IGDS9-SF score	0.203 (0.047)/0.295 ***	0.188 (0.039)/0.325 ***	0.220 (0.043)/0.339 ***	0.052 (0.023)/0.157 *
BSMAS score	0.250 (0.067)/0.235 ***	0.196 (0.057)/0.219 **	0.264 (0.063)/0.262 ***	0.150 (0.033)/0.292 ***
Age	−0.356 (0.167)/−0.121 *	−0.144 (0.140)/−0.058	−0.171 (0.154)/−0.061	−0.037 (0.082)/−0.026
Gender	0.251 (0.528)/0.028	0.375 (0.444)/0.050	1.030 (0.489)/0.121 *	0.069 (0.259)/0.016
Time on smartphone	0.215 (0.169)/0.102	0.094 (0.143)/0.053	0.125 (0.157)/0.062	−0.021 (0.083)/−0.020
Time gaming on the internet	−0.249 (0.216)/−0.085	−0.165 (0.182)/−0.067	−0.354 (0.200)/−0.128	0.052 (0.106)/0.037
Time on social media	0.039 (0.187)/0.016	0.117 (0.157)/0.057	0.043 (0.173)/0.018	0.121 (0.092)/0.103
Smoking status	1.731 (4.131)/0.023	2.42 (3.479)/0.039	6.44 (3.827)/0.092	−2.055 (2.027)/−0.058
Model summary				
F-value	8.501 ***	8.459 ***	10.323 ***	6.916 ***
R^2	0.202	0.201	0.235	0.171
Adjusted R^2	0.178	0.177	0.212	0.146

IGDS9-SF = Internet Gaming Disorder Scale- Short Form; BSMAS= Bergen Social Media Addiction Scale; PSQI = Depression, anxiety, and stress were subdomains of the Depression Anxiety Stress Scales; sleep quality was assessed using Pittsburgh Sleep Quality Index. * $p < 0.05$; ** $p < 0.01$; *** $p < 0.001$.

4. Discussion

This study found that participants with greater IGD and/or SMA severities had more depression, anxiety, and stress. Moreover, participants' sleep quality was poorer with greater severities of

IGD or SMA. According to our Pearson's correlation and multiple regression results, sleep quality demonstrated a numerically more robust association with SMA severity as compared to IGD severity. On the other hand, similar to findings from Pontes [32], our findings showed that psychological distress demonstrated a numerically more robust association with IGD severity, as compared SMA severity. Although no significant differences were found in the comparisons of Pearson's correlation coefficients, regression analyses revealed that some relationships were significantly different in the association magnitudes and some were not. Specifically, the sleep quality had a significantly stronger association with SMA severity (β = 0.292) than with IGD severity (β = 0.157); psychological distress had similar magnitudes of association with both SMA severity (β = 0.219 to 0.262) and IGD severity (β = 0.295 to 0.339). We believe that the results of comparing regression coefficients are more robust than those of comparing Pearson's correlation coefficients, because Pearson's correlation did not control confounders' effects, whereas regression analysis did. Therefore, we tentatively conclude that severities of IGD and SMA share similar associations with psychological distress; SMA severity had stronger association with sleep quality than did IGD severity.

Our sample had comparable or higher IGDS9-SF scores (Mean score = 16.98) than those from the general population in Italy (Mean score = 15.93; n = 687) [43]. Our sample also had comparable or higher BSMAS scores (Mean score = 15.37) than those from the general population in Italy (Mean score = 14.20; n = 734) [48]. When comparing scores to similar ethnic populations, our sample had similar IGDS9-SF scores relative to a sample comprised of young adults from Hong Kong and Taiwan (Mean score = 16.92; n = 640) [46] and comparable or slightly higher BSMAS scores (Mean score = 14.46; n = 640) [46].

Associations between IGD severity and psychological distress found in the present study are in line with previous studies [2,4,22]. Adolescents with anxiety, depression, or stress may spend excessive time on gaming on the internet as a coping mechanism, to escape from worries and difficulties in reality [22,59]. Unfortunately, gaming may not help people cope with psychological distress in a positive way. Spending more time gaming may provoke more emotional difficulties, and subsequently lead to IGD and related problems [59]. This cycle could further exacerbate symptoms of IGD and psychological distress [59]. Additionally, people with IGD have exhibited relatively less cognitive reappraisal and more expressive suppression, and these tendencies may prevent emotional difficulties from being resolved and the potential for depression to develop or worsen [59].

The present study also found a positive correlation between IGD severity and poor sleep quality, consistent with prior studies. Achab et al. suggested that people with IGD tend to have sleep deprivation or diurnal sleepiness [12], in line with findings that people who engage frequently in gaming are likely to delay their bedtimes and shorten their total time spent in bed [14]. Internet gaming may also arouse central and autonomic nervous systems, which may subsequently lead to increases in sleep latency [20]. Prolonged gaming may lead to physical discomfort, such as muscular pain and headache, which may impact sleep quality [13]. As a result, engaging more frequently in internet gaming may lead to poorer sleep.

The present study found a significantly positive association between SMA severity and psychological distress, in line with previous studies that people with SMA are prone to depressive and anxiety symptoms [4,21]. A sense of loss of control may underlie this phenomenon [9]. Individuals with more problematic smartphone use may experience more functional impairment, and this may interfere with their school/work and family life and eventually lead to increased stress [9]. Individuals with SMA may also be less physically active and have poorer sleep, which may predispose to psychological distress. Social networking provides a platform for persons to escape from negative emotions. However, excessive escapism may disrupt sleep and eventually induce more stress and depressive symptoms [21]. Negative social comparison may also contribute. Feelings of inferiority may be elicited if individuals engage in self-comparison with idealized representations often communicated on social media [4].

The present study found that SMA severity was positively correlated with sleep disturbance. This observation supports prior findings that suggest that time spent on social media is positively associated to sleep problems, such as insomnia, daytime sleepiness, and evening chronotype [13]. A phase delay in the circadian clock could be a reason for the association between SMA severity and sleep quality [13]. Using social media, especially before bed, may lead to difficulties falling asleep and bedtime delay [13]. The relationship between SMA severity and sleep quality may reflect cognitive and emotional arousal when using social media before sleep, with increased arousal preventing sleep [60]. Additionally, blue light from the screen may activate circadian clocks and generate delays in sleep latency [15].

Although both severities of both IGD and SMA were associated with poor sleep, SMA severity was more strongly related. Different strengths of associations could involve multiple possible mechanisms. First, the use of social media may constitute a more on-going process than internet gaming, which may have more well-defined beginnings and endings for each gaming task or component. The sleep patterns of users may be disrupted when they are preoccupied and waiting for replies from others on social media, which may not be well limited in time [14]. Being offline from interactions on social media may generate greater preoccupation and withdrawal when compared to gaming, potentially leading to greater disturbance in sleep quality [35]. Second, different levels and natures of interactions between social media and internet gaming may also explain differences in strengths of associations. Internet gaming may contain similar stimuli within games with main goals involving winning. In contrast, interactions on social media may be more complex, although this may be debatable given the complexities and varieties of games. Individuals may have a variety of goals and aims when using social media, involving multiple interpersonal relations which may require more mental or emotional effort that could lead to poorer sleep. However, as these factors were not assessed in the present study, further investigation is needed to test these presently speculative possibilities.

IGD severity showed associations with psychological distress that were comparable to those between SMA severity and psychological distress. Aspects of gaming and social media warrant consideration in relationships to psychological distress. Internet gaming often involves activities in multi-player chat rooms. Online gamers may thus form a team with individuals they have never physically contacted before when they engage in online games [61]. The teammates may share a goal in the game, and they may discuss their teamwork strategy to win the game. With the mindset of winning and within a virtual competitive environment, these individuals may become aggressive as they focus on winning [61]. Therefore, online gaming may not be an ideal platform for disclosing inner feelings, while social media may be used as a platform to express emotions [62]. Indeed, people with psychological distress can upload a new post on social media to share their current feelings or have an online discussion regarding their work or academic issues in *WhatsApp*. Therefore, the reasons may be different for the associations between IGD/SMA severity and psychological distress; however, both may share similar magnitudes of association with psychological distress. Additional research is needed to examine possible mechanisms linking IGD and SMA severities with psychological distress.

The present findings suggest that teaching faculty and healthcare providers in universities should attend to students' online gaming behaviors and social media use, especially as IGD and SMA may interact in mutually reinforcing ways [63]. Future research should investigate overlapping and unique factors relating to IGD and SMA. For example, interventions related to SMA may wish to focus on sleeping habits, although given the associations between SMA and IGD with sleep disturbances, the specificity may not be robust.

Study Limitations and Future Research

This study has several limitations. First, convenience and snowball sampling were used to collect data. Therefore, the representativeness of the collected sample is limited. Specifically, as participants were approached on the basis of availability and questionnaires were distributed to familiar people who may share similar characteristics, the potential bias of self-selection exists and it reduces the representativeness of sample. Thus, generalizability is reduced. Second, the sample size was small, especially as we recruited participants from the general population instead of clinical settings (i.e., those who with diagnosed IGD or SMA); therefore, the findings may not generalize to clinical samples. Third, all study variables (i.e., psychological distress, sleep, and behavioral addiction) were assessed using self-report instruments. Therefore, effects of social desirability or recall biases cannot be excluded. Fourth, the present study cannot make causal inferences given its cross-sectional design. Fifth, we did not explore gender-related differences. Given that males and females may have different propensities for IGD, SMA, and other domains assessed in the present study (e.g., psychological distress that is affective in nature), future studies should systematically examine these relationships in females and males. In such studies, examining motivations (e.g., fear of missing out for SMA) will be important [64]. Lastly, diverse findings in significance testing were observed when we compared the associations between sleep quality and severities of IGD and SMA. Pearson correlation did not support that sleep quality had different levels of associations with severities of IGD and SMA. However, the regression coefficient between sleep quality and SMA severity was significantly stronger than that between sleep quality and IGD severity. Although we believed that the findings from regression analyses are more robust than those from Pearson correlations, future studies are needed to investigate further the robustness of potential differences.

5. Conclusions

In conclusion, the present study assessed associations between severities of IGD and SMA and two health outcomes (i.e., psychological health and sleep quality) among Hong Kong university students. The results showed that both severities of IGD and SMA were positively associated with psychological distress and sleep disruption. In addition, although severities of IGD and SMA show similar associations with psychological distress, SMA severity was more strongly associated with poor sleep relative to IGD severity (Table 4). Thus, healthcare providers should consider both domains (psychological distress and sleep) when encountering IGD or SMA, with consideration of the potentially greater impact of SMA on sleep. More research is needed into specific interventions to improve health and sleep in individuals with features of IGD or SMA.

Table 4. Summary of associations between severities of internet gaming disorder (IGD)/social media addiction (SMA) and health measures.

	Depression	Anxiety	Stress	Sleep Quality
Severities of IGD	o	o	o	–
Severities of SMA	o	o	o	+
t (p) [a]	0.574 (0.57)	0.116 (0.91)	0.577 (0.56)	2.436 (0.01)

+ indicates a stronger association; – indicates a weaker association; o indicates a similar association. [a] T-tests that compared unstandardized coefficient of IGD severity on health outcomes and that of SMA severity on health outcomes.

Author Contributions: Conceptualization, C.-Y.L. and A.H.P.; methodology, C.-Y.L.; software, H.Y.W., H.Y.M., M.N.M.C., W.M.L., and T.K.C.; validation, H.Y.W., H.Y.M., M.N.M.C., W.M.L. and T.K.C.; formal analysis, C.-Y.L., H.Y.W., and H.Y.M.; investigation, C.-Y.L.; resources, C.-Y.L.; data curation, H.Y.W., H.Y.M., M.N.M.C., W.M.L., and T.K.C.; writing—original draft preparation, H.Y.W., H.Y.M., M.N.M.C., W.M.L. and T.K.C.; writing—review and editing, C.-Y.L., H.Y.W., M.N.P. and A.H.P.; visualization, M.N.M.C. and W.M.L.; supervision, C.-Y.L. and A.H.P.; project administration, C.-Y.L.; funding acquisition, C.-Y.L. All authors have read and agreed to the published version of the manuscript.

Acknowledgments: We thank all the participants.

References

1. Van den Eijnden, R.J.; Meerkerk, G.J.; Vermulst, A.A.; Spijkerman, R.; Engels, R.C. Online communication, compulsive Internet use, and psychosocial well-being among adolescents: A longitudinal study. *Dev. Psychol.* **2008**, *44*, 655–665. [CrossRef] [PubMed]
2. Weinstein, A.; Dorani, D.; Elhadif, R.; Bukovza, Y.; Yarmulnik, A.; Dannon, P. Internet addiction is associated with social anxiety in young adults. *Ann. Clin. Psychiatry* **2015**, *27*, 4–9. [PubMed]
3. Internet Users by Region and Country, 2010–2016. Available online: https://www.itu.int/en/ITUD/Statistics/Pages/stat/Treemap.aspx (accessed on 20 December 2019).
4. Tang, C.S.K.; Wu, A.M.S.; Yan, E.C.W.; Ko, J.H.C.; Kwon, J.H.; Yogo, M.; Gan, Y.Q.; Koh, Y.Y.W. Relative risks of Internet-related addictions and mood disturbances among college students: A 7-country/region comparison. *Public Health* **2018**, *165*, 16–25. [CrossRef] [PubMed]
5. Smith, A.; Anderson, M. *Social Media Use in 2018: A Majority of Americans Use Facebook and YouTube, but Young Adults Are Especially Heavy Users of Snapchat and Instagram*; Pew Reserch Center: Washington, DC, USA, 2018.
6. American Society of Addiction Medicine (ASAM). Available online: https://www.asam.org/Quality-Science/publications/magazine/public-policy-statements/2019/10/21/short-definition-of-addiction (accessed on 10 March 2020).
7. American Psychiatric Association. *Diagnostic and Statistical Manual of Mental Disorders DSM-5®*, 5th ed.; American Psychiatric Association Publishing: Washington, DC, USA, 2013.
8. ICD-11 for Mortality and Morbidity Statistics—Gaming Disorder (6C51). Available online: https://icd.who.int/browse11/l-m/en#/http://id.who.int/icd/entity/1448597234 (accessed on 20 December 2019).
9. Alhassan, A.A.; Alqadhib, E.M.; Taha, N.W.; Alahmari, R.A.; Salam, M.; Almutairi, A.F. The relationship between addiction to smartphone usage and depression among adults: A cross sectional study. *BMC Psychiatry* **2018**, *18*, 148. [CrossRef] [PubMed]
10. Griffiths, M.D.; Pontes, H.M. Internet Addiction Disorder and Internet Gaming Disorder are Not the Same. *J. Addict. Res.* **2014**, *5*, e124. [CrossRef]
11. Griffiths, M.D.; Szabo, A. Is excessive online usage a function of medium or activity? An empirical pilot study. *J. Behav. Addict.* **2013**, *3*, 74–77. [CrossRef]
12. Achab, S.; Nicolier, M.; Mauny, F.; Monnin, J.; Trojak, B.; Vandel, P.; Sechter, D.; Gorwood, P.; Haffen, E. Massively multiplayer online role-playing games: Comparing characteristics of addict vs non-addict online recruited gamers in a French adult population. *BMC Psychiatry* **2011**, *11*, 144. [CrossRef]
13. Fossum, I.N.; Nordnes, L.T.; Storemark, S.S.; Bjorvatn, B.; Pallesen, S. The association between use of electronic media in bed before going to sleep and insomnia symptoms, daytime sleepiness, morningness, and chronotype. *Behav. Sleep Med.* **2014**, *12*, 343–357. [CrossRef]
14. Van den Bulck, J. Television viewing, computer game playing, and Internet use and self-reported time to bed and time out of bed in secondary-school children. *Sleep* **2004**, *27*, 101–104. [CrossRef]
15. Touitou, Y.; Touitou, D.; Reinberg, A. Disruption of adolescents' circadian clock: The vicious circle of media use, exposure to light at night, sleep loss and risk behaviors. *J. Physiol. Paris* **2016**, *110*, 467–479. [CrossRef]
16. Hale, L.; Kirschen, G.W.; LeBourgeois, M.K.; Gradisar, M.; Garrison, M.M.; Montgomery-Downs, H.; Kirschen, H.; McHale, S.M.; Chang, A.M.; Buxton, O.M. Youth Screen Media Habits and Sleep: Sleep-Friendly Screen Behavior Recommendations for Clinicians, Educators, and Parents. *Child Adolesc. Psychiatr. Clin. N. Am.* **2018**, *27*, 229–245. [CrossRef] [PubMed]
17. van der Lely, S.; Frey, S.; Garbazza, C.; Wirz-Justice, A.; Jenni, O.G.; Steiner, R.; Wolf, S.; Cajochen, C.; Bromundt, V.; Schmidt, C. Blue blocker glasses as a countermeasure for alerting effects of evening light-emitting diode screen exposure in male teenagers. *J. Adolesc. Health* **2015**, *56*, 113–119. [CrossRef] [PubMed]
18. Alimoradi, Z.; Lin, C.-Y.; Broström, A.; Bülow, P.H.; Bajalan, Z.; Griffiths, M.D.; Ohayon, M.M.; Pakpour, A.H. Internet addiction and sleep disorders: A systematic review and meta-analysis. *Sleep Med. Rev.* **2019**, *47*, 51–61. [CrossRef] [PubMed]
19. Rehbein, F.; Kliem, S.; Baier, D.; Mößle, T.; Petry, N.M. Prevalence of internet gaming disorder in German adolescents: Diagnostic contribution of the nine DSM-5 criteria in a state-wide representative sample. *Addiction* **2015**, *110*, 842–851. [CrossRef] [PubMed]

20. Higuchi, S.; Motohashi, Y.; Liu, Y.; Maeda, A. Effects of playing a computer game using a bright display on presleep physiological variables, sleep latency, slow wave sleep and REM sleep. *J. Sleep Res.* **2005**, *14*, 267–273. [CrossRef] [PubMed]
21. Elhai, J.D.; Dvorak, R.D.; Levine, J.C.; Hall, B.J. Problematic smartphone use: A conceptual overview and systematic review of relations with anxiety and depression psychopathology. *J. Affect. Disord.* **2017**, *207*, 251–259. [CrossRef]
22. Ho, R.C.; Zhang, M.W.; Tsang, T.Y.; Toh, A.H.; Pan, F.; Lu, Y.; Cheng, C.; Yip, P.S.; Lam, L.T.; Watanabe, H.; et al. The association between internet addiction and psychiatric co-morbidity: A meta-analysis. *BMC Psychiatry* **2014**, *14*, 183. [CrossRef]
23. Chan, W.S.; Fu, K.W.; Wong, P.W.; Yip, P.S. Internet addiction: Prevalence, discriminant validity and correlates among adolescents in Hong Kong. *Br. J. Psychiatry* **2010**, *196*, 486–492.
24. Huang, C. Internet use and psychological well-being: A meta-analysis. *Cyberpsychol. Behav. Soc. Netw.* **2010**, *13*, 241–249. [CrossRef]
25. Griffiths, M.D.; Kuss, D.J.; Demetrovics, Z. Behavioral addictions: Criteria, evidence and treatment. In *Social Networking Addiction: An Overview of Preliminary Findings*; Rosenberg, K., Feder, L., Eds.; Elsevier Inc.: New York, NY, USA, 2014; pp. 119–141.
26. Griffiths, M.D.; Kuss, D. Adolescent social media addiction (revisited). *Educ. Health* **2017**, *35*, 49–52.
27. Kuss, D.J.; Griffiths, M.D. Excessive online social networking: Can adolescents become addicted to Facebook? *Educ. Health* **2011**, *29*, 68–71.
28. Kuss, D.J.; Griffiths, M.D. Online social networking and addiction—A review of the psychological literature. *Int. J. Environ. Res. Public Health* **2011**, *8*, 3528–3552. [CrossRef] [PubMed]
29. Kuss, D.J.; Griffiths, M.D. Social networking sites and addiction: Ten lessons learned. *Int. J. Environ. Res. Public Health* **2017**, *14*, 311. [CrossRef] [PubMed]
30. Griffiths, M.D.; Kuss, D.J.; King, D.L. Video game addiction: Past, present and future. *Curr. Psychiatry Rev.* **2012**, *8*, 308–318. [CrossRef]
31. Kuss, D.J.; Griffiths, M.D. Internet gaming addiction: A systematic review of empirical research. *Int. J. Ment. Health Addict.* **2012**, *10*, 278–296. [CrossRef]
32. Pontes, H.M. Investigating the differential effects of social networking site addiction and Internet gaming disorder on psychological health. *J. Behav. Addict.* **2017**, *6*, 601–610. [CrossRef]
33. Andreassen, C.S.; Billieux, J.; Griffiths, M.D.; Kuss, D.J.; Demetrovics, Z.; Mazzoni, E.; Pallesen, S. The relationship between addictive use of social media and video games and symptoms of psychiatric disorders: A large-scale cross-sectional study. *Psychol. Addict. Behav.* **2016**, *30*, 252–262. [CrossRef]
34. Yam, C.W.; Pakpour, A.H.; Griffiths, M.D.; Yau, W.Y.; Lo, C.M.; Ng, J.M.T.; Lin, C.Y.; Leung, H. Psychometric testing of three Chinese online-related addictive behavior instruments among Hong Kong university students. *Psychiatr. Q.* **2019**, *90*, 117–128. [CrossRef]
35. Leung, L. Predicting Internet risks: A longitudinal panel study of gratifications-sought, Internet addiction symptoms, and social media use among children and adolescents. *Health Psychol. Behav. Med.* **2014**, *2*, 424–439. [CrossRef]
36. Arıcak, O.T.; Dinç, M.; Yay, M.; Griffiths, M.D. Adapting the Short Form of the Internet Gaming Disorder Scale into Turkish: Validity and reliability. *Addicta Turk. J. Addict.* **2019**, *6*, 15–22.
37. de Palo, V.; Monacis, L.; Sinatra, M.; Griffiths, M.D.; Pontes, H.M.; Petro, M.; Miceli, S. Measurement invariance of the nine-item Internet Gaming Disorder Scale across Albania, United States of America, United Kingdom, and Italy. *Int. J. Ment. Health Addict.* **2019**, *17*, 935–946. [CrossRef]
38. Evren, C.; Dalbudak, E.; Topcu, M.; Kutlu, N.; Evren, B.; Pontes, H.M. Psychometric validation of the Turkish nine-item Internet Gaming Disorder Scale-Short Form (IGDS9-SF). *Psychiatry Res.* **2018**, *265*, 349–354. [CrossRef] [PubMed]
39. Pontes, H.M.; Griffiths, M.D. Portuguese validation of the Internet Gaming Disorder Scale-Short-Form. *Cyberpsychol. Behav. Soc. Netw.* **2016**, *19*, 288–293. [CrossRef] [PubMed]
40. Pontes, H.M.; Stavropoulos, V.; Griffiths, M.D. Measurement Invariance of the Internet Gaming Disorder Scale–Short-Form (IGDS9-SF) between the United States of America, India and the United Kingdom. *Psychiatry Res.* **2017**, *257*, 472–478. [CrossRef] [PubMed]

41. chivinski, B.; Brzozowska-Woś, M.; Buchanan, E.M.; Griffiths, M.D.; Pontes, H.M. Psychometric assessment of the Internet Gaming Disorder diagnostic criteria: An Item Response Theory study. *Addict. Behav. Rep.* **2018**, *8*, 176–184. [CrossRef]
42. Wu, T.-Y.; Lin, C.-Y.; Årestedt, K.; Griffiths, M.D.; Broström, A.; Pakpour, A.H. Psychometric validation of the Persian nine-item Internet Gaming Disorder Scale—Short Form: Does gender and hours spent online gaming affect the interpretations of item descriptions? *J. Behav. Addict.* **2017**, *6*, 256–263. [CrossRef]
43. Monacis, L.; Palo, V.; Griffiths, M.D.; Sinatra, M. Validation of the Internet Gaming Disorder Scale-Short-Form (IGDS9-SF) in an Italian-speaking sample. *J. Behav. Addict.* **2016**, *5*, 683–690. [CrossRef]
44. Pontes, H.M.; Griffiths, M.D. Measuring DSM-5 Internet gaming disorder: Development and validation of a short psychometric scale. *Comput. Hum. Behav.* **2015**, *45*, 137–143. [CrossRef]
45. Leung, H.; Pakpour, A.H.; Strong, C.; Lin, Y.C.; Tsai, M.C.; Griffiths, M.D.; Lin, C.Y.; Chen, I.H. Measurement invariance across young adults from Hong Kong and Taiwan among three internet-related addiction scales: Bergen Social Media Addiction Scale (BSMAS), Smartphone Application-Based Addiction Scale (SABAS), and Internet Gaming Disorder Scale-Short Form (IGDS-SF9) (Study Part A). *Addict. Behav.* **2020**, *101*, 105969.
46. Chen, I.-H.; Strong, C.; Lin, Y.-C.; Tsai, M.-C.; Leung, H.; Lin, C.-Y.; Pakpour, A.H.; Griffiths, M.D. Time invariance of three ultra-brief internet-related instruments: Smartphone Application-Based Addiction Scale (SABAS), Bergen Social Media Addiction Scale (BSMAS), and the nine-item Internet Gaming Disorder Scale- Short Form (IGDS-SF9) (Study Part B). *Addict. Behav.* **2020**, *101*, 105960. [CrossRef]
47. Lin, C.-Y.; Broström, A.; Nilsen, P.; Griffiths, M.D.; Pakpour, A.H. Psychometric validation of the Persian Bergen Social Media Addiction Scale using classic test theory and Rasch models. *J. Behav. Addict.* **2017**, *6*, 620–629. [CrossRef] [PubMed]
48. Monacis, L.; De Palo, V.; Griffiths, M.D.; Sinatra, M. Social networking addiction, attachment style, and validation of the Italian version of the Bergen Social Media Addiction Scale. *J. Behav. Addict.* **2017**, *6*, 178–186. [CrossRef] [PubMed]
49. Pontes, H.M.; Andreassen, C.S.; Griffiths, M.D. Portuguese validation of the Bergen Facebook Addiction Scale: An empirical study. *Int. J. Ment. Health Addict.* **2016**, *14*, 1062–1073. [CrossRef]
50. Griffiths, M. A 'components' model of addiction within a biopsychosocial framework. *J. Subst. Use* **2005**, *10*, 191–197. [CrossRef]
51. Bányai, F.; Zsila, Á.; Király, O.; Maraz, A.; Elekes, Z.; Griffiths, M.D.; Andreassen, C.S.; Demetrovics, Z. Problematic social media use: Results from a large-scale nationally representative adolescent sample. *PLoS ONE* **2017**, *12*, e0169839. [CrossRef] [PubMed]
52. Taouk, M.; Lovibond, P.F.; Laube, R. *Report for New South Wales Transcultural Mental Health Centre*; Cumberland Hospital: Sydney, Australia, 2001.
53. Nieuwenhuijsen, K.; De Boer, A.; Verbeek, J.; Blonk, R.; Van Dijk, F. The Depression Anxiety Stress Scales (DASS): Detecting anxiety disorder and depression in employees absent from work because of mental health problems. *Occup. Environ. Med.* **2003**, *60*, I77–I82. [CrossRef]
54. Buysse, D.J.; Reynolds, C.F., III; Monk, T.H.; Berman, S.R.; Kupfer, D.J. The Pittsburgh Sleep Quality Index: A new instrument for psychiatric practice and research. *Psychiatry Res.* **1989**, *28*, 193–213. [CrossRef]
55. Khayat, M.A.; Qari, M.H.; Almutairi, B.S.; Rambo, M.Z.; Alrogi, M.J.; Alkhattabi, S.Z.; Alqarni, D.A. Sleep Quality and Internet Addiction Level among University Students. *Egypt J. Hosp. Med.* **2018**, *73*, 7042–7047.
56. Dietch, J.R.; Taylor, D.J.; Sethi, K.; Kelly, K.; Bramoweth, A.D.; Roane, B.M. Psychometric evaluation of the PSQI in US college students. *J. Clin. Sleep Med.* **2016**, *12*, 1121–1129. [CrossRef]
57. Ho, R.T.; Fong, T.C. Factor structure of the Chinese version of the Pittsburgh Sleep Quality Index in breast cancer patients. *Sleep Med.* **2014**, *15*, 565–569. [CrossRef]
58. Wong, W.S.; Fielding, R. Prevalence of insomnia among Chinese adults in Hong Kong: A population-based study. *J. Sleep Res.* **2011**, *20*, 117–126. [CrossRef] [PubMed]
59. Yen, J.; Lin, H.; Chou, W.; Liu, T.; Ko, C. Associations Among Resilience, Stress, Depression, and Internet Gaming Disorder in Young Adults. *Int. J. Environ. Res. Public Health* **2019**, *16*, 318. [CrossRef]
60. Levenson, J.C.; Shensa, A.; Sidani, J.E.; Colditz, K.B.; Primack, B.A. The association between social media use and sleep disturbance among young adults. *Prev. Med.* **2016**, *85*, 36–41. [CrossRef] [PubMed]

61. Ko, C.H.; Yen, J.Y.; Liu, S.C.; Hunag, C.F.; Yen, C.F. The associations between aggressive behaviours and Internet addiction and online activities in adolescents. *J. Adolesc. Health* **2009**, *44*, 598–605. [CrossRef] [PubMed]
62. Steinkuehler, C.A.; Williams, D. Where Everybody Knows Your (Screen) Name: Online Games as "Third Places". *J. Comput. Mediat. Commun.* **2006**, *11*, 885–909. [CrossRef]
63. Ostovar, S.; Allahyar, N.; Aminpoor, H.; Moafian, F.; Mariani, M.N.; Griffiths, M.D. Internet addiction and its psychosocial risks among Iranian adolescents and young adults: A structural equation model in a cross-sectional study. *Int. J. Ment. Health Addict.* **2016**, *14*, 257–267. [CrossRef]
64. Wegmann, E.; Oberst, U.; Stodt, B.; Brand, M. Online-specific fear of missing out and Internet-use expectancies contribute to symptoms of Internet-communication disorder. *Addict. Behav. Rep.* **2017**, *5*, 33–42. [CrossRef]

8

The Assessment of Problematic Internet Pornography Use: A Comparison of Three Scales with Mixed Methods

Lijun Chen * and Xiaoliu Jiang

Department of Psychology, School of Humanities and Social Sciences, Fuzhou University, Fuzhou 350108, China; psyjxl@126.com
* Correspondence: qqkx159@126.com

Abstract: The primary aim of this study was to compare different screening tools for problematic internet pornography use (IPU) and identify the most accurate measure. The reliability and validity of three scales, namely, the Problematic Pornography Consumption Scale (PPCS), Problematic Pornography Use Scale (PPUS), and Short Internet Addiction Test Adapted to Online Sexual Activities(s-IAT-sex), were examined using three homogeneous groups, respectively. A total of 972 adults (mean age = 24.8) from 28 provinces/regions in China participated in the quantitative part (QUAN). The Brief Pornography Screener served as the reference standard. The PPCS demonstrated stronger reliability and validity, including criterion validity, as well as greater sensitivity and acceptable specificity; therefore, it was considered to be the more accurate screening instrument. In the qualitative part (QUAL), we interviewed 22 volunteers and 11 therapists (who had worked with individuals with problematic IPU) to examine their perspectives on the core features of problematic IPU and dimensions of the PPCS. Almost all the interviewees endorsed the structure of the PPCS. These findings encourage the use of the PPCS in future research studies and underscore its screening applications because of its ability to classify IPU as problematic or nonproblematic.

Keywords: problematic pornography use; internet pornography use; problematic pornography consumption scale; problematic pornography use scale; the short internet addiction test adapted to online sexual activities

---

1. Introduction

Internet pornography use (IPU) is a sexual behavior [1], corresponding to the use of internet to engage in various gratifying sexual activities also known as online pornography use or cybersex [2–4]. It comprises a variety of online sexual activities (OSAs), including watching pornography, online pornography exchange, engaging in sex chats, using sex webcams, searching for sexual partners, or engaging in sexual role playing, among which stands the watching pornography, which is the most popular activity [5]. According to the past findings, engaging in IPU sometimes derives various negative consequences, such as financial, legal, occupational, and relationship trouble or personal problems [6]. Feelings of loss of control and persistent use despite these adverse outcomes constitute compulsive cybersex or problematic IPU. To date, no consensus exists regarding the conceptualization and diagnosis of problematic IPU. For instance, numerous terms have been used to describe the phenomenon (e.g., internet sex addiction [7,8], problematic online sexual activities [9], cybersex addiction [10], and problematic internet pornography use [6]). Although these concepts are slightly different, they all comprise three crucial components: the medium (the internet), the content (sexual behavior), and the problematic use (the compulsive behavior). Regardless of the debate, it is now acknowledged that excessive involvement in IPU or cybersex may become dysfunctional and associated with addiction symptoms (e.g., loss of control, compulsive use). Considering these inconsistent terms sharing crucial components, problematic IPU may be regarded as a subtypes of problematic internet use from a classification perspective, which may help advance clinical and research efforts into its prevalence and impact.

Nevertheless, evidence regarding the problematic IPU is inconsistent, due to the heterogeneity of assessment tool. The fundamental reason is that the definition and diagnostic criteria of problematic IPU is still unclear. In order to address these conceptual ambiguities, researchers have developed several scales that measure different aspects of pornography use [11]. Some briefer scales are more convenient to administer, but they underscore the self-perceived addiction (e.g., Cyber-Pornography Use Inventory-9). Some of these scales have been designed to assess the motivations underlying pornography use among hypersexual men (e.g., Pornography Consumption Inventory) [12]. Some scales fail to capture the different aspects of problematic IPU and focus solely on specific dimensions (e.g., the Pornography Craving Questionnaire, PCQ). Additionally, some globally accessible websites host the Cybersex Addiction Test, Sexaholics Anonymity Test, Sex Addicts Anonymous, and Sexual Addiction Screening Test, which assess difficulties in exercising self-control, its negative consequences, and the social problems that are associated with sexual activities. Furthermore, assessing IPU, using measures of sexual addiction, entails a few challenges. Specifically, these assessments may not be able to capture the characteristics of the activities (e.g., chat-based cybersex, sexual video games that cannot be played offline) and symptoms (e.g., separation from reality due to immersion in the virtual world that are unique to IPU. To address this gap in the literature and conduct further research in this domain, assessments with strong psychometric properties are much needed [5,7].

Several scales of problematic IPU are available to researchers and clinicians. Indeed, a recent meta-analysis identified 22 psychometric instruments that assess problematic pornography use [11]. Otherwise, most of the studies that have been conducted during the past decade had used self-developed items and a few of these measures have been subsequently revalidated [4,5,13]. Therefore, it is difficult to compare the results of different studies because there is a lack of concordance in the assessments that have been used. In order to select suitable tools for comparison from the existing scales, a systematic review was conducted. The following terms and their derivatives were used in multiple combinations: (Cybersex* OR internet porn* OR hypersex*) AND (addict* OR compulsiv* OR problem*) AND (assessment OR scale OR instrument OR measure*), to identify relevant studies in order to address the questions related to assessment and available screening questionnaires. The selection criteria of the literature search were limited to articles focusing specifically on cybersex and/or internet pornography consumption and dysfunctional cybersex, and also describe the development and adaptation of self-reported psychometric instruments that assesses at least one aspect of problematic pornography use. Finally, we found a total of 27 instruments on assess the problematic IPU (cybersex). Through the systematic review process conducted, we decided to retain three scales that were developed to measure problematic pornography use, even if not all of the three scales were specifically designed to measure internet pornography, as a large majority of participants used online pornography, and the developers of these scales suggested that they could be used to measure problematic IPU [14,15], additionally we replaced "pornography" into "internet pornography" in the Chinese version. We selected these three scales for the following reasons: (1) they include fewer items and are thus easily administered measures, (2) all of them cover the core characteristics of IPU, such as loss control, (3) they are grounded in addiction components such as impaired control, conflict, salience [11], (4) they are applicable within the Chinese culture [16–19], and (5) they display strong test-retest (i.e., two weeks) reliability; consequently, these three previously validated scales were identified for further examination. First, the Short Internet Addiction Test Adapted to OSAs (s-IAT-sex), which has demonstrated satisfactory psychometric properties [9]. However, this scale has been validated only among men [5], and a large number of studies have shown that there are substantial gender differences in IPU [18,20,21]. Second, the Problematic Pornography Use Scale (PPUS) [15], which has been validated using a large sample; unfortunately, however, a valid cutoff score has not been specified for this measure. Third, the Problematic Pornography Consumption Scale (PPCS); this scale is founded upon the theoretical framework of Griffiths's components model of addiction [22]. All three scales include strong internal consistency and a valid factorial structure, which has been supported by the results of confirmatory factor analysis (CFA) [9,14,15,19]. Nevertheless, it is difficult to compare the findings of studies that have used these scales because they entail different factor structures. Therefore, it is necessary to select reliable indicators and methods, and identify the most accurate instrument.

In order to effectively compare different scales, a unifying and reliable standard should first be established. The Brief Pornography Screener (BPS), which is a screening tool that measures loss of self-control, overuse of problematic pornography use, may be useful in identifying individuals who are at risk for problematic pornography use or can serve as a proxy measure [23]. Kraus et al., who developed the BPS, have proposed that the diagnostic criteria for compulsive sexual behavior (CSB) should be included in the new International Classification of Diseases (ICD-11) [24], and this proposal has been accepted. According to the upcoming ICD-11's diagnostic criteria for impulse control disorder [25], patterns of failure to control intense sexual impulses or urges and the resultant repetitive sexual behaviors are considered to be the characteristic features of the disorder. The BPS considers compulsive pornography to be the core component of problematic pornography use. Moreover, the BPS has been used with different samples, and it has demonstrated satisfactory psychometric properties among American and Polish pornography users [26]. Many past studies have used the BPS to identify pornography addicts. Furthermore, it has also been used to ascertain the severity of problematic pornography use among men who seek pharmacologic or psychological treatment as a result of their loss of control over their sexual behaviors [27–29]. Therefore, in this study, the BPS scores were used as the reference standard against which the sensitivity and specificity of the three aforementioned scales were ascertained.

Several recent reviews have focused specifically on the conceptualization and assessment of problematic pornography use [4,11,30,31]. Some reviews have briefly summarized and commented on the included instruments [5], whereas others have evaluated their ability to assess the core components of problematic pornography use [11]. However, no past study has compared the different scales and identified the most accurate measure of problematic pornography use using a same standard or indicator. Measures of problematic IPU are heterogeneous, and each scale focuses on a different aspect of problematic IPU. Furthermore, because these scales have not been extensively validated, it is difficult to compare the findings of the studies that have used them. In addition, the sensitivity of the different scales that assess problematic IPU have not been adequately compared. Therefore, in the present study, a QUAN→QUAL mixed-methods design was conducted, including (1) using quantitative methods to identify a scale with a higher sensitivity index from three selected scales (PPCS, PPUS, s-IAT-sex) for assessing problematic IPU. Moreover, the duration of usage, frequency of engagement in OSAs, sexual compulsivity, and pornography cravings were used to examine the criterion validity of the assessments. Subsequently, (2) qualitative interviews were conducted with volunteers and therapists who have serviced the individuals in trouble of problematic IPU to further examine the appropriateness of the "more accurate" scale from the service providers' perspectives, whereby the qualitative part helps to evaluate and interpret the results obtained from the main quantitative study.

2. The Quantitative Part: A Comparison of the Three Retained Scales

2.1. Materials and Methods

2.1.1. Sample

The study sample consisted of 560 men and 412 women, and the mean age of the sample was 24.8 years [*standard deviation (SD)* = 7.2 years; range = 18–48 years]. The group comparisons of the demographic characteristics of the three study samples can be inferred from Table 1.

Table 1. Group comparisons of the demographic characteristics of the three study samples.

The Scales		PPCS [1] (*n* = 317)	PPUS [2] (*n* = 332)	s-IAT-Sex [3] (*n* = 323)	χ^2 (*F*)	*p*
Gender ratio (men/women)		1.39	1.39	1.48	6.92	0.31
Age	Mean ± SD [4]	24.64 ± 7.39	24.47 ± 7.27	25.31 ± 6.93	1.24	0.29
	Range	18–48	18–45	18–45		
Sexual orientation	Homosexual	1.31%	1.76%	0.91%	2.61	0.11
	Heterosexual	91.52%	91.97%	94.69%		
	Bisexual	7.17%	6.37%	4.40%		
Relationship status	Single	46.78%	42.52%	40.64%	12.85	0.23
	Partnered	14.81%	21.41%	22.90%		
	Engaged	0.90%	1.20%	0.96%		
	Married	37.51%	34.91%	35.60%		
Educational level	Primary school or below	0	0	0	2.99	0.08
	Vocational school	1.24%	0.35%	0.34%		
	Middle school	1.55%	0.67%	0.91%		
	University or college	97.21%	99.08%	98.75%		
Work	Full time	46.10%	45.51%	47.43%	0.39	0.53
	Part time	2.51%	2.68%	4.57%		
	Short-term hired labor	1.64%	1.21%	0.56%		
	Unemployed	49.75%	50.60%	47.54%		
Place of residence	Capital	36.01%	47.37%	43.69%	11.70	0.07
	County town	40.38%	31.02%	35.04%		
	Town	12.01%	10.51%	8.36%		
	Village	11.70%	11.10%	13.01%		
Age of first exposure to pornography		16.21 ± 4.27	16.62 ± 4.69	16.62 ± 4.81	75.86	0.08

[1] PPCS = Problematic Pornography Consumption Scale, [2] PPUS = Problematic Pornography Use Scale, [3] s-IAT-sex = Short Internet Addiction Test Adapted to Online Sexual Activities, [4] SD = standard deviation.

2.1.2. Instruments

Three Main IPU Measurements

PPUS. The PPUS is a 12-item self-report scale that assesses four dimensions of IPU [15]: distress and functional problems, excessive use, difficulties in self-control, and IPU to escape or avoid negative emotions. In the Chinese version of the assessment, the term "pornography," which was used in the original scale, was modified as "internet pornography" in all instances (e.g., "I spend too much time being involved in thoughts about internet pornography"). The participants were required to indicate the frequency with which they had engaged in IPU during the past 6 months on a six-point scale that ranged from 0 (never) to 5 (all the time). Higher scores were indicative of a greater severity of engagement in IPU. The Cronbach's alpha of the total scale was 0.95 in this study.

PPCS. The PPCS was used to measure problematic IPU [14]. Responses were recorded on the following 7-point scale: 1 = never, 2 = rarely, 3 = occasionally, 4 = sometimes, 5 = often, 6 = very often, 7 = all the time. PPCS consists of 18 items, and assesses the six core components of addiction: salience, mood modification, conflict, tolerance, relapse, and withdrawal. Each factor is measured by three items (e.g., "I felt that I had to watch more and more internet porn for satisfaction" is an item of measure "tolerance"); the Cronbach's alphas of the aforementioned six factors were 0.77, 0.84, 0.71, 0.78, 0.86, and 0.86, respectively, in the study. The Cronbach's alpha of the total PPCS was 0.96. A cutoff score of 76 was used to ascertain normal and problematic use; specifically, scores that were greater than 76 were indicative of problematic use.

s-IAT-sex. Responses to each of the 12 items of the s-IAT-sex are recorded on a five-point scale that ranges from 1 (never) to 5 (always) [9]. The scale consists of two dimensions. The first factor assesses poor self-control and difficulties in reducing the amount of time that is spent online (six items, e.g., "How often do you find that you stay on Internet sex sites longer than you intended?"), whereas the second factor measures the functional impairments that are associated with engagement in cybersex (six items, e.g., "How often do you feel depressed, moody, or nervous when you are offline, which goes away once you are back on internet sex sites?"). The composite score, which can be computed by summing the individual item scores, can range from 12 to 60; higher scores are indicative of greater problems. The internal consistency (Cronbach's alpha) coefficients of the total scale and first and second factors were 0.89, 0.77, and 0.88, respectively, in this study.

Criterion Validity Questionnaires

PCQ. This 12-item questionnaire is a unidimensional assessment [32,33]. The following are a few sample items: "If the situation permitted, I would watch pornography right now" and "If I were to watch pornography right now, I would have difficulty stopping." The respondents were required to indicate how strongly they agreed with each item using the following seven response options (presented without numerals): "completely disagree," "somewhat disagree," "disagree a little," "neither agree nor disagree," "agree a little," "somewhat agree," and "completely agree." Higher scores are indicative of a greater craving for pornography. The Cronbach's alpha of this scale was 0.92 in the current study. The instructions of the PCQ present a craving-for-pornography vignette, which requires the respondent to imagine that they are alone in their room and seated in front of their computer and that they have a strong urge to watch their favorite type of pornography.

The Sexual Compulsivity Scale (SCS). The extent to which participants exhibit the characteristics of compulsive pornography use was assessed using the 10-item SCS that has been developed by Kalichman et al. [34]. Responses were recorded on a four-point rating scale (1 = not at all like me, 2 = slightly like me, 3 = mainly like me, 4 = very much like me, e.g., "I have to struggle to control my sexual thoughts and behavior"). In this study, the Cronbach's alpha of this scale was 0.86.

Questionnaire of OSAs. Thirteen items were used to measure participants' use of the internet for the following purposes: (1) viewing sexual explicit materials (SEM), (2) seeking sexual partners, (3) cybersex, and (4) flirting and sexual relationship maintenance [35]. Viewing SEM was assessed using five items (e.g., visiting erotic/pornographic websites, viewing and downloading erotic/pornographic videos from the internet, reading erotic/pornographic material online), each of which required responses to be rated on a nine-point scale that ranged from 1 (never) to 9 (at least once a day). The other three subscales assessed frequency using a nine-point scale that ranged from 1 (0 times) to 9 (20 or more times). Two items measured the frequency with which the respondents had sought sexual partners as well as the number of sexual partners that they had sought and found online. The frequency of engagement in cybersex was assessed using four items (e.g., masturbating or viewing strangers masturbating in front of a webcam, describing sexual fantasies either through texts or orally). Internet use for the purposes of flirting and sexual relationship maintenance was measured using two items. The Cronbach's alpha of the entire scale was 0.88 in the study. Higher scores were indicative of more frequent engagement in OSAs.

Additional Questions about IPU. In addition to items that assessed demographic characteristics, a few questions that were related to IPU were also posed to the participants. After providing them with a clear definition of internet pornography, the participants were asked to indicate their age of first exposure to pornography and the duration of time that they typically spent watching internet pornography every week.

The Reference Standard—BPS

The BPS, which has been developed by Kraus et al. [26], was used to assess pornography use during the past 6 months. This five-item assessment uses a three-point rating scale (0 = never, 1 = occasionally, 2 = always, e.g., "You find it difficult to resist strong urges to use sexually explicit material."); a cutoff score of 4 was used to detect problematic pornography use (absolute range = 0–10). Higher scores are indicative of more problematic pornography use. The Cronbach's alpha of the BPS was 0.84.

2.1.3. Procedure

This online study was conducted through a popular Chinese survey website, namely, Wenjuanxing (www.sojump.com). Adult members of the website received an email with a link that redirected them to the survey website and a brief introduction to our survey. This brief introduction informed the recipients that they were eligible for participation if they had engaged in IPU during the past 6 months (e.g., reading online pornographic content, browsing pornographic websites, sharing/watching pornographic videos or pictures, interacting and flirting with others) and were interested in participating in the survey. A total of 972 valid responses were collected from participants from 110 cities in 28 of the 34 provinces/regions in China (i.e., identified using the internet protocol addresses). As expected, all participants obtained scores that were equal to or greater than 14 on the measure of OSAs (the lowest possible score is 13, and it indicates no prior IPU); this indicated that all of them had engaged in at least one OSA during the past 6 months. Three highly homogeneous samples were required to respond to the three measures of problematic IPU, namely, the PPCS, PPUS, and s-IAT-sex, respectively. Each sample also completed the aforementioned mentioned assessments against which their criterion validity was to be examined. This study was conducted in accordance with the Declaration of Helsinki, and the protocol was approved by the Ethics Committee of the Department of Psychology, Fuzhou University (date of approval, 7 April 2019).

2.2. Analysis

Statistical analyses were conducted using SPSS 19.0 (IBM, Armonk, NY, USA) and Mplus version 7 [36]. Item-total correlations were computed to identify items that functioned poorly. CFA was used to test the factor structures of the scales of interest. Maximum likelihood estimation with the Satorra-Bentler correction was used to determine the fit between the data and the factor structures. Model fit was tested by inspecting the following indices: root mean square error of approximation (RMSEA; good: $\leq$0.06, acceptable: $\leq$0.08), comparative fit index (CFI; good: $\geq$0.95, acceptable: $\geq$0.90), and Tucker-Lewis index (TLI; good: $\geq$0.95, acceptable: $\geq$0.90). The reliability of the scales was assessed by computing Cronbach's alpha coefficients.

To identify possible groups of at-risk pornography users, latent profile analysis (LPA) was used. LPA was conducted using the original dimensions of each scale as explicit variables, and different groups of individuals with problematic IPU were successively divided into two to four categories for model fitting estimation. Sensitivity was defined as the proportion of persons with positive symptoms (as detected by the BPS) and members of the at-risk group (identified through LPA), whereas specificity was defined as the proportion of persons with negative symptoms and the nonproblematic group [37].

2.3. Results and Discussion

2.3.1. Validation of the Three Scales

The results of item analysis, CFA, and tests of reliability and convergent validity are shown in Table 2. Item-sum correlations were computed to examine item functioning. The PPCS and PPUS yielded higher coefficients, and both these scales also yielded good fit indices (i.e., CFA) and stronger reliability coefficients. PPCS, PPUS, and s-IAT-sex significantly positively related with SCS, PCQ, OSAs and usage time severally, and PPCS demonstrated stronger convergent validity.

Table 2. Reliability and validity of the three scales.

Scales	Item Analysis	Confirmatory Factor Analysis				α	External and Convergent Validity			
	rs (Item-Sum Correlation)	χ^2/df	CFI [4]	TLI [5]	RMSEA [6] [90% CI [7]]		SCS [8]	PCQ [9]	OSAs [10]	UT [11]
PPCS [1]	0.62 ***–0.82 ***	210.70/120	0.963	0.952	0.049 [0.038, 0.060]	0.96	0.67 ***	0.70 ***	0.67 ***	0.28 ***
PPUS [2]	0.66 ***–0.85 ***	90.30/48	0.966	0.953	0.052 [0.035, 0.068]	0.95	0.71 ***	0.66 ***	0.56 ***	0.17 ***
s-IAT-sex [3]	0.60 ***–0.79 ***	155.55/52	0.923	0.902	0.079 [0.082, 0.109]	0.89	0.73 ***	0.66 ***	0.46 ***	0.22 ***

[1] PPCS = Problematic Pornography Consumption Scale, [2] PPUS = Problematic Pornography Use Scale, [3] s-IAT-sex = Short Internet Addiction Test Adapted to Online Sexual Activities, [4] CFI = comparative fit index, [5] TLI = Tucker-Lewis index, [6] RMSEA = root mean square error of approximation, [7] CI = confidence interval, [8] SCS = Sexual Compulsivity Scale, [9] PCQ = Pornography Craving Questionnaire, [10] OSAs = online sexual activities, [11] UT = usage time. *** $p < 0.001$.

2.3.2. LPA

The results of LPA are shown in Table 3. For PPCS, the Lo-Mendell-Rubin adjusted likelihood ratio test (LMRT) results were significant when the number of classes was 4, and the entropy value was lower. Thus, the classification accuracy was not as high as that of the three-class solution; accordingly, the three-class solution was selected. For PPUS, when the model consisted of three classes, the LMRT results were significant; furthermore, the entropy value was evidently higher than that of the four-class solution. With regard to the s-IAT-sex, the nonsignificant *p*-value that emerged for the LMRT results suggested that the three- and four-class solutions should be rejected in favor of the two-class solution.

Table 3. Fit indices for latent profile analysis of the three scales assessing problematic internet pornography use.

Scales	Classes [4]	AIC [5]	BIC [6]	SSABIC [7]	Entropy	LMRT [8]
PPCS [1] (*n* = 317)	2	9298.755	9370.174	9309.910	0.959	1154.76 ***
	3	**8898.213**	**8995.944**	**8913.478**	**0.940**	**404.51 ***
	4	8746.574	8870.618	8765.950	0.899	161.63 *
PPUS [2] (*n* = 332)	2	5718.021	5767.488	5726.251	0.953	799.82 ***
	3	**5424.503**	**5492.995**	**5435.899**	**0.924**	**293.41 ****
	4	5348.339	5435.857	5362.900	0.931	83.29
s-IAT-sex [3] (*n* = 323)	2	**3652.433**	**3678.877**	**3656.674**	**0.845**	**205.41 *****
	3	3588.004	3625.780	3594.062	0.771	66.59
	4	3538.775	3587.884	3546.650	0.824	52.22

[1] PPCS = Problematic Pornography Consumption Scale, [2] PPUS = Problematic Pornography Use Scale, [3] s-IAT-sex = Short Internet Addiction Test Adapted to Online Sexual Activities, [4] classes = number of latent classes, [5] AIC = Akaike information criterion, [6] BIC = Bayesian information criterion, [7] SSABIC = sample-size-adjusted Bayesian information criterion, [8] LMRT = Lo-Mendell-Rubin adjusted likelihood ratio test, p = p-value associated with the LMRT results. Bold text is the finally selected models. * $p < 0.05$, ** $p < 0.01$, *** $p < 0.001$.

With regard to the three groups that emerged for the PPCS and PPUS, the first class obtained the lowest averages across all the scale dimensions; thus, this group was referred to as nonproblematic consumption. The second class obtained moderate scores on all the scale dimensions; therefore, these group members were referred to as low-risk pornography users. The third class obtained the highest scores on all the scale dimensions; thus, this group was referred to as at-risk users. As shown in Table 4, with regard to the two classes that emerged for the s-IAT-sex, class 1 obtained lower scores than class 2 on both the scale dimensions; therefore, they were referred to as the nonproblematic and at-risk groups, respectively (group differences in scores on the specific dimensions are shown in Appendix A).

Table 4. Comparisons of the accuracy of the three scales.

Scale	Group	Scores on the BPS					Mean	Range
		<4	4 ≤ x < 6	≥6	Sensitivity [4]	Specificity [5]		
PPCS [1] (*n* = 317)	At-risk (*n* = 29)	3	11	15	89.66%	-	4.60 ± 0.59	1–7
	Low-risk (*n* = 90)	28	34	28	-	-	2.89 ± 0.46	1–7
	Nonproblematic (*n* = 198)	170	23	5	-	85.86%	1.41 ± 0.39	1–7
PPUS [2] (*n* = 332)	At-risk (*n* = 48)	9	8	31	81.25%	-	2.43 ± 0.48	0–5
	Low-risk (*n* = 86)	43	25	18	-	-	1.12 ± 0.29	0–5
	Nonproblematic (*n* = 198)	188	8	2	-	94.95%	0.75 ± 0.84	0–5
s-IAT-sex [3] (*n* = 323)	At-risk (*n* = 99)	28	26	45	71.72%	-	2.84 ± 0.44	1–5
	Nonproblematic (*n* = 224)	195	19	10	-	87.05%	1.54 ± 0.42	1–5

[1] PPCS = Problematic Pornography Consumption Scale, [2] PPUS = Problematic Pornography Use Scale, [3] s-IAT-sex = Short Internet Addiction Test Adapted to Online Sexual Activities, [4] Sensitivity = the proportion of persons with positive symptoms and members of the at-risk group that was identified through LPA, [5] Specificity = the proportion of persons with negative symptoms and the nonproblematic group.

2.3.3. Sensitivity and Specificity Analysis

The results showed that the sensitivity of the PPCS was 89.66%, which is higher than the values that emerged for the PPUS (i.e., 81.25%) and the s-IAT-sex (i.e., 71.72%). There were differences in the specificity of the three scales, and the values ranged from 85.86% to 94.95%. The PPCS demonstrated greater sensitivity (89.66%), and its specificity was 85.86%. This indicates that approximately 10% of problematic users had been classified as nonproblematic users and that approximately 14% of nonproblematic users had not been identified. In general, the PPCS and PPUS performed better than the s-IAT-sex. Since this study aimed to identify the scale with greater sensitivity in detecting problematic IPU, the PPCS was investigated in greater detail.

3. The Qualitative Part: Identification of the Most Accurate Scale

3.1. Methods

3.1.1. Sample

We interviewed 22 (20 men; mean age = 27.2) problematic IPU service volunteers (who provide online services on the following website: http://www.ryeboy.org/; average service time = 3.3 years) and 11 therapists (who have worked with individuals with problematic IPU and had more than 3 years of clinical experience).

3.1.2. The Interview Outline

Since the used scales were easy to administer and consisted of close-ended questions, interviews were conducted to examine participants' perspectives more deeply and comprehensively. The interview guide primarily sought to explore interviewees' understanding of problematic IPU/addiction and their evaluations of the dimensions of the selected scale. The interviewees were required to rate the importance of the dimensions on a scale that ranged from 1 (not at all important) to 7 (very important).

3.1.3. Procedure

In this study, we primarily explored their understanding of the concept of problematic IPU and the dimensions of the recommended scale. Two psychology graduate students served as the interviewers. At the beginning of the interview, the interviewees were informed about the purpose and significance of the interview and assured of the anonymity and strict confidentiality of their interview data; the interviews were recorded with their permission.

3.2. Analysis

The interview recordings were transcribed into verbatim scripts, and participants' identifying information was concealed. Next, we undertook thematic analysis of the text; in other words, we collated different interviewees' responses to the same question to create new text. Tree Nodes were established based on the dimensions of the selected scale, and interviewees' original statements were identified and summarized as a named code. Through this process, NVivo automatically generated statistics for all the references of the texts.

3.3. Results

With regard to the characteristics of problematic IPU, we generated a total of 20 codes by analyzing the interview data. Among these features, preoccupation with IPU (22 mentions), IPU to escape or avoid a negative emotional state (21 mentions), interpersonal conflict (22 mentions), and physiological and psychological symptoms (45 mentions) were most commonly mentioned. Furthermore, the 20 codes were summarized into the six dimensions of the PPCS (see Figure 1).

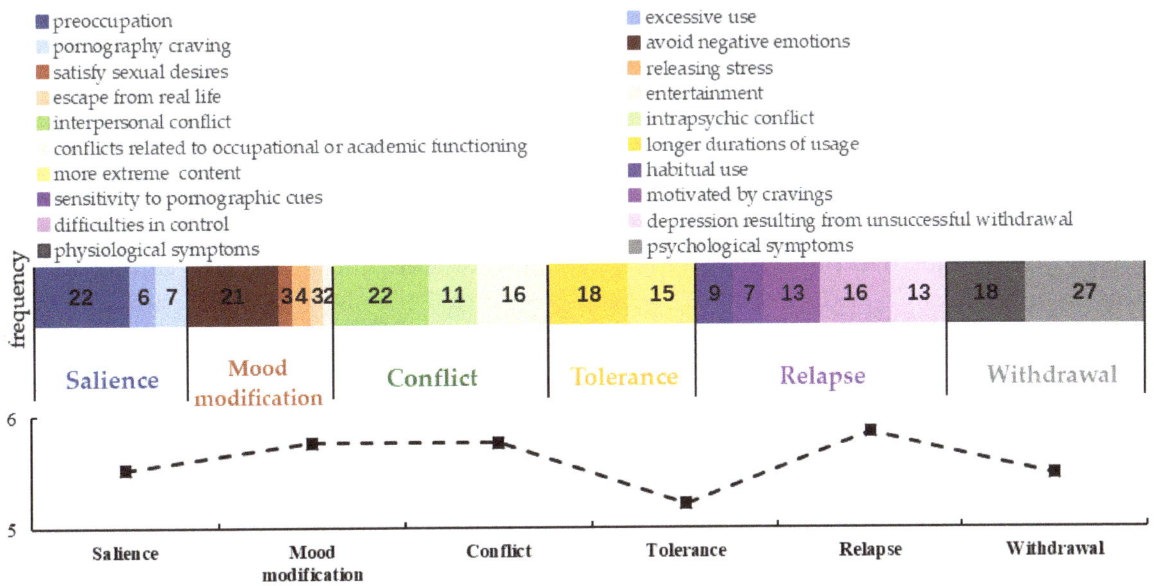

Figure 1. Volunteers and therapists' frequency of mentioning the dimensions of the Problematic Pornography Consumption Scale, features, and importance ratings for the six dimensions (average scores across 33 interviewees). Note: the numbers in the color blocks represent the frequency of mentions, whereas the polyline represents importance ratings for the six dimensions (range = 1–7).

Instance of the interview:

Interviewer: According to your service experience, what do you think is problematic internet pornography use? In other words, what are the expressions/symptoms of problematic internet pornography use?

Interviewee (service volunteer): They (problematic users) show difficulty controlling the craving for internet pornography (code: pornography carving), they are unable to control their own behavior, for instance, browsing pornographic websites, masturbating while watching porn frequently (code: difficulties in control). Their brains are constantly bombarded with sexual materials (code: preoccupation). If they are not exposed to internet pornography, they will feel uncomfortable, or feel that their heart is empty (code: depression resulting from unsuccessful withdrawal).

After presenting interviewees with the definitions of the six components of problematic IPU and further clarifying their meaning using examples, we presented them with questions "Based on your service experience, do you endorse this structure? Which dimension or dimensions do you think are particularly central to IPU?" Most (>95%) participants endorsed the six dimensions. It also can be inferred from Figure 1 that both volunteers and therapists emphasized the centrality of conflict, relapse and withdrawal in IPU (basing the frequency of mentions); at the same time, they weighted the mood modification, relapse and withdrawal as more important features in the problematic use (basing the important rating).

4. General Discussion

Problematic IPU is still a controversial issue; notably, it appears that no real consensus exists regarding the conceptualization and screening tool of problematic IPU. Several scales are available; thus, the assessment of problematic IPU is inconsistent, indicating that findings in this area are not readily comparable. The present study aimed to selected a more sensitive scale to screen problematic IPU, because higher sensitivity implies lower rate of missed diagnosis (i.e., problematic users who have been incorrectly screened as nonproblematic users). Basing on a systematic literature review, three scales were retained. Considering that research with mixed methods combining quantitative and qualitative analyses can enrich and improve our understanding of complicated phenomena [38,39], a quantitative method was used to identify a "more accurate" analysis from the three retained scales. Results of CFA showed that all three scales have good applicability in the wide range of adult groups (age in this case ranged from 18 to 45 years) in three highly homogeneous samples; compared to the other two scales, the PPCS demonstrated greater sensitivity and comparative specificity among samples drawn from the general population (results of the QUAN). Considering that the expression of questionnaire survey is brief and closed, and that the interview can understand the participants' undefined views more deeply and comprehensively, subsequently, results of QUAL showed that symptoms of problematic IPU proposed by the servers (volunteers and therapists) can be grouped into the six dimensions of PPCS and most of the servers supported the six-factor structure of PPCS.

Among the three scales, the PPCS score was most robustly related to the duration of usage, frequency of engagement in OSAs, and pornography cravings. Problematic IPU can appear under the umbrella of hypersexuality similarly to frequent engaging in various forms of cybersex, intense craving for pornography, and compulsive sexual behaviors [40], insofar that the robust relationship not only demonstrated a higher criterion validity, but also implied that co-screening instruments (i.e., pornography craving, frequency and duration of use, compulsive use) are expected to work as auxiliary screening indicators. Recent studies have revealed that for some people, pornographic use gave rise to their feeling of discord and shame contributing to their conflict of actual sexual materials consumption and their belief; in turn, these feelings of distress and shame may drive a morbid self-perception that they are addicted, but this may not be a real behavioral disorder [41,42]. In order to avoid misjudgment due to the self-perceived problematic use, it is more advisable to combine other supporting scales, and the combination diagnosis indexes of the diversity were selected to screen the prevalence of problematic IPU. In this study, with the higher correlation of PPCS with frequency of OSAs, the PCQ showed that combined with other indicators, it can better screen out problematic use and is more likely to avoid the misjudgment caused by subjective self-perceived addiction.

The more robust psychometric properties and higher recognition accuracy of the PPCS may be attributable to the fact that it has been developed in accordance with Griffiths's six-component structural theory of addiction (i.e., in contrast to the PPUS and s-IAT-sex). The PPCS has a very strong theoretical framework, and it assesses more components of addiction [11]. In particular, tolerance and withdrawal are the important dimensions of problematic IPU that are not assessed by the PPUS and s-IAT-sex; PPCS is the only instrument that explicitly assesses the "tolerance" component [11,14]. According to the "two-phased" internet pornography addiction model, in which the first step is characterized by an excessive use to internet pornography, and the second functions as a marker by repeated failures to break free from excessive use, despite negative consequences [43]. Items related to information about salience, carving, and tolerance reflect the engagement in internet pornography, corresponding to the first step, whereas items related to withdrawal, relapse, and conflict measure addiction more, corresponding to the second step. Obviously, components of PPCS includes both engagement in pornography and addiction of IPU, which has an intact theoretical framework of addiction.

The PPCS appears to be a more valid instrument for assessing problematic pornography use, has potential application in detecting prevalence concerning problematic IPU or cybersex addiction, and may be useful in assessing treatment outcomes. Our findings indicate that individuals who score high on the PPCS also report frequent engaging in various forms of online sexual activities, intense craving for pornography, and compulsive sexual behaviors. Thus, it appears important for clinicians to be aware of problematic pornography use and its related associations such as pornography craving, compulsive use. Moreover, it is important to note that the scale PPCS is recommended as a screening instruments to identify problematic users in the public and assess the prevalence rather than a diagnostic tool; future studies should further research its validity and cutoff in clinical sample; we also encourage individuals to visit a clinical therapist after being identified with problematic IPU by the use of PPCS.

This study has several limitations. First, data were collected using self-report measures; therefore, the reliability of the results depends on the respondents' honesty and accuracy of their comprehension of the scale items. Second, the study sample was recruited through an online survey company; therefore, the participants of this study may have been more educated and affluent than the average Chinese person. Furthermore, the study participants primarily lived in the capital/provincial capital, cities, and towns. Third, because the sample consisted of only a small number of non-heterosexual subjects, it was not possible to examine whether the factor structure and meaning of the contents of the PPCS differed across individuals with different sexual orientations.

5. Conclusions

The present study showed that the PPUS, PPCS, and s-IAT-sex are promising measures of problematic IPU. However, when sensitivity and specificity were simultaneously examined, the PPCS emerged as a more suitable measure of problematic IPU. The qualitative findings further confirmed that service providers endorsed the underlying structure of the PPCS.

Author Contributions: Conceptualization, L.C.; Data curation, L.C.; Formal analysis, X.J.; Funding acquisition, L.C.; Investigation, X.J.; Methodology, L.C.; Project administration, L.C.; Resources, L.C.; Supervision, L.C.; Visualization, X.J.; Writing—original draft, L.C.; Writing—review and editing, L.C. and X.J. All authors have read and agreed to the published version of the manuscript.

Acknowledgments: We would like to acknowledge Bin Wu and Yan Zhao (the founders of the "*Reyboys*", a non-governmental organization focusing on helping the problematic internet pornography users) for their help to recruit volunteers who serviced the addicts in the qualitative step, and pay tribute to them for their effort in helping problematic users.

Appendix A

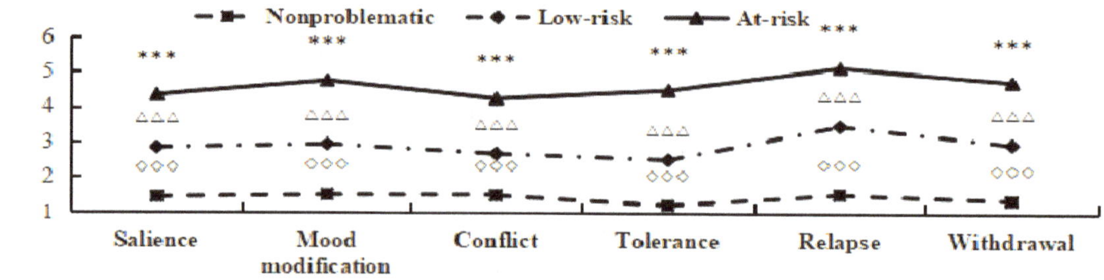

Figure A1. The average scores of the three latent classes based on the dimensions of PPCS. Note: PPCS = Problematic Pornography Consumption Scale, range = 1–7; *** $p < 0.001$ indicate that the score of at-risk group was significantly higher than that of low-risk group; $^{\triangle\triangle\triangle}$ $p < 0.001$ indicate that the score of low-risk group was significantly higher than that of non-problematic group; $^{\diamond\diamond\diamond}$ $p < 0.001$ indicate that the score of at-risk group was significantly higher than that of non-problematic group. The same below.

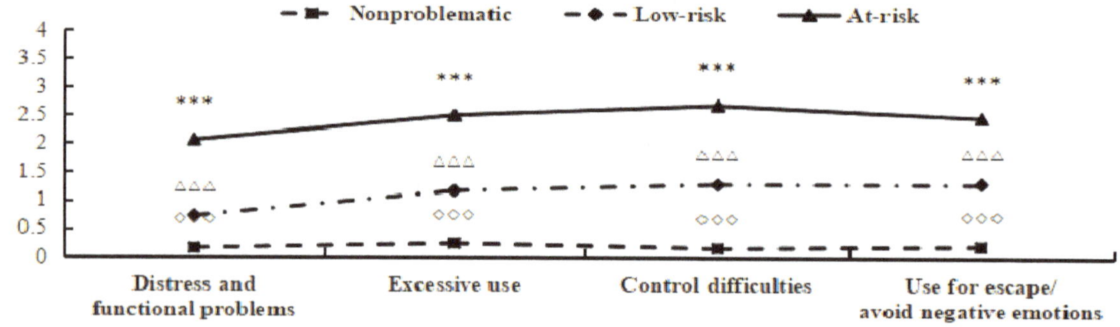

Figure A2. The average scores of the three latent classes based on the dimensions of PPUS. Note: PPUS = Problematic Pornography Use Scale, range = 0–5.

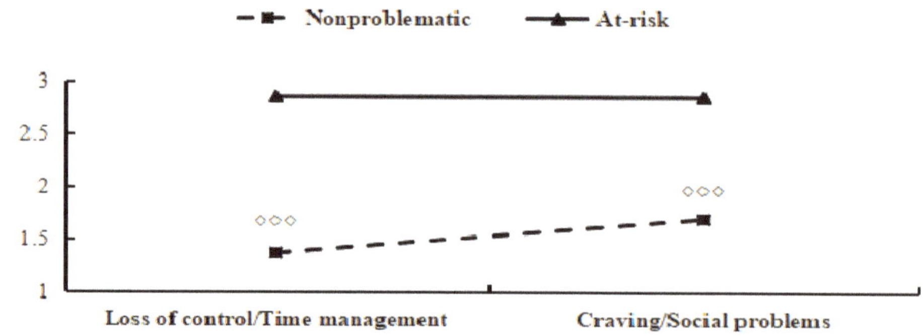

Figure A3. The average scores of the tow latent classes based on the dimensions of s-IAT-sex. Note: s-IAT-sex = short version of the Internet Addiction Test adapted to online sexual activities, range = 1–5.

References

1. Grubbs, J.B.; Wright, P.J.; Braden, A.L.; Wilt, J.A.; Kraus, S.W. Internet pornography use and sexual motivation: A systematic review and integration. *Ann. Int. Commun. Assoc.* **2019**, *43*, 117–155. [CrossRef]
2. Delmonico, D.L. Cybersex: High tech sex addiction. *Sex. Addict. Compulsivity J. Treat. Prev.* **1997**, *4*, 159–167. [CrossRef]
3. Cooper, A.L.; Delmonico, D.L.; Griffin-Shelley, E.; Mathy, R.M. Online sexual activity: An examination of potentially problematic behaviors. *Sex. Addict. Compulsivity* **2004**, *11*, 129–143. [CrossRef]
4. De Alarcón, R.; de la Iglesia, J.I.; Casado, N.M.; Montejo, A.L. Online Porn Addiction: What We Know and What We Don't—A Systematic Review. *Clin. Med.* **2019**, *8*, 91. [CrossRef]

5. Wéry, A.; Billieux, J. Problematic cybersex: Conceptualization, assessment, and treatment. *Addict. Behav.* **2017**, *64*, 238–246. [CrossRef] [PubMed]
6. Grubbs, J.B.; Volk, F.; Exline, J.J.; Pargament, K.I. Internet pornography use: Perceived addiction, psychological distress, and the validation of a brief measure. *Sex. Marital. Ther.* **2015**, *41*, 83–106. [CrossRef]
7. Griffiths, M.D. Internet sex addiction: A review of empirical research. *Addict. Res. Theory* **2012**, *20*, 111–124. [CrossRef]
8. Young, K.S. Internet sex addiction: Risk factors, stages of development, and treatment. *Am. Behav. Sci.* **2008**, *52*, 21–37. [CrossRef]
9. Wéry, A.; Burnay, J.; Karila, L.; Billieux, J. The Short French Internet Addiction Test adapted to online sexual activities: Validation and links with online sexual preferences and addiction symptoms. *Sex Res.* **2015**, *53*, 701–710. [CrossRef]
10. López-Fernández, O. How has internet addiction research evolved since the advent of internet gaming disorder? An overview of cyberaddictions from a psychological perspective. *Curr. Addict. Rep.* **2015**, *2*, 263. [CrossRef]
11. Fernandez, D.P.; Griffiths, M.D. Psychometric Instruments for Problematic Pornography Use: A Systematic Review. *Eval. Health Prof.* **2019**. [CrossRef] [PubMed]
12. Reid, R.C.; Li, D.S.; Gilliland, R.; Stein, J.A.; Fong, T. Reliability, validity, and psychometric development of the Pornography Consumption Inventory in a sample of hypersexual men. *J. Sex Marital Ther.* **2011**, *37*, 359–385. [CrossRef] [PubMed]
13. Short, M.B.; Black, L.; Smith, A.H.; Wetterneck, C.T.; Wells, D.E. A review of Internet pornography use research: Methodology and content from the past 10 years. *Cyberpsychol. Behav. Soc. Netw.* **2012**, *15*, 13–23. [CrossRef] [PubMed]
14. Bőthe, B.; Tóth-Király, I.; Zsila, Á.; Griffiths, M.D.; Demetrovics, Z.; Orosz, G. The development of the problematic pornography consumption scale (PPCS). *Sex Res.* **2018**, *55*, 395–406. [CrossRef] [PubMed]
15. Kor, A.; Zilcha-Mano, S.; Fogel, Y.A.; Mikulincer, M.; Reid, R.C.; Potenza, M.N. Psychometric development of the Problematic Pornography Use Scale. *Addict. Behav.* **2014**, *39*, 861–868. [CrossRef] [PubMed]
16. Chen, L.; Demetrovics, Z.; Potenza, M.N. Does mate preference predict problematic online pornography? Cross-cultural findings. *Behav. Addict.* **2019**, *8*, 63. [CrossRef]
17. Chen, L.; Ding, C.; Jiang, X.; Potenza, M.N. Frequency and duration of use, craving and negative emotions in problematic online sexual activities. *Sex. Addict. Compulsivity* **2018**, *25*, 396–414. [CrossRef]
18. Chen, L.; Yang, Y.; Su, W.; Zheng, L.; Ding, C.; Potenza, M.N. The relationship between sexual sensation seeking and problematic Internet pornography use: A moderated mediation model examining roles of online sexual activities and the third-person effect. *Behav. Addict.* **2018**, *7*, 565–573. [CrossRef]
19. Chen, L.; Wang, X.; Chen, S.M.; Jiang, C.H.; Wang, J.X. Reliability and validity of the Problematic Internet Pornography Use Scale in Chinese college students. *Chin. J. Public Health* **2018**, *34*, 1034–1038. [CrossRef]
20. Ševčíková, A.; Šerek, J.; Barbovschi, M.; Daneback, K. The roles of individual characteristics and liberalism in intentional and unintentional exposure to online sexual material among European youth: A multilevel approach. *Sex. Res. Soc. Policy* **2014**, *11*, 104–115. [CrossRef]
21. Cooper, A.; Delmonico, D.L.; Burg, R. Cybersex users, abusers, and compulsives: New findings and implications. *Sex. Addict. Compulsivity J. Treat. Prev.* **2000**, *7*, 5–29. [CrossRef]
22. Griffiths, M. A 'components' model of addiction within a biopsychosocial framework. *Subst. Use* **2005**, *10*, 191–197. [CrossRef]
23. Sklenarik, S.; Potenza, M.N.; Gola, M.; Kor, A.; Kraus, S.W.; Astur, R.S. Approach bias for erotic stimuli in heterosexual male college students who use pornography. *Behav. Addict.* **2019**, *8*, 234–241. [CrossRef] [PubMed]
24. Kraus, S.W.; Krueger, R.B.; Briken, P.; First, M.B.; Stein, D.J.; Kaplan, M.S.; Voon, V.; Abdo, C.; Grant, J.E.; Atalla, E.; et al. Compulsive sexual behaviour disorder in the ICD-11. *World Psychiatry* **2018**, *17*, 109–110. [CrossRef]
25. Efrati, Y.; Gola, M. Treating Compulsive Sexual Behavior. *Curr. Sex. Health Rep.* **2018**, *10*, 57–64. [CrossRef]
26. Kraus, S.W.; Gola, M.; Kowalewska, E.; Lew-Starowicz, M.; Hoff, R.A.; Porter, E.; Potenza, M.N. Brief Pornography Screener: A comparison of US and Polish pornography users. *J. Behav. Addict.* **2017**, *6*, 27–28. [CrossRef]

27. Kowalewska, E.; Kraus, S.W.; Lew-Starowicz, M.; Gustavsson, K.; Gola, M. Which dimensions of human sexuality are related to compulsive sexual behavior disorder (CSBD)? Study using a multidimensional sexuality questionnaire on a sample of Polish males. *J. Sex. Med.* **2019**, *16*, 1264–1273. [CrossRef]
28. Gola, M.; Wordecha, M.; Sescousse, G.; Lew-Starowicz, M.; Kossowski, B.; Wypych, M.; Makeig, S.; Potenza, M.N.; Marchewka, A. Can pornography be addictive? An fMRI study of men seeking treatment for problematic pornography use. *Neuropsychopharmacology* **2017**, *42*, 2021–2031. [CrossRef]
29. Wordecha, M.; Wilk, M.; Kowalewska, E.; Skorko, M.; Łapiński, A.; Gola, M. "Pornographic binges" as a key characteristic of males seeking treatment for compulsive sexual behaviors: Qualitative and quantitative 10-week-long diary assessment. *Behav. Addict.* **2018**, *7*, 433–444. [CrossRef]
30. Duffy, A.; Dawson, D.L.; Das Nair, R. Pornography addiction in adults: A systematic review of definitions and reported impact. *J. Sex. Med.* **2016**, *13*, 760–777. [CrossRef]
31. Eleuteri, S.; Tripodi, F.; Petruccelli, I.; Rossi, R.; Simonelli, C. Questionnaires and scales for the evaluation of the online sexual activities: A review of 20 years of research. *Cyberpsychol. J. Psychosoc. Res. Cyberspace* **2014**, *8*. [CrossRef]
32. Kraus, S.; Rosenberg, H. The pornography craving questionnaire: Psychometric properties. *Arch. Sex. Behav.* **2014**, *43*, 451–462. [CrossRef] [PubMed]
33. Rosenberg, H.; Kraus, S. The relationship of "passionate attachment" for pornography with sexual compulsivity, frequency of use, and craving for pornography. *Addict. Behav.* **2014**, *39*, 1012–1017. [CrossRef] [PubMed]
34. Kalichman, S.C.; Rompa, D. Sexual sensation seeking and sexual compulsivity scales: Validity, and predicting HIV risk behavior. *J. Personal. Assess* **1995**, *65*, 586–601. [CrossRef]
35. Zheng, L.; Zheng, Y. Online sexual activity in Mainland China: Relationship to sexual sensation seeking and sociosexuality. *Comput. Hum. Behav.* **2014**, *36*, 323–329. [CrossRef]
36. Muthen, L. *Mplus Version 7 User's Guide: Version 7*; Muthen & Muthen: Los Angeles, CA, USA, 2012.
37. Orford, J. *Excessive Appetites: A Psychological View of Addictions*; John Wiley & Sons Ltd.: Hoboken, NJ, USA, 2001.
38. López-Fernández, O.; Molina Azorín, J.F. The use of mixed methods research in the behavioral sciences field. *Qual Quant* **2011**, *45*, 1459–1472. [CrossRef]
39. López-Fernández, O.; Molina-Azorín, J.F. The use of mixed methods research in interdisciplinary educational journals. *Int. J. Mult. Res. Approaches* **2011**, *5*, 269–283. [CrossRef]
40. Kafka, M.P. Hypersexual disorder: A proposed diagnosis for DSM-V. *Arch. Sex. Behav.* **2010**, *39*, 377–400. [CrossRef]
41. Grubbs, J.B.; Perry, S.L.; Wilt, J.A.; Reid, R.C. Pornography problems due to moral incongruence: An integrative model with a systematic review and meta-analysis. *Arch. Sex. Behav.* **2019**, *48*, 397–415. [CrossRef]
42. Grubbs, J.B.; Kraus, S.W.; Perry, S.L. Self-reported addiction to pornography in a nationally representative sample: The roles of use habits, religiousness, and moral incongruence. *Behav. Addict.* **2019**, *8*, 88–93. [CrossRef]
43. Bensimon, P. The role of pornography in sexual offending. *Sex. Addict. Compulsivity* **2007**, *14*, 95–114. [CrossRef]

9

Mobile Phone Dependence, Social Support and Impulsivity in Chinese University Students

Songli Mei [1], Jingxin Chai [2,*], Shi-Bin Wang [3], Chee H. Ng [4], Gabor S. Ungvari [5,6] and Yu-Tao Xiang [7,*]

1 School of Public Health, Jilin University, Changchun 130021, China; meisongli@sina.com
2 Hepin Street, Dongcheng District, Beijing Center for Disease Prevention and Control, Beijing 100013, China
3 Guangdong Mental Health Center, Guangdong General Hospital and Guangdong Academy of Medical Sciences, Guangzhou 510120, China; spiriorwang@126.com
4 Department of Psychiatry, University of Melbourne, Melbourne, VIC 3050, Australia; cng@unimelb.edu.au
5 Division of Psychiatry, Notre Dame university Australia, Fremantle, WA 6160, Australia; sungvari@e.cuhk.edu.hk
6 Graylands Hospital, Claremont, WA 6010, Australia
7 Unit of Psychiatry, Faculty of Health Sciences, University of Macau, Avenida da Universidade, Taipa, Macau, China
* Correspondence: chaitong2008@163.com (J.C.); xyutly@gmail.com (Y.-T.X.)

Abstract: This study examined the frequency of mobile phone dependence in Chinese university students and explored its association with social support and impulsivity. Altogether, 909 university students were consecutively recruited from a large university in China. Mobile phone use, mobile phone dependence, impulsivity, and social support were measured with standardized instruments. The frequency of possible mobile phone use and mobile phone dependence was 78.3% and 7.4%, respectively. Multinomial logistic regression analyses revealed that compared with no mobile phone dependence, possible mobile phone dependence was significantly associated with being male ($p = 0.04$, OR = 0.7, 95% CI: 0.4–0.98), excessive mobile phone use ($p < 0.001$, OR = 1.2, 95% CI: 1.09–1.2), and impulsivity ($p < 0.001$, OR = 1.05, 95% CI: 1.03–1.06), while mobile phone dependence was associated with length of weekly phone use ($p = 0.01$, OR = 2.5, 95% CI: 1.2–5.0), excessive mobile phone use ($p < 0.001$, OR = 1.3, 95% CI: 1.2–1.4), and impulsivity ($p < 0.001$, OR = 1.08, 95% CI: 1.05–1.1). The frequency of possible mobile phone dependence and mobile phone dependence was high in this sample of Chinese university students. A significant positive association with impulsivity was found, but not with social support.

Keywords: mobile phone dependence; mobile phone use; impulsivity; China

---

1. Introduction

Mobile phone dependence, defined as inapt use of a mobile phone, is broadly viewed as a subset of behavioral or technological addiction [1] which could lead to significant social and emotional impairment [2]. Excessive mobile phone use is common among young people and is negatively associated with academic performance [3], interpersonal relationships, self-esteem, self-regulation, and life satisfaction [4].

High level of impulsivity appears to be closely associated with excessive mobile phone use and dependence [5,6]. For example, Smetaniuk [7] reported that mobile phone dependence could be considered as an impulse control disorder. Those with a high level of impulsivity often prefer mobile phone use as a choice of gratification without fully thinking through consequences of the action [6].

In addition, social extraversion has been shown to have a positive association with mobile phone addiction, while self-esteem has a negative association [8]. Furthermore, social support is negatively associated with mobile phone use [9], but frequent social networking could increase the risk of mobile phone addiction [10].

China has become the largest mobile phone market worldwide and mobile phone use has increased dramatically in Chinese university students in recent years [11]. Better understanding of the frequency of mobile phone dependence and its associated factors is important to develop effective strategies to reduce its harmful impact. To date, few studies have examined the association of mobile phone dependence with impulsivity and social support. In this study, we aimed to examine the frequency of mobile phone dependence in Chinese university students and explore its association with demographic variables, impulsivity, and social support.

2. Materials and Methods

2.1. Study Design and Participants

This cross-sectional study was conducted in a large university in Jilin province, China between 1 September and 30 November 2013. Students who fulfilled the following inclusion criteria were recruited: (1) being registered as undergraduate students; (2) having a mobile phone; (3) having the ability to complete the assessment; (4) having the willingness to participate in the study and provide informed consent. The study protocol was approved by the Human Ethical Committee of the Jilin University School of Public Health (BSERE-APP002-FHS).

Three of the six campuses in the University were randomly selected and students who were enrolled in the selected campuses were consecutively screened for eligibility during the study period following a detailed explanation about the study protocol. The questionnaires were distributed to all eligible students in person by the research team members after they provided informed consent. Completed questionnaires were collected on a voluntary basis on the same day. The survey was completed anonymously and confidentially.

2.2. Assessment Instruments

Basic demographic characteristics were recorded on a standard study form. At the time of the study, no validated standardized questionnaires on mobile phone use were available in China. Therefore a self-reported questionnaire entitled "Mobile Phone Use Questionnaire (MPUQ)" was developed based on the recommendation of the China Internet Network Information Center [12]. The MPUQ consists of two parts. In the first part, respondents were screened for smart phone use by asking: "Do you own and use a smart phone?" If the answer was "yes", then the respondent was required to complete the second part. In the second part, the frequency of mobile phone use was assessed in two domains: (1) "use for networking purposes", including voice calling, sending short messages, using communication programs, watching internet news and blogs; (2) "use for entertainment purposes", including listening to music, watching videos, playing online games, and reading internet novels. Each domain includes four items with each item scoring from 1 (never) to 4 (frequently). The MPUQ total score ranges from 8 to 32, with a higher score indicating more frequent mobile phone use. The details of MPUQ items are presented in Supplementary Materials Table S1. The internal consistency of the MPUQ was fair: Cronbach's $\alpha = 0.66$ for the whole scale, and 0.68 and 0.58 for the two parts, respectively.

The Chinese version of the Barratt Impulsiveness Scale (BIS-11) was used to measure impulsivity trait [13]. The BIS-11 is a 30-item self-reported questionnaire with three subscales: attention impulsivity, motor impulsivity, and non-planning impulsivity. Each item is scored from 1 (never) to 5 (always). The Chinese version of the BIS-11 has been validated with good reliability and validity in China [14]. The internal consistency of the BIS-11 was satisfactory (Cronbach's $\alpha = 0.87$) in this study.

The factor structure of Chinese version of the BIS-11 was tested using the confirmatory factor analysis (CFA) with the AMOS 18.0 program. The model was acceptable if the value of χ^2/df was less than 8, the goodness of fit index (GFI) was greater than 0.90, the comparative fit index (CFI) was greater than 0.90, or the root mean square of approximation (RMSEA) was less than 0.08 [15]. The factor structure of Chinese version of the BIS-11 was found to be acceptable (χ^2/df = 7.42, GFI = 0.95, CFI = 0.89, $RMSEA$ = 0.08).

The multidimensional scale of perceived social support (MSPSS) is a self-reported questionnaire measuring perceived social support. There are three subscales with a total of 12 items: family members' support, friends' support, and others' support. The items is scored from 1 (strongly disagree) to 7 (strongly agree). The Chinese version of the MSPSS has been validated in China [16]. The internal consistency of the MSPSS in this study was satisfactory (Cronbach's α = 0.83). The factor structure of Chinese version of the MSPSS was found to be acceptable (χ^2/df = 7.81, GFI = 0.93, CFI = 0.94, $RMSEA$ = 0.08).

Mobile phone addiction was assessed using the mobile phone addiction scale for college students (MPAS) [17]. The MPAS comprises 16 items in four areas: withdrawal symptoms, salience, social comfort, and mood changes. Each item is rated on a five-point (1–5) scale with higher scores indicating higher level of mobile phone addiction. A total score of 16–31 indicates "no mobile phone addiction", while the score of 32–56 indicates "possible mobile phone addiction", and 57 or above indicates "mobile phone addiction" [9]. This definition of mobile phone addiction was also used in a previous study [16]. The factor structure of the MPAS was found to be acceptable (χ^2/df = 2.92, NFI = 0.94, CFI = 0.96, $RMSEA$ = 0.07).

2.3. Statistical Analysis

The database was established using EpiData 3.2 (Epidata Assoc., Odense, Denmark). The data were analyzed with SPSS 18.0 (SPSS, Chicago, IL, USA) for Windows. Comparisons between no dependence, possible dependence, and mobile phone dependence individuals with respect to demographic and mental variables were conducted with chi-square and analysis of variance (ANOVA), as appropriate. Multinomial logistic regression analysis was used to determine the independent correlates significantly associated with mobile phone dependence. Mobile phone dependence was the dependent variable, while the demographic and clinical characteristics that significantly differed in the univariate analyses were entered as independent variables. Statistical significance was set at 0.05 (two-tailed).

3. Results

Out of 946 students who were approached, 909 students consented to the study and completed the questionnaire, giving a response rate of 96.1%. The frequency of having no mobile phone dependence, possible mobile phone dependence, and mobile phone dependence was 14.3% (n = 130), 78.3% (n = 712), and 7.4% (n = 67), respectively.

Table 1 presents the socio-demographic and clinical characteristics of the whole sample and separately by groups of mobile phone dependence. Univariate analyses revealed that being a single child, weekly mobile phone use time, and the total scores of the MPUQ and BIS were significantly different between the three groups.

Table 1. Comparison of socio-demographic and clinical characteristics between different groups of phone dependence.

	Whole Sample (n = 909)		No Phone Dependence (n = 130)		Possible Phone Dependence (n = 712)		Phone Dependence (n = 67)		Statistics [a]		
	n	%	n	%	n	%	n	%	χ^2	df	p
Male	404	44.4	70	53.8	302	42.5	31	46.3	5.9	2	0.053
Grade											
UG1-UG4	644	70.8	88	67.7	508	71.3	48	71.6	3.7	4	0.4

Table 1. *Cont.*

	Whole Sample (n = 909)		No Phone Dependence (n = 130)		Possible Phone Dependence (n = 712)		Phone Dependence (n = 67)		Statistics [a]		
	n	%	n	%	n	%	n	%	χ^2	df	p
UG5	132	14.5	24	18.5	96	13.5	12	17.9			
PG	133	14.6	18	13.8	108	15.2	7	10.4			
Urban	426	46.9	63	48.5	330	46.3	33	49.3	0.4	2	0.8
Single child	485	53.4	66	50.8	373	52.4	46	68.7	6.9	2	**0.03**
Length of phone use >3 years	647	71.2	95	73.1	503	70.6	49	73.1	0.45	2	0.8
Length of weekly phone use >24 h	512	56.4	55	42.3	407	57.2	50	74.6	19.8	2	**<0.001**
	Mean	**SD**	**Mean**	**SD**	**Mean**	**SD**	**Mean**	**SD**	f	df	p
MPUQ total	26.0	5.1	23.0	5.2	26.2	4.8	29.7	5.6	44.7	2	**<0.001**
BIS total	73.8	12.9	67.7	13.2	74.4	12.7	78.8	11.5	21.0	2	**<0.001**
PSS total	64.4	11.1	64.0	13.1	64.2	10.8	66.8	9.9	1.8	2	0.2

Bolded values: <0.05; [a] comparison between no, possible and phone dependence; BIS = Barratt Impulsiveness Scale; PSS = perceived social support; PG = postgraduate; MPUQ = Mobile Phone Use Questionnaire; UG = under graduate.

Multinomial logistic regression analyses revealed that compared with no mobile phone dependence, possible mobile phone dependence was significantly associated with male gender (p = 0.04, OR = 0.7, 95% CI: 0.4–0.98) and MPUQ (p < 0.001, OR = 1.2, 95% CI: 1.09–1.2) and BIS total scores (p < 0.001, OR = 1.05, 95% CI: 1.03–1.06), while mobile phone dependence was associated with length of weekly phone use (p = 0.01, OR = 2.5, 95% CI: 1.2–5.0) and MPUQ (p < 0.001, OR = 1.3, 95% CI: 1.2–1.4) and BIS total scores (p < 0.001, OR = 1.08, 95% CI: 1.05–1.1) (see Table 2). Supplementary Materials Table S1 shows the details regarding the purpose of mobile phone use.

Table 2. Factors independently associated with phone dependence (multinomial logistic regression analysis with no dependence as the reference group).

	Possible Phone Dependence vs. No Dependence			Phone Dependence vs. No Dependence		
	p	OR	95% CI	p	OR	95% CI
Male	**0.04**	**0.7**	**0.4, 0.98**	0.6	0.8	0.5, 1.6
Single child	0.9	1.0	0.7, 1.5	0.2	1.6	0.8, 3.2
Length of weekly phone use >24 h	0.1	1.4	0.9, 2.1	**0.01**	**2.5**	**1.2, 5.0**
MPUQ total	**<0.001**	**1.2**	**1.09, 1.20**	**<0.001**	**1.3**	**1.2, 1.4**
BIS total	**<0.001**	**1.05**	**1.03, 1.06**	**<0.001**	**1.08**	**1.05, 1.1**

Bolded value: <0.05; BIS = Barratt Impulsiveness Scale; MPUQ = Mobile Phone Use Questionnaire; OR = odds ratio.

4. Discussion

In this study, 78.3% and 7.4% of university students reported possible mobile phone dependence and mobile phone dependence, respectively, which is inconsistent with previous findings using the MPAS in Chinese young adults (possible mobile phone dependence: 56.4%; mobile phone dependence: 36.4%) [9] and British and American college students (mobile phone dependence 10–25%) [7,18]. The discrepancy in the results across studies could be due to different socioeconomic and cultural factors, such as age group [7], type of university [11], and religion [19]. The major purpose of mobile phone use in this sample was voice calling and sending short messages, followed by using communication programs, watching internet news, reading blogs, listening music, watching video, playing online games, and reading internet novels.

Compared to male students, female students reported more frequent possible mobile phone dependence, but there was no significant gender difference in mobile phone dependence, which is partly supported by earlier findings in other settings [20,21]. This could be related to gender preferences in the use of mobile phones for maintaining interpersonal relationship [19]. Similar to previous studies [19,22] although different measures were used, we found that excessive use of mobile phones was positively associated with mobile phone dependence.

We found that impulsivity was positively associated with both possible mobile phone dependence and mobile phone dependence, which is in line with previous studies. For example, Smetaniuk [7] found a positive relationship between problematic mobile phone use and impulse control. Roberts et al. [23] found that attention impulsivity is predictive of mobile phone addiction. Further qualitative and empirical studies are warranted to explore the association between mobile phone behavior and impulsivity.

A mobile phone is a communication tool that can enhance social support. Therefore, greater family support could increase the likelihood of excessive mobile phone use [24], which may increase the risk of mobile phone dependence. For example, Crosswhite et al. [25] found that young adults prefer texting to engaging in general conversation with their parents. On the other hand, mobile phone dependence could negatively affect social relationships which in turn may have a negative impact on academic performance [26]. However, our study found no significant association between social support and mobile phone dependence in this study.

There are several limitations in this study. First, this was a cross-sectional study, therefore the causality between mobile phone dependence and other variables could be not examined. Second, the study was conducted only in one university so the findings could not be generalized to all Chinese university students. Multicenter studies involving different regions across China are needed. Third, other important information related to mobile phone dependence—such as depressive and anxiety symptoms—were not recorded. Fourth, second-digital divide and third-digital divide which may affect individual behavior including impulsiveness, was not examined in this study. Fifth, the mediating effects of various purposes of mobile phone use on impulsiveness could not be examined due to the current study design. Finally, the Cronbach's α of the MPUQ was relatively low.

5. Conclusions

In conclusion, the frequency of possible mobile phone dependence and mobile phone dependence in this sample of Chinese university students was relatively high. A significant positive association between mobile phone dependence and impulsivity was found. Further longitudinal research is needed to explore the relationship between mobile phone dependence and impulsivity, and how the different purposes for mobile phone use could mediate their interaction.

Acknowledgments: The authors are grateful to all the participants who were involved in this study. This study was supported by the Science and Technology International Cooperation Project of Jilin province (20160414035GH).

Author Contributions: Study design: Songli Mei, Jingxin Chai, and Yu-Tao Xiang Data collection, analysis, and interpretation of data: Jingxin Chai and Songli Mei Drafting of the manuscript: Jingxin Chai, Shi-Bin Wang, and Yu-Tao Xiang Critical revision of the manuscript: Chee H. Ng and Gabor S. Ungvari. Approval of the final version for publication: all co-authors.

References

1. Billieux, J. Problematic Use of the Mobile Phone: A Literature Review and a Pathways Model. *Curr. Psychiatry Rev.* **2012**, *8*, 299–307. [CrossRef]
2. Yen, C.F.; Tang, T.C.; Yen, J.Y.; Lin, H.C.; Huang, C.F.; Liu, S.C.; Ko, C.H. Symptoms of problematic cellular phone use, functional impairment and its association with depression among adolescents in Southern Taiwan. *J. Adolesc.* **2009**, *32*, 863–873. [CrossRef] [PubMed]
3. Lepp, A.; Barkley, J.E.; Karpinski, A.C. The Relationship Between Cell Phone Use and Academic Performance in a Sample of U.S. College Students. *SAGE Open* **2015**, *5*. [CrossRef]
4. Lepp, A.; Barkley, J.E.; Karpinski, A.C. The relationship between cell phone use, academic performance, anxiety, and Satisfaction with Life in college students. *Comput. Hum. Behav.* **2014**, *31*, 343–350. [CrossRef]
5. Billieux, J.; Van der Linden, M.; Rochat, L. The role of impulsivity in actual and problematic use of the mobile phone. *Appl. Cogn. Psychol.* **2008**, *22*, 1195–1210. [CrossRef]
6. Mitchell, M.R.; Potenza, M.N. Addictions and Personality Traits: Impulsivity and Related Constructs. *Curr. Behav. Neurosci. Rep.* **2014**, *1*, 1–12. [CrossRef] [PubMed]
7. Smetaniuk, P. A preliminary investigation into the prevalence and prediction of problematic cell phone use. *J. Behav. Addict.* **2014**, *3*, 41–53. [CrossRef] [PubMed]
8. Hong, F.-Y.; Chiu, S.-I.; Huang, D.-H. A model of the relationship between psychological characteristics, mobile phone addiction and use of mobile phones by Taiwanese university female students. *Comput. Hum. Behav.* **2012**, *28*, 2152–2159. [CrossRef]
9. Hoffner, C.A.; Lee, S. Mobile Phone Use, Emotion Regulation, and Well-Being. *Cyberpsychol. Behav. Soc. Netw.* **2015**, *18*, 411–416. [CrossRef] [PubMed]
10. Salehan, M.; Negahban, A. Social networking on smartphones: When mobile phones become addictive. *Comput. Hum. Behav.* **2013**, *29*, 2632–2639. [CrossRef]
11. Chen, L.; Yan, Z.; Tang, W.; Yang, F.; Xie, X.; He, J. Mobile phone addiction levels and negative emotions among Chinese young adults: The mediating role of interpersonal problems. *Comput. Hum. Behav.* **2016**, *55*, 856–866. [CrossRef]
12. China Internet Network Information Center (CNNIC). *The 2013 Statistics Report the Development of China Internet Network*; China Internet Network Information Center (CNNIC): Beijing, China, 2013; Available online: http://www.cnnic.net.cn/hlwfzyj/hlwxzbg/hlwtjbg/201307/P020130717505343100851.pdf (accessed on 17 July 2017). (In Chinese)
13. Patton, J.M.; Stanford, M.S.; Barratt, E.S. Factor structure of the Barratt Impulsiveness Scale. *J. Clin. Psychol.* **1995**, *51*, 768–774. [CrossRef]
14. Li, X.Y.; Phillips, M.R.; Xu, D.; Zhang, Y.L.; Yang, S.J.; Tong, Y.S.; Wang, Z.Q.; Niu, Y.J. Reliability and validity of an adapted Chinese version of Barratt Impulsiveness Scale. *Chin. Ment. Health J.* **2011**, *25*, 610–615.
15. Bentler, P.M. On the fit of models to covariances and methodology to the Bulletin. *Psychol. Bull.* **1992**, *112*, 400–404. [CrossRef] [PubMed]
16. Wang, X.D.; Jiang, C.Q.; Ma, H. *Rating Scales for Mental Health*; Mental Health in Chinese Press: Beijing, China, 1999.
17. Xiong, J.; Zhou, Z.K.; Chen, W.; You, Z.Q.; Zhai, Z.Y. Development of the Mobile Phone Addiction Tendency Scale for College Students. *Chin. Ment. Health J.* **2012**, *26*, 222–225.
18. Lopez-Fernandez, O.; Honrubia-Serrano, L.; Freixa-Blanxart, M.; Gibson, W. Prevalence of problematic mobile phone use in British adolescents. *Cyberpsychol. Behav. Soc. Netw.* **2014**, *17*, 91–98. [CrossRef] [PubMed]
19. Jiang, Z.; Zhao, X. Self-control and problematic mobile phone use in Chinese college students: The mediating role of mobile phone use patterns. *BMC Psychiatry* **2016**, *16*, 416. [CrossRef] [PubMed]
20. Lee, Y.-K.; Chang, C.-T.; Lin, Y.; Cheng, Z.-H. The dark side of smartphone usage: Psychological traits, compulsive behavior and technostress. *Comput. Hum. Behav.* **2014**, *31*, 373–383. [CrossRef]
21. Toda, M.; Ezoe, S. Multifactorial study of mobile phone dependence in medical students: Relationship to health-related lifestyle, Type A behavior, and depressive state. *Open J. Prev. Med.* **2013**, *3*, 99–103. [CrossRef]
22. Liu, H.; Yu, H.-L. The Relationship among University Students' Mobile Phone Addiction and Mobile Phone Motive, Loneliness. *J. Psychol. Sci.* **2011**, *34*, 1453–1457.
23. Roberts, J.A.; Pullig, C.; Manolis, C. I need my smartphone: A hierarchical model of personality and cell-phone addiction. *Personal. Individ. Differ.* **2015**, *79*, 13–19. [CrossRef]

24. Pourrazavi, S.; Allahverdipour, H.; Jafarabadi, M.A.; Matlabi, H. A socio-cognitive inquiry of excessive mobile phone use. *Asian J. Psychiatry* **2014**, *10*, 84–89. [CrossRef] [PubMed]
25. Crosswhite, J.M.; Rice, D.; Asay, S.M. Texting among United States young adults: An exploratory study on texting and its use within families. *Soc. Sci. J.* **2014**, *51*, 70–78. [CrossRef]
26. Dong, G.S.; Park, Y.; Min, K.K.; Park, J. Mobile phone dependency and its impacts on adolescents' social and academic behaviors. *Comput. Hum. Behav.* **2016**, *63*, 282–292.

10

Self-Exclusion among Online Poker Gamblers: Effects on Expenditure in Time and Money as Compared to Matched Controls

Amandine Luquiens [1,2,3,4,*], Aline Dugravot [3], Henri Panjo [3], Amine Benyamina [1], Stéphane Gaïffas [2,5] and Emmanuel Bacry [2,6]

1 Hôpital Paul Brousse, APHP Villejuif, France. Université Paris-Saclay, 94800 Villejuif, France; amine.benyamina@aphp.fr
2 CMAP, Ecole Polytechnique, 91128 Palaiseau Cedex, France; stephane.gaiffas@polytechnique.edu (S.G.); emmanuel.bacry@polytechnique.edu (E.B.)
3 Université Paris-Sud membre de Université Paris-Saclay, UVSQ, CESP, INSERM, 94800 Villejuif, France; aline.dugravot@inserm.fr (A.D.); henri.panjo@inserm.fr (H.P.)
4 Addictions Department, Nîmes University Hospital, 30000 Nîmes, France
5 LPSM UMR 8001, Université Paris Diderot, 8001 Paris, France
6 CEREMADE UMR 7534 CNRS, Université Paris-Dauphine PSL, 75765 Paris Cedex 16, France
* Correspondence: amandineluquiens@gmail.com

Abstract: *Background:* No comparative data is available to report on the effect of online self-exclusion. The aim of this study was to assess the effect of self-exclusion in online poker gambling as compared to matched controls, after the end of the self-exclusion period. *Methods:* We included all gamblers who were first-time self-excluders over a 7-year period ($n = 4887$) on a poker website, and gamblers matched for gender, age and account duration ($n = 4451$). We report the effects over time of self-exclusion after it ended, on money (net losses) and time spent (session duration) using an analysis of variance procedure between mixed models with and without the interaction of time and self-exclusion. Analyzes were performed on the whole sample, on the sub-groups that were the most heavily involved in terms of time or money (higher quartiles) and among short-duration self-excluders (<3 months). *Results:* Significant effects of self-exclusion and short-duration self-exclusion were found for money and time spent over 12 months. Among the gamblers that were the most heavily involved financially, no significant effect on the amount spent was found. Among the gamblers who were the most heavily involved in terms of time, a significant effect was found on time spent. Short-duration self-exclusions showed no significant effect on the most heavily involved gamblers. *Conclusions:* Self-exclusion seems efficient in the long term. However, the effect on money spent of self-exclusions and of short-duration self-exclusions should be further explored among the most heavily involved gamblers.

Keywords: online gambling; self-exclusion; responsible gambling; comparative study; poker

---

1. Introduction

Harmful gambling behaviors are widespread and treatment-seeking is still very low among problem gamblers. Self-exclusion processes could be seen as an accessible tool for problem gamblers who are not ready to seek treatment. In France, gamblers can apply for online self-exclusion per website, for the length of their choice from one week to three years. During this period, they cannot access their gambling account on the website and receive no commercial offer from the gambling service provider. At the end of the period, they can gamble back on the website with no additional procedure. No help is provided nor any counselling during the self-exclusion period.

It has been consistently demonstrated that most self-excluders were indeed heavy gamblers and probably problem gamblers [1,2]. A recent meta-analysis describing gamblers who self-excluded highlighted that this tool, perceived as one of the main "responsible gambling" tools, is still considerably under-used [3]. Main barriers for self-exclusion has been described: complicated enrollment processes, lack of complete exclusion from all venues, little support from venue staff, and lack of adequate information on self-exclusion programs. The proportion of self-excluders could be particularly low among problem internet gamblers [4]. Regulators have reached the conclusion that this tool should be promoted to increase its use. Promoting the use of a potentially therapeutic tool needs to rely on robust efficacy data and not only on empirical data or mere common sense. A recent systematic review of the literature demonstrated that the impact of responsible gambling tools is still poorly supported by scientific evidence [5]. In particular, efficacy data for the effect of self-exclusion on gambling behaviors remains scarce [5]: several studies have shown reduced gambling after a self-exclusion period on both online and offline environments, with variable durations of follow-up, sometimes including the self-exclusion period itself [1,6,7]. Follow-up after online self-exclusion has been reported in only two studies [7,8]. The first one included a limited sample of 20 gamblers, with no control group, and assessed psychosocial outcomes [8]. The other one reported that the majority of online self-excluders returned to gambling after the self-exclusion period expired (n = 1996) [7], and that most of them self-excluded a second time, after another period of more intensive gambling than the first [1]. Only one study has reported follow-up data from matched controls with a comparative research design (n = 86) [5]. One study reported that gambling outcomes did not differ between self-exclusion alone vs self-exclusion combined with counseling or counseling only [9]. No study has reported efficacy data on spontaneous voluntary self-exclusion as compared to no intervention (i.e., no self-exclusion). One experimental study randomized volunteering problem gamblers (but not pathological gamblers, who were excluded) to either a very short 7-day period of self-exclusion or no self-exclusion [10]. The authors reported no significant between-group differences in terms of changes regarding money and time spent gambling at two months.

Skills are important in poker gambling and poker gamblers have been demonstrated to have particular thoughts about their own gambling behavior and to be particularly sensitive to feedbacks on their own practice [11]. Illusion of control could be high in poker gamblers [12] and perception of their own skills could be amplified [13]. The prevalence of problem gambling among online poker gamblers is particularly high, consistently reported between 15% and 20% of active gamblers [14,15]. Several factors predicting excessive gambling in poker gamblers were identified: stress, internal attribution, dissociation, boredom, negative emotions, irrational beliefs, anxiety, and impulsivity [16], lower performance in the emotional intelligence competences (Emotional Quotient inventory Short) and, in particular, those grouped in the Intrapersonal scale (emotional self-awareness, assertiveness, self-regard, independence and self-actualization). Classical financial moderators' relevance have been consistently discussed in poker gambling as financial involvement of problem gamblers can be very low and time involved is critical to take into account [14]. No time moderator is mandatory for online gamblers in France [17]. Self-exclusion could then be one of the most relevant tools currently available for poker online gamblers in France. Poker gamblers are then a particularly interesting population to study to assess the efficacy of self-exclusion.

The aim of the present study was to document the long-term effects of self-exclusion from a poker website as compared to no self-exclusion, using matched controls. Our hypothesis was that self-exclusion would have an effect on time and money spent after the exclusion ended compared to no self-exclusion.

2. Methods

2.1. Population

We included all gamblers who self-excluded for the first time over a 7-year period from June 2010 up to October 2016 (n = 4887) on a poker website, Winamax ®, and1:1 matched gamblers who had never self-excluded up to the time of data collection, matched for gender, age and account duration automatically extracted from the account database following a structured query language (SQL) request. For technical reasons we could not match gamblers for the level of gambling involvement in terms of money/time, which were constructed variables not available from the SQL database. From the matched control group, we removed doubloons where one and the same gambler was matched to several self-excluders (n= 436). In France, self-exclusion is a voluntary process; its duration is fixed by the player from 1 day up to a maximum of 3 years. At the end of the self-exclusion period, the gamblers are notified by email by the provider, and they are then allowed to gamble again on the platform without any additional procedure. At no point during the self-exclusion process is guidance or any kind of help offered. Self-exclusion prevents the gambler from any kind of gambling activity on the website during the chosen period of time.

2.2. Measures

We collected data retrospectively from different prospective databases systematically recorded by the gambling service provider: (a) Gambler data: self-excluders' basic demographics (gender, age, date of opening of the account), characteristics of self-exclusions (date, duration) and detailed gambling variables in the month prior to self-exclusion: cash game winnings, prize amounts for tournaments, buy-in-plus-rake for tournaments, session characteristics (starting date, end date, duration). Sessions were defined as gambling with no period under 10 min without action. This measure was based on our clinical experience and on the information provided by the provider of no systematic disconnection when leaving from the website or the application on wireless devices especially. This measure was built on the experience of difficulty in extracting and interpretation of sessions duration when taking into account connection time only in a previous study [14]. We chose to explore 4-week periods because most employed people in France receive their income once a month. It is therefore important to capture at least 4 weeks per period to avoid any artificially enhanced gambling activity resulting from a possible effect following receipt of income.

Money and time spent in the preceding 4 weeks were the 2 outcomes of interest and were defined as follows: (a): time spent was obtained by summing all session durations in the last 4 weeks. Session duration was obtained by subtracting session end date from session starting date. Money spent in the last 4 weeks was defined as the net losses in the previous 4 weeks, obtained from all cash game and tournament gambling data at table level for players using real money. Table net loss was obtained from the reverse of winnings. Winnings were computed from table data (cash game winnings + prize amount for tournaments-buy-in-plus-rake for tournaments). Account-duration was defined as the time between opening the account on the website and the self-exclusion date, or the self-exclusion date of the matched self-excluders for matched gamblers. Money and time spent in the last 4 weeks on poker on the website were calculated at the self-exclusion date (or self-exclusion date of the matched self-excluders for matched gamblers), and at 3, 4, 6 and 12 months after the end of the self-exclusion period (or after self-exclusion date of the matched self-excluders for matched gamblers). We intentionally took the 12 months period after the end of the self-exclusion period into account to explore any possible changes in patterns over time when gambling was again accessible on the website, the self-exclusion period itself being of no interest for the variables studied, since gamblers were prevented from gambling. There was no missing data.

2.3. Sub-Groups

As we could not match our sample for gambling involvement, we chose to additionally analyze subgroups with similar levels of involvement in terms of money and time. Sub-groups of the gamblers who were the most heavily involved were defined as follows: gamblers from the highest quartile for amounts of money/time spent in the last 4 weeks, respectively >170 €/23 hours. In this sub-group analysis, the matching ratio of 1:1 could not be maintained, and gamblers could no longer be matched on age, sex and account duration. However, the mean age and the proportion of males remained very close across groups: 32.13 years (sd = 9.68) and 86% male among the self-excluders who were the most heavily involved in terms of money (n = 2265) vs 33.08 years (sd = 10.15) and 86% male among the gamblers who were the most heavily involved in money in the matched group (n = 79) and 32.05 years (sd= 9.74) and 87% male among the self-excluders who were the most heavily involved in terms of time (n = 2150) vs 32.73 years (sd = 9.72) and 86% male among the gamblers in the matched group who were the most heavily involved in terms of time (n = 185).

Short-duration self-exclusion was defined as <90 days (n = 1460). In this group, money and time spent in the last 4 weeks were collected at 4, 6 and 12 months after the start of self-exclusion.

2.4. Statistical Analysis

The money and time spent over 12 months after the end of the self-exclusion period were analyzed using a mixed model with the subjects as a random effect. The fixed effects were self-exclusion, time as a categorical variable, and their interaction. This interaction of self-exclusion and time provides a test for the null hypothesis that "the reduction in money/time spent over the 12 months after the end of the self-exclusion would not be different between the two groups": we report here only the p-value of the ANalysis Of Variance (ANOVA) between the mixed models with and without the interaction (i.e., the "null" model), which is in accordance with our hypothesis, testing for an effect of self-exclusion on time/ money spent at any time point over the 12 months. A significant interaction effect means that there are significant differences between groups and over time. In other words, the change in scores over time is different depending on group membership. Analyzes were performed on the whole sample, on the sub-groups with the greatest time or money involvement and on short-duration self-excluders. As sample sizes were smaller in the subgroups of gamblers who were the most heavily involved and led to a lack of power, we completed our analysis with the calculation of effect sizes for self-exclusion at 12 months in these subgroups. We use the Morris d_2 which is a standardized measure of effect size suitable for groups with unequal sample sizes within a pre-post-control design [18]. Additionally, we calculated the effect size for short self-exclusions (< 90 days) at month 12 after self-exclusion among the gamblers who were the most heavily involved (respectively in terms of money / time, self-excluders and matched: n = 683 and 18/n = 665 and 35).The strength of the effect sizes was determined using descriptors of magnitudes of d = 0.01 to 2.0, as initially suggested by Cohen and expanded by Sawilowsky [19].

All tests were 2-sided and performed with R software V3.5.1. (R core Team, free collaborative software).

2.5. Ethics

Gamblers were informed of, and consented to, personal and gambling data collection and analysis in the general conditions of use when opening an account on the website. Data collection and analysis by Winamax were authorized by the "Comité National Informatique et Libertés" (CNIL) and registered with CNIL declaration n° 1430126, which allows the analysis of the routinely recorded data for public health purposes.

The study respected the STrengthening the Reporting of OBservational studies in Epidemiology (STROBE) statement checklist items [20].

3. Results

3.1. Matched Gamblers

The matched gamblers were aged 31.5 (*sd* = 9.5) on average and predominantly male (87%). Money/time spent by the matched gamblers in the preceding 4 weeks amounted to 12.9€ (*sd* = 145.5)/ 3.5h (*sd* = 12.9) on average before the self-exclusion day of their matched self-excluders, and 4.2€ (*sd* = 72.5)/ 1.3h (*sd* = 7.2) at12 months after the end of the self-exclusion period of their matched self-excluders. Account age was 322.33 days on average (*sd* = 445.83).

3.2. Self-Excluders

The characteristics of the first-time self-excluders and short-duration first-time self-excluders are presented in Table 1. The self-excluders were aged 31 on average and predominantly male. The short-duration first-time self-excluders amounted to 30% of all first-time self-excluders over the 7 years. Money/time spent by self-excluders in the last 4 weeks was 398.5€ (*sd* = 1221.4)/ 32.8h (*sd* = 40.1) before self-exclusion, and 32.3€ (*sd*= 386.6)/6.3h (*sd* = 20.0) at12 months after the end of the self-exclusion period. The mean length of self-exclusion was 614 days (*sd* = 499). Short-duration first-time self-excluders were younger and had a greater financial and time involvement in gambling; their account was one month older on average than in the overall sample.

Table 1. Characteristics of first-time self-excluders, and short-duration first-time self-excluders subgroup.

Characteristics	All 1st Self-Exclusions n = 4887	Short Self-Exclusions n = 1460
Account age (days), mean (sd)	272.4 (407.1)	307.59 (415.63)
Age (years), mean (sd)	31.4 (9.6)	30.48 (9.21)
Gender(male), n(%)	4252 (87.0)	1270 (87.99)
Money spent in the last 4 weeks before self-exclusion (€), mean (sd)	398.5 (1221.4)	445.96 (1350.21)
Time spent in the last 4 weeks before self-exclusion (minutes), mean (sd)	1969.8 (2406.0)	2791.3 (2706.4)
Self-exclusion period duration, days, mean (sd)	614.0(499.0)	32.0 (23.0)

3.3. Effects of Self-Exclusion over 12 Months after the End of the Self-Exclusion Period

A significant effect of self-exclusion was found for money and time spent over the 12 months after the end of the self-exclusion period (p-value for both models < 2.2e−16) using mixed models with a subject random effect (Figure 1).

3.4. Effect of Self-Exclusion over 12 Months after the End of the Self-Exclusion Period among the Most Heavily Involved Gamblers

The average amount of money spent in the four weeks before and after the self-exclusion period among the gamblers who were the most heavily involved in terms of money, among self-excluders (n = 2255) and in the matched group (n = 79) are shown in Figure 2. No significant effect of self-exclusions was found on the amounts of money spent (p = 0.072) and the effect size was very small (d = 0.18).

The average amount of time spent in the 4 weeks before and after the self-exclusion period among the gamblers who were the most heavily involved in terms of time among self-excluders (n = 2150) and in the matched group (n = 185) are shown in Figure 3. A significant effect of self-exclusion was found for time spent (p < 2.2e−16) and the effect size was small (d = 0.34).

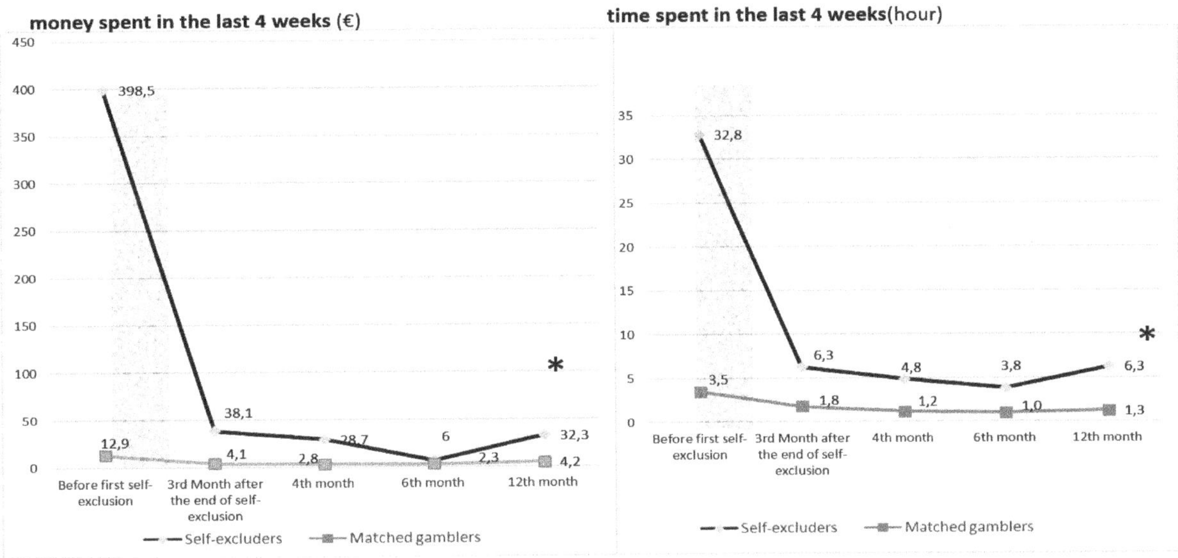

Figure 1. Evolution of money/time spent in the last 4 weeks (€/hours) at baseline and after the end of self-exclusion period (n = 4887 and n = 4451). (* = p-value < 0.05—ANOVA between the mixed model with and the null model without the interaction of self-exclusion X time).

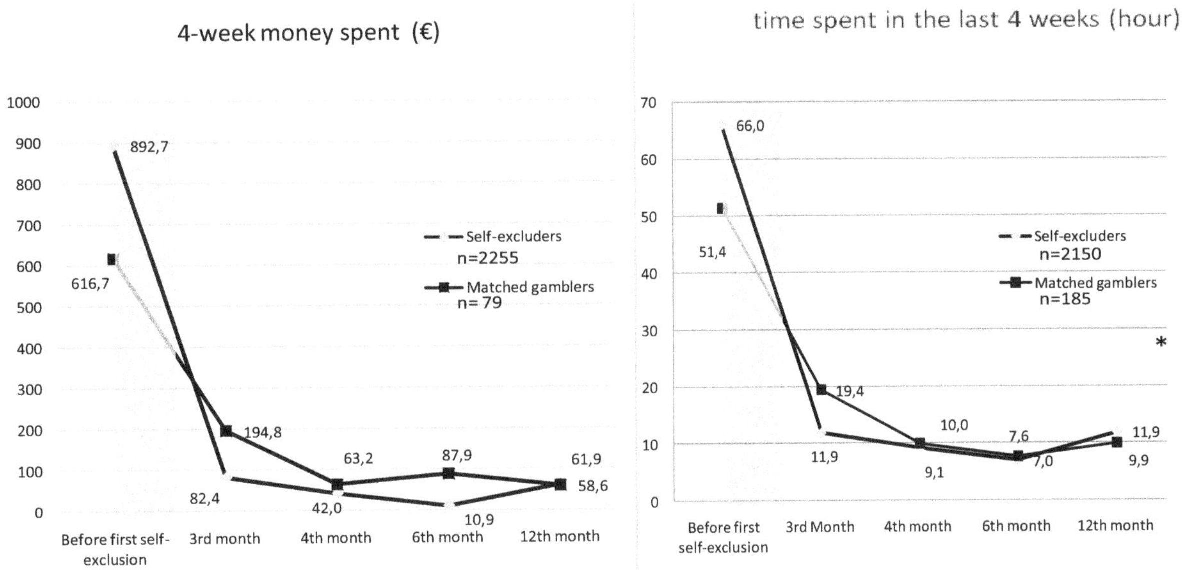

Figure 2. Evolution of money spent (net loss) in the last 4 weeks before and after the self-exclusion period among the gamblers who were the most heavily involved in terms of money (n = 2255 and 79 respectively for the self-excluders and the control group of matched gamblers) and time (n = 2150 and 185 respectively for the self-excluders and the control group of matched gamblers) (* = p-value < 0.05 —ANOVA between the mixed model with and the null model without the interaction of self-exclusion X time). (* = *p-value < 0.05* - ANOVA between the mixed model with and the null model without the interaction of self-exclusion X time).

3.5. Short Self-Exclusions

Significant effect of short self-exclusion was found for money and time spent over the 12 months after a short self-exclusion (p-value in both models <2.2e−16) using mixed models with a subject random effect (Figure 3).

No significant effect of short self-exclusions was found on money/ time spent gambling among the gamblers who were the most heavily involved in terms of money/time (respective p-values = 0.873

and 0.491) (Figure 4) but the sizes of the control groups were very small (respectively $n = 683$ vs 18, and $n = 665$ vs 35). The effect size was very small for money spent ($d = 0.17$), and negative and below the very small level for time spent ($d = -0.09$).

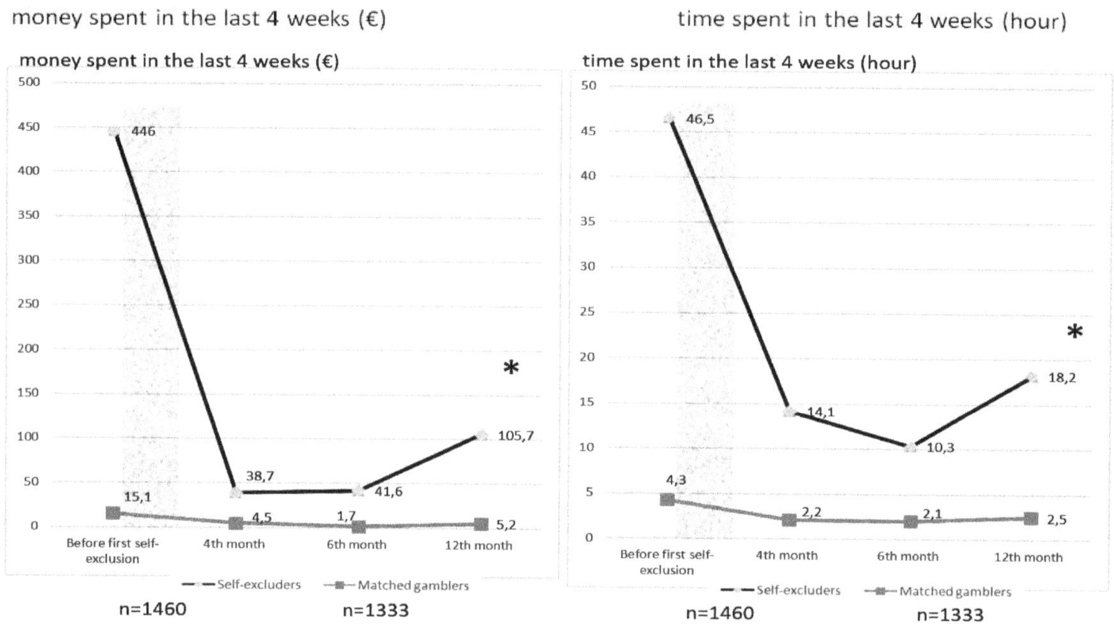

Figure 3. Evolution of money / time spent in the last 4 weeks (€/hours) before and after a short self-exclusion ($n = 1460$ and 1333). (* = p-value < 0.05—ANOVA between the mixed model with and the null model without the interaction of self-exclusion X time).

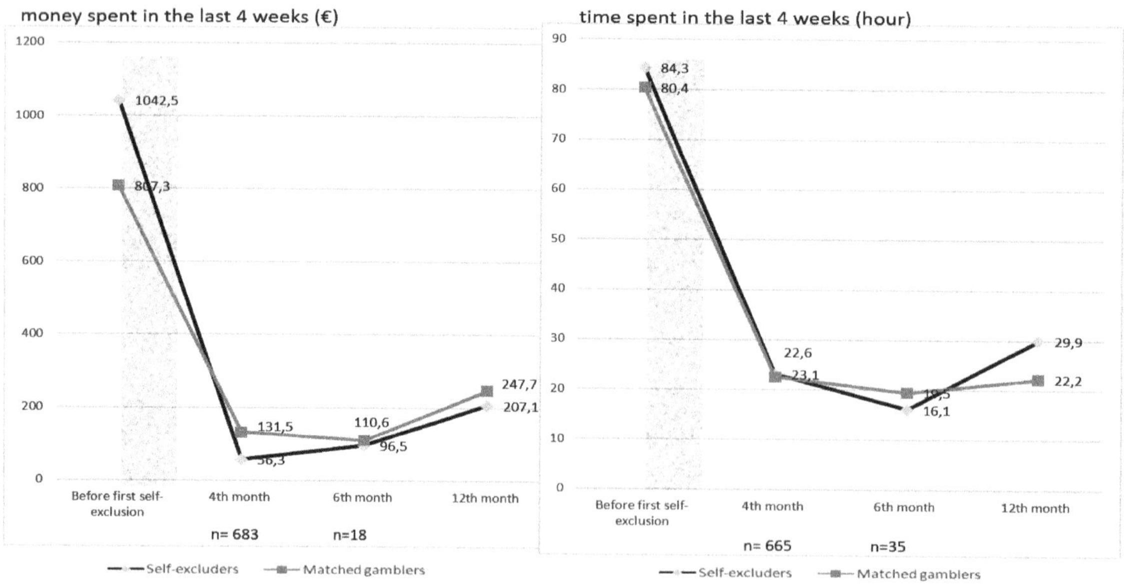

Figure 4. Evolution of money spent (net loss) in the last 4 weeks before and after a short self-exclusion among the gamblers who were the most heavily involved in terms of money ($n = 683$ and 18 respectively for the self-excluders and the control group of matched gamblers) and in terms of time ($n = 665$ and 35 respectively for the self-excluders and the control group of matched gamblers). (* = p-value < 0.05—ANOVA between the mixed model with and the null model without the interaction of self-exclusion X time).

4. Discussion

This is the first real life study, reporting comparative follow-up data on voluntary self-exclusion on the initiative of gamblers and including non-self-selected gamblers. This retrospective study analyzed prospectively registered account -based gambling data. The aim was to assess the efficacy of self-exclusion in the long term in term of time and money involvement.

The analysis of account-based gambling data for all first-time self-excluders on a website over 7 years confirmed the efficacy of self-exclusion on gambling outcomes in the long term. The exhaustiveness of this data is a strength that ensures representativeness and power for the statistical analyzes. However, the effect of self-exclusion among the most heavily involved gamblers was found only for the time spent, and not for the money spent, despite a very high level of expenditure before self-exclusion in this subgroup [14]. One important piece of information here is the spontaneous decrease in gambling involvement among gamblers who were the most heavily involved and who did not self-exclude. This result is congruent with a high rate of spontaneous remissions observed in gambling disorder [21]. This result shows the need to provide comparative data, more informative than a tool that is de facto considered to be efficient and promoted by the regulatory authorities [17]. Another interpretation of this decrease among heavy gamblers who did not self-exclude is that the gamblers were not randomized here, and could have chosen to self-exclude if they lacked confidence in their ability to bring about a change in their gambling without an external constraint such as self-exclusion, the reverse being true for non-self-excluders. The efficacy of short self-exclusions among the most heavily involved gamblers was not supported by our data. This is in line with recent experimental data among problem gamblers suggesting no efficacy of very short self-exclusions on gambling outcomes [10]. Another qualitative study reported a preferred duration to ensure efficacy of 12 months from the perspective of problem gamblers who self-excluded [22].

This study presents some important limitations. First, we included only poker gamblers. As discussed in the introduction, poker gamblers present particular cognitive profiles. Moreover, online poker gamblers are younger than other gamblers [4,12], and their history of gambling and associated damages could differ, as well as their motivation to change. The presented results could reflect some of these particularities and not be true in other gambling activities. No data was available on gambling on other online or offline gambling service providers. Gamblers could have just switched from one website to another during the exclusion period. However, all follow-up data reported here concerns gambling after the end of the exclusion period. Gamblers can gamble back on the website after this period and are commercially encouraged and sometimes offered incentives to do so. Moreover, we have already documented in another study that most gamblers return to the initial website to gamble after a self-exclusion [1]. On the other hand, as gambling is regulated in France, gamblers have to provide their Identity Card when opening an account; this measure theoretically prevents from gambling from an account opened under a false identity. The gambling profiles observed are still informative as such, even if not representative of all gambling activities. The use of account-based gambling data is a strength of the study because it enables objective data to be reported. However, it would be interesting to document the effect of self-exclusion on non-gambling outcomes, such as quality of life. No formal diagnosis of gambling disorder and no information on mental disorders or comorbidities were available. We could not, for technical reasons, match the gamblers for the level of gambling involvement in terms of time and money. Our statistical analysis allows for comparisons between the groups by adjusting the mixed model on the subject, which takes into account all subject characteristics including gambling involvement; however, it does not replace a control group with similar involvement in gambling in term of time and money spent. In addition, self-excluders could be different from non-self-excluders in term of the degree of motivation to change, as self-exclusion is a voluntary process in France. Finally, the naturalistic and ecological design of this study of course prevented any randomization process. We therefore report here results on the effect of self-exclusion rather than on efficacy. Further studies could inform on possible response factors to self-exclusion. No information was available on the health care resources used by the gamblers included.

5. Conclusions

Self-exclusion seems efficient in the long term (i.e., 12 months after the end of the self-exclusion period). However, the effects on money spent as a result of self-exclusion or short self-exclusion should be further explored among the online poker gamblers who are the most heavily involved. A spontaneous, clinically-relevant decrease in gambling activities was demonstrated among most involved gamblers who did not self-exclude. Further study with a randomized design and non-gambling outcomes should be conducted to conclude robustly on the efficacy of short and long self-exclusions in problem gambling, and on response factors.

Author Contributions: Conceptualization, A.L., A.D., H.P., S.G. and E.B.; Methodology, A.L., A.D., H.P., S.G. and E.B.; Software, A.L., A.D., H.P., S.G. and E.B.; Validation, A.L.; Formal Analysis, A.L.,A.D., H.P., S.G. and E.B.; Investigation, A.L.; Resources, A.L.; Data Curation, A.L.; Writing—Original Draft Preparation, A.L.; Writing—Review & Editing, A.L., A.B., A.D., H.P., S.G. and E.B.; Supervision, A.B., S.G. and E.B.; Project Administration, A.L.; Funding Acquisition, A.L.

Acknowledgments: We would like to thank Winamax for allowing access to data through an agreement allowing free analysis and interpretation by our academic team.

References

1. Luquiens, A.; Vendryes, D.; Aubin, H.J.; Benyamina, A.; Gaiffas, S.; Bacry, E. Description and assessment of trustability of motives for self-exclusion reported by online poker gamblers in a cohort using account-based gambling data. *BMJ Open* **2018**, *8*, 022541. [CrossRef] [PubMed]
2. Ladouceur, R.; Sylvain, C.; Gosselin, P. Self-exclusion program: A longitudinal evaluation study. *J. Gambl. Stud.* **2007**, *23*, 85–94. [CrossRef] [PubMed]
3. Motka, F.; Grune, B.; Sleczka, P.; Braun, B.; Ornberg, J.C.; Kraus, L. Who uses self-exclusion to regulate problem gambling? A systematic literature review. *J. Behav. Addict.* **2018**, *7*, 903–916. [CrossRef] [PubMed]
4. Hing, N.; Russell, A.M.; Gainsbury, S.M.; Blaszczynski, A. Characteristics and help-seeking behaviors of Internet gamblers based on most problematic mode of gambling. *J. Med. Internet Res.* **2015**, *17*, 13. [CrossRef] [PubMed]
5. Shaffer, P.; Blaszczynski, A.; Shaffer, H.J. Responsible gambling: A synthesis of the empirical evidence AU-Ladouceur, Robert. *Addict. Res. Theory* **2017**, *25*, 225–235. [CrossRef]
6. Kotter, R.; Kraplin, A.; Buhringer, G. Casino Self-and Forced Excluders' Gambling Behavior Before and After Exclusion. *J. Gambl. Stud.* **2018**, *34*, 597–615. [CrossRef] [PubMed]
7. Drawson, A.S.; Tanner, J.; Mushquash, C.J.; Mushquash, A.; Mazmanian, D. The Use of Protective Behavioural Strategies in Gambling: A Systematic Review. *Int. J. Ment. Health Addict.* **2017**, *15*, 1302–1319. [CrossRef]
8. Hayer, T.; Meyer, G. Internet Self-Exclusion: Characteristics of Self-Excluded Gamblers and Preliminary Evidence for Its Effectiveness. *Int. J. Ment. Health Addict.* **2010**, *9*, 296–307. [CrossRef]
9. Hing, N.; Russell, A.; Tolchard, B. Internet Self-Exclusion: Characteristics of Self-Excluded Gamblers and Preliminary Evidence for Its Effectiveness. *Int. J. Ment. Health Addict.* **2015**, *13*, 296–307. [CrossRef]
10. Caillon, J.; Grall-Bronnec, M.; Perrot, B.; Leboucher, J.; Donnio, Y.; Romo, L.; Challet-Bouju, G. Effectiveness of At-Risk Gamblers' Temporary Self-Exclusion from Internet Gambling Sites. *J. Gambl. Stud.* **2018**, *35*, 601–615. [CrossRef] [PubMed]
11. Gainsbury, S.M.; Abarbanel, B.L.L.; Philander, K.S.; Butler, J.V. Strategies to customize responsible gambling messages: A review and focus group study. *BMC Public Health* **2018**, *18*, 1381. [CrossRef] [PubMed]
12. Barrault, S.; Varescon, I. Cognitive distortions, anxiety, and depression among regular and pathological gambling online poker players. *Cyberpsychol. Behav. Soc. Netw.* **2013**, *16*, 183–188. [CrossRef] [PubMed]
13. MacKay, T.L.; Bard, N.; Bowling, M.; Hodgins, D.C. Do pokers players know how good they are? Accuracy of poker skill estimation in online and offline players. *Comput. Hum. Behav.* **2014**, *31*, 419–424. [CrossRef]
14. Luquiens, A.; Tanguy, M.L.; Benyamina, A.; Lagadec, M.; Aubin, H.J.; Reynaud, M. Tracking online poker problem gamblers with player account-based gambling data only. *Int. J. Methods Psychiatr. Res.* **2016**, *25*, 333–342. [CrossRef] [PubMed]

15. Halme, J. Overseas Internet poker and problem gambling in Finland 2007: A secondary data analysis of a Finnish population survey. *Nord. Stud. Alcohol Drugs* **2011**, *28*, 51–64. [CrossRef]
16. Moreau, A.; Chabrol, H.; Chauchard, E. Psychopathology of Online Poker Players: Review of Literature. *J. Behav. Addict.* **2016**, *5*, 155–168. [CrossRef] [PubMed]
17. *LOI n° 2010-476 du 12 Mai 2010 Relative à L'ouverture à la Concurrence et à la Régulation du Secteur des Jeux D'argent et de Hasard en Ligne-Article 26, 26. Sect. Chapitre Vii: La Lutte Contre Le Jeu Excessif Ou Pathologique*, France, 2010.
18. Morris, S.B. Estimating Effect Sizes From Pretest-Posttest-Control Group Designs. *Organ. Res. Methods* **2008**, *11*, 364–386. [CrossRef]
19. Sawilowsky, S. New effect size rules of thumb. *J. Mod. Appl. Stat. Methods* **2009**, *8*, 467–474. [CrossRef]
20. STROBE Statement. Available online: https://strobe-statement.org/index.php?id=strobe-home (accessed on 6 November 2019).
21. Froberg, F.; Rosendahl, I.K.; Abbott, M.; Romild, U.; Tengstrom, A.; Hallqvist, J. The Incidence of Problem Gambling in a Representative Cohort of Swedish Female and Male 16-24 Year-Olds by Socio-demographic Characteristics, in Comparison with 25-44 Year-Olds. *J. Gambl. Stud.* **2015**, *31*, 621–641. [CrossRef] [PubMed]
22. Ly, C. *Investigating the Use and Effectiveness of the Tasmanian Gambling (Self) Exclusion Programme*; Tasmanian Government: Hobart, Australia, 2010.

11

Comparison of Behavioral Changes and Brain Activity between Adolescents with Internet Gaming Disorder and Student Pro-Gamers

Ki Hyeon Kwak, Hyun Chan Hwang, Sun Mi Kim and Doug Hyun Han *

Department of Psychiatry, Chung Ang University Hospital, 102 Heuk seok ro, Dongjak gu, Seoul 06973, Korea; letter2kh@naver.com (K.H.K.); mossflower28@naver.com (H.C.H.); cryslake@naver.com (S.M.K.)
* Correspondence: hduk70@gmail.com

Abstract: While pro-gamers play according to defined living habits and planned schedules, adolescents with internet gaming disorder (IGD) exhibit irregular lifestyles and unregulated impulsive gaming behavior. Fourteen IGD adolescents and 12 pro-gaming students participated in this study. At baseline and after one year, demographic data, the Child Behavior Check List (CBCL), depressed mood, anxiety, and resting-state functional magnetic resonance imaging were assessed. Over the year, IGD adolescents played games as per their usual schedule, while pro-gamer students played according to their school's team schedule. After one year, the pro-gamers' scores had decreased in the CBCL-total (total problematic behaviors), CBCL-externalizing (under-controlled behavior, like impulsivity and aggression), and CBCL-internalizing (over-controlled behavior like depression and anxiety) compared to those of the IGD adolescents. Both groups displayed increased brain activity in the parietal lobe (a component of the attention network) over the years. Compared to pro-gamers, IGD adolescents showed higher brain activity within the left orbitofrontal cortex. Brain activity within the orbitofrontal cortex was associated with CBCL-externalizing scores. These results suggest that gaming had increased the attention network's brain activity, but a well-organized support system could lead to different results, in terms of improved behaviors and suppressing brain activity within the orbitofrontal cortex.

Keywords: internet gaming disorder; pro-gamers; Child Behavior Check List; resting-state functional magnetic resonance imaging

---

1. Introduction

1.1. Debates on Internet Gaming Disorder

Over the last two decades, many studies have suggested that excessive and problematic online gaming should be defined as a psychiatric disorder along with other addictive behaviors and functional impairments [1–3]. In a national survey of 1178 Americans aged between 8 and 18 years old, Gentile et al. [4] reported that patients with internet gaming disorder (IGD) performed poorly at school and suffered from attentional problems. Stockdale and Coyne [5] asserted that patients with IGD had poor mental health and cognitive functions, including poorer impulse control and attentional problems, compared to healthy controls. Hull et al. [6] reported that mature-rated, risk-glorifying gameplay was associated with substance use (including alcohol and cigarettes), aggression, delinquency, and risky sex. Since 2014, the World Health Organization (WHO) has regarded internet gaming addiction as a significant public health problem. In 2018, the International Classification of Diseases version 11 (ICD-11) defined gaming disorder as a medical disease with a pattern of repetitive or persistent gaming behavior [2,3].

Several studies have suggested that the psychobiological mechanisms underlying behavioral addiction resemble those of chemical addiction, such as that of alcohol and other drugs [7]. Moreover, it is believed that those with IGD share similar characteristics in neural activity and cognitive dysfunctions with those with a gambling disorder [8].

Based on previous correlational studies, the brain neurobiology of IGD can be summarized as increased activity within the orbitofrontal cortex and decreased activity within the dorsolateral prefrontal cortex [9,10]. Kim and Kang [9] found that IGD patients, compared to other gamers, showed a stronger functional connectivity (FC) within the orbitofrontal cortex, which is involved in motivational salience, and a decreased FC within the dorsolateral prefrontal cortex, which is involved in learning and attention. Additionally, Wang et al. [10] reported a decreased cortical thickness within the dorsolateral prefrontal cortex, related to cognitive control, decision making, and reward and loss processing. Motivational salience was thought to be associated with continuous and repetitive behaviors in various addictive diseases [11]. The dorsolateral prefrontal cortex was reported to control the orbitofrontal cortex [12]. In many addictive behaviors, the dorsolateral prefrontal cortex can fail to control the hyper-activated orbitofrontal cortex [12].

However, there is some debate about whether IGD or gaming disorder can be classified as a medical disease [1,13,14]. The American Psychiatric Association (APA) included IGD in Section III of the Diagnostic and Statistical Manual of mental disorders (DSM-5), as it requires further research and data accumulation, due to a lack of IGD cases, high prevalence of non-formal diagnostic criteria, and an unbalanced prevalence rate [1]. Several studies have also suggested that IGD might just be a social phenomenon induced by environmental and social stress [13,14]. Jeong et al. [13] suggested that adolescents excessively played internet games when they were under academic stress or lost self-control. The period of adolescence was known as a particularly at-risk developmental stage for problematic internet game playing [15,16], because individuals were prone to impulsivity and uncontrolled, unplanned internet game play [16,17]. Large, accumulating literature suggests that the prevalence of IGD is dominant in the male population [16]. The initial onset of IGD is not associated with gaming time or the game's genre [13]. Pang et al. [14] reported that gaming motivation in adolescents with IGD was associated with social anxiety and psychological stress.

Several studies expressed opposing opinions regarding the cognitive dysfunction induced by internet gameplay [18–20]. Latham et al. [18] asserted that video gaming could result in extensive improvements in various cognitive functions. Pallavicini et al. [20] suggested that video games could be used as a tool to improve the patient's wellbeing through cognitive and emotional training. Mentiplay et al. [19] also showed that video games could help improve symptoms of patients with developmental coordination disorders. Ballesteros et al. [21] suggested that the working memory and selective attention of older adults could be improved through video games.

1.2. Pro-Gamers vs. Patients with IGD

It's already known that IGD patients not only display excessive internet gameplay, but also have unplanned and irregular lifestyles, and impulsive, unregulated behavior in the absence of support systems [5,22,23]. Kim et al. [24] reported that most IGD patients were unable to control their impulses and displayed delinquent behavior. In a two-year follow up study, Baysak et al. [22] reported that social support systems could be a protective factor for IGD.

There is another population in South Korea that also displays excessive internet gameplay but does not meet the criteria of IGD, called professional gamers (pro-gamers). Pro-gamers belong to the internet game league and have contracts with teams that result in a salary and potential prizes. To perform well, pro-gamers practice for about 10 h a day within a defined schedule [25]. This schedule includes practicing, physical exercise, team strategy conferences, resting, and mealtimes.

For several years, A-hyun High School has recruited students who want to become professional gamers. Before going to A-hyun High School, all adolescents must complete the second grade at a general high school. In their schooling, they have a similar curriculum to third grade general high school students, such as Korean, English, mathematics, and sciences. In addition, they also play internet games for 4–5 h a day, following a schedule the game teacher suggests.

1.3. Resting-State Functional Magnetic Resonance Imaging (MRI) and Fractional Amplitude of Low-Frequency Fluctuation

Resting-state functional MRI (rs-fMRI) is thought to measure spontaneous brain activity, representing brain function [26]. Low-frequency (0.009–0.08 Hz) fluctuations (ALFF) of the blood oxygen level-dependent signal were thought to be related to spontaneous neural activity in rs-fMRI [27]. The fractional amplitude of low-frequency fluctuations (fALFF) is an advanced version of the original ALFF and helps to detect spontaneous brain activity more sensitively [28]. Changes in the fALFF have already been reported in several studies of psychiatric diseases, including schizophrenia [29], autism [30], and attention deficit hyperactivity disorders (ADHD) [31]. Moreover, Kim et al. [32] observed correlations between changes of fALFF within the inferior frontal gyrus and changes in delinquency and externalizing behaviors.

1.4. Hypothesis

We hypothesized that long term internet game play would increase the brain activity within the attentional system in both groups. However, the existence of a support system, including a regular schedule and a supervisor, would lead to different results in terms of behaviors and brain activity. Student pro-gamers with a good support system would show improved behavioral scores compared to IGD patients. In addition, a good support system would prevent the hyperactivity within the orbitofrontal cortex in student pro-gamers, while a poor support system would not prevent hyperactivity within the orbitofrontal cortex in response to impulsive internet game play.

2. Methods

2.1. Participants

The participants in the current study were classified into two groups; pro-gamer students and IGD adolescents. The two groups were both engaged in excessive internet game play. However, the pro-gaming students with a support system had characteristics of a regular lifestyle, while IGD adolescents, without a support system, showed an irregular lifestyle.

The institutional review board of the Chung-Ang University Hospital approved the research protocol for this study. All adolescents were informed about the study's procedures and signed a written informed consent form. Their parents also provided written informed consent. The diagnostic criteria of IGD were based on the DSM-5 [1].

From September 2016 to December 2017, 121 IGD adolescents visited the Department of Psychiatry at the OO University hospital for diagnosis and treatment. In contrast to the systematic caring group (student pro-gamer group), IGD patients who visited for an initial assessment but received no treatment (non-systematic caring group) were regarded as the compared group.

Of the 121 IGD adolescents, we found 27 adolescents who completed psychological and brain-imaging assessments at their first and second visits, but they had not received any treatment or interventions, such as cognitive behavior therapy or psychiatric medications, over the years. Although parents and caretakers had asked that the adolescents receive treatment for IGD, those adolescents refused treatment due to no interest in treatment, no insight of problematic behaviors, and laziness to come to the treatment center. On January 2018, we contacted 27 adolescents via phone to introduce our study, and 14 adolescents and their parents agreed to participate. The other 13 adolescents or their parents were not willing or able to participate in study.

In 2017, 55 adolescents who wanted to be professional gamers applied to A-hyun High School's Pro-Gamer Department. With a ranking from the internet game "League of Legend" competition and a basic academic ability test, 12 adolescents qualified and were accepted to be admitted to the school.

After listening to the purpose of our research, all pro-gaming students and their parents agreed to participate in our study.

The pro-gamer students had school schedules, including regular academic classes (4 h/day), physical sports class, strategy meetings, mealtimes, and game training time (3 h/day in school). Two teachers managed and checked the schedules, while the parents of the IGD adolescents observed the life patterns of the adolescents and reported it. At a baseline and after a year, both groups were asked to give their demographic data, including age, educational year, and internet gameplay time ("How many hours per day do you play internet game?") as well as a number of psychological scales, including the Young Internet Addiction Scale (YIAS), Child Behavior Checklist (CBCL), Child Depressive Inventory (CDI), Beck Anxiety Inventory (BAI), and Korean ADHD Rating Scale (K-ARS). Resting-state functional MRI (rs-fMRI) was also undertaken.

2.2. Clinical Scales

The CBCL is known as a screening tool for assessing problem behaviors in children and adolescents based on the parent's self-report [33,34]. The Korean version of the CBCL (K-CBCL) has standardized reliability and validity [33,34]. Parents assessed their children and adolescents, aged between 4 and 18, using the K-CBCL, in terms of social adaptation and problem behavior. It consisted of 117 questions, with three subscales including a total problem score, as well as externalizing and internalizing scores. Higher scores indicated a greater degree of behavioral and emotional problems [33,34]

The Young Internet Addiction Scale (YIAS), proposed by Young in 1998, is a self-reporting measure for routine internet use [35]. The YIAS consists of 20 self-assessment questions, each graded on a scale of 1 to 5 ("rarely" to "always"). YIAS scores above 50 are considered to reflect problematic internet use. The Korean version of YIAS was verified by Lee et al. The YIAS' internal consistency has been reported to be in the range of 0.90 to 0.91 [36].

The Children's Depression Inventory (CDI), developed in 1977 by Kovacs (1985), is a self-reported measure of depression in children and adolescents aged 7 to 17 years old [37]. The 27 items of the Korean version of CDI, with internal consistency of Cronbach's $\alpha = 0.88$, was verified by Cho and Lee [38].

The Beck Anxiety Inventory (BAI), with 21 questions, is used to measure anxiety severity [39]. The BAI is scored on a scale of 0 to 3 and has a maximum score of 63 points. The Korean version of the BAI, with an internal consistency of Cronbach's $\alpha = 0.93$, was verified by Kwon et al. [40].

The Korean ADHD Rating Scale (K-ARS) is an ADHD symptom severity scale composed of 18 items (9 items for inattentive evaluation and 9 items for hyperactivity evaluation) designed by Dupaul [41]. The Korean version of the ARS, with an internal consistency of 0.77 to 0.89, has been verified by So et al. [42].

2.3. Brain Image Acquisition and Processing

All MRIs were acquired using a 3.0 T Philips Achieva scanner. All participants laid down with their eyes closed and were asked to stay awake. The heads of the participants were stabilized with cushions and taped for severe head movement prevention. Resting-state (Rs-fMRI) images were acquired axially, with an echo-planar imaging sequence, using the following parameters: TR/TE = 3000/40 ms, 40 slices, 64×64 matrix, 90° flip angle, 230 mm field of view (FOV), and 3 mm section thickness without a gap. Each scan lasted 720 s, and 230 volumes were obtained. The first 10 volumes were removed for gradient field stabilization.

Data preprocessing and processing were carried out using the Data Processing Assistant for Rs-fMRI (DPARSFA-http://www.restfmri.net), which is a plug-in software that works with Statistical Parametric Mapping (SPM12; http://www.fil.ion.ucl.ac.uk/spm/software/spm12/) and the Rs-fMRI Data Analysis Toolkit (REST; http://resting-fmri.sourceforge.net). Images were corrected for slice acquisition time differences, realigned, normalized, spatially smoothed with a 6 mm full-width half maximum kernel, de-trended, and temporally band-pass filtered to 0.01–0.08 Hz. Based on the results from the realignment processing by SPM, subjects that had a translation or a rotating motion greater than 3 mm or 2°, respectively, in any direction, were excluded from the study. No subject was excluded because of excessive head motion.

To assess brain activity among the groups at baseline, fALFF was performed using the REST software before treatment was administered. During preprocessing, Fisher-transformed correlation coefficients were measured for each pair of the regions of interest (ROIs) in each participant. The fALFF between the ROIs was calculated using the CONN-fMRI FC toolbox (version 15; https://www.nitrc.org/projects/conn). The fALFF method was used to find the regions where the local connectivity was correlated to the clinical scores. As an indicator of fALFF value, Kendall's coefficient of concordance of a given voxel was calculated using the surrounding 26 voxels to evaluate the similarity of the time series. These were then standardized using Z-scores to perform group analyses.

2.4. Statistics

Demographic and psychological data between the pro-gamer group and the IGD adolescent group were analyzed using the Mann–Whitney U test. The changes in the psychological scales were assessed with the Kruskal–Wallis test. The differences in the psychological scales' changes were also evaluated with an analysis of variance (ANOVA).

At baseline, the fALFF between the student pro-gamers and the IGD adolescents was compared using an independent t-test with the SPM12 software package. We performed a paired t-test, using the SPM12 software, to investigate fALFF changes in both the student pro-gamers and the IGD adolescents. Additionally, the difference in fALFF changes between the student pro-gamers and IGD adolescents were measured with an ANOVA using the SPM12 software package. The correlation was calculated between the fALFF map and the CBCL using SPM12. The resulting maps were set to a threshold using a p-value of <0.05, and false discovery rate correction was made for multiple comparisons with an extent of more than 20 contiguous voxels.

3. Results

3.1. Comparison of Demographic and Psychological Data

There were no significant differences in age, intelligence quotient (IQ), internet gaming time, CDI, BAI, K-ARS, CBCL-T, and CBCL-E scores between the student pro-gamer and IGD adolescent groups. However, the IGD adolescents showed increased YIAS and CBCL-I scores compared to the student pro-gamer group (Table 1).

After a year, no difference was seen in the YIAS (F = 1.12, $p = 0.30$), internet game playing time (F = 0.62, $p = 0.44$), CDI (F = 3.50, $p = 0.07$), BAI (F = 0.02, $p = 0.89$), and K-ARS (F = 0.46, $p = 0.51$) scores between the two groups. However, the CBCL-total scores (F = 12.76, $p < 0.01$) and CBCL-externalizing (F = 19.81, $p < 0.01$) and CBCL-internalizing (F = 11.09, $p < 0.01$) scores decreased in the student pro-gamer group but did not change in the IGD adolescent group (Figure 1).

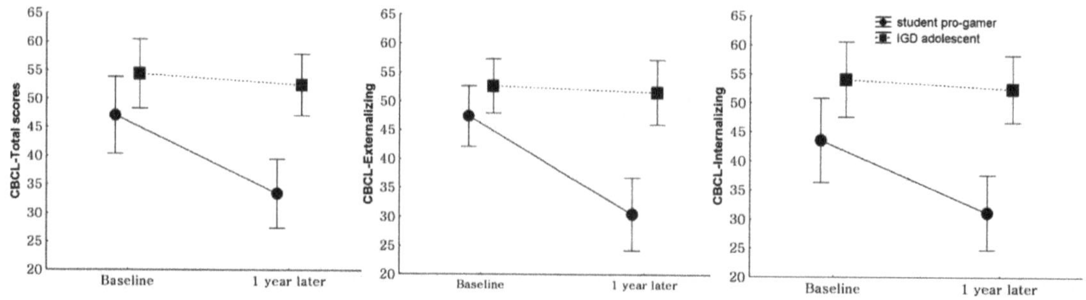

Figure 1. Comparison of the changes in the CBCL between student pro-gamer and IGD adolescent groups.

Table 1. Demographic and psychological data.

		Student Pro-Gamers	IGD Adolescents	Statistics
Age (years)		17.1 ± 0.3	16.5 ± 1.2	z = 1.07, p = 0.28
Education (years)		11.1 ± 0.3	9.7 ± 2.7	z = 1.63, p = 0.10
IQ		86.8 ± 6.3	90.4 ± 10.3	z = −1.29, p = 0.19
YIAS	B	56.3 ± 7.5	65.3 ± 7.5	z = −2.24, p = 0.02 *
	F	55.8 ± 13.0	61.4 ± 11.0	z = −1.46, p = 0.14
Game time (hours/day)	B	6.7 ± 1.4	7.0 ± 1.7	z = −0.24, p = 0.81
	F	7.2 ± 1.2	6.7 ± 2.0	z = 1.19, p = 0.23
CDI	B	7.8 ± 4.7	11.4 ± 5.6	z = −1.73, p = 0.08
	F	5.4 ± 3.9	12.2 ± 6.0	z = −3.10, p < 0.01 *
BAI	B	6.4 ± 2.9	7.9 ± 3.7	z = −1.07, p = 0.28
	F	6.2 ± 2.0	7.8 ± 3.3	z = −1.21, p = 0.81
K-ARS	B	12.5 ± 5.5	12.9 ± 5.8	z = −0.29, p = 0.22
	F	13.1 ± 3.8	12.7 ± 6.5	z = 0.22, p = 0.83
CBCL-T	B	47.1 ± 6.8	54.4 ± 13.9	z = −1.43, p = 0.15
	F	33.4 ± 8.9	52.5 ± 10.9	z = −3.53, p < 0.01 *
CBCL-E	B	47.4 ± 3.9	52.7 ± 11.3	z = −1.82, p = 0.07
	F	30.5 ± 7.8	51.6 ± 12.2	z = −3.81, p < 0.01 *
CBCL-I	B	43.6 ± 8.6	54.1 ± 14.4	z = −2.37, p = 0.02 *
	F	31.2 ± 7.6	52.4 ± 12.9	z = −3.93, p < 0.01 *

Notes: IGD adolescents: adolescents with internet gaming disorder (IGD), B: baseline, F: follow up; Young Internet Addiction Scale (YIAS), Child Behavior Checklist (CBCL), CBCL-T: total, CBCL-E: externalizing, CBCL-I: internalizing; Children's Depressive Inventory (CDI), Beck Anxiety Inventory (BAI), Korean ADHD Rating Scale (K-ARS). * Statistically significant.

The Children Behavior Check List (CBCL) total (F = 12.76, $p < 0.01$), CBCL-externalizing (F = 19.81, $p < 0.01$), and CBCL-internalizing (F = 11.09, $p < 0.01$) scores in student pro-gamers decreased while all CBCL scores in IGD adolescents were unchanged.

3.2. Comparison of the Changes in fALFF between Student Pro-Gamers and IGD Adolescents after a Year

At baseline, there were no regions with different brain activity at resting state between the IGD adolescents and the student pro-gamers.

After a year, both groups showed increased brain activity within the attention networks (parietal lobe). The details were as follows: The fALFF within the parietal lobe (x, y, z, 42, −66, 36, voxels = 26, T = 4.61, uncorrected $p < 0.001$) in the student pro-gamer group and the fALFF within the parietal lobe gyrus (x, y, z, 36, −24, 45, voxels = 25, T = 4.52, uncorrected $p < 0.001$) in the IGD adolescents increased.

Only in the IGD adolescents, orbitofrontal cortex activity increased after a year. The details are as follows: IGD adolescents showed an increased fALFF within the left orbitofrontal cortex, including the left subcallosal gyrus (x, y, z, −6, 12, −12, voxels = 121, T = 6.37, uncorrected $p < 0.001$), left orbital gyrus (x, y, z, −15, 33, −24, voxels = 121, T = 5.99, uncorrected $p < 0.001$), and left inferior frontal gyrus (x, y, z, −21, 27, −21, voxels = 121, T = 6.37, uncorrected $p < 0.001$), compared with those of the student pro-gamers (Figure 2).

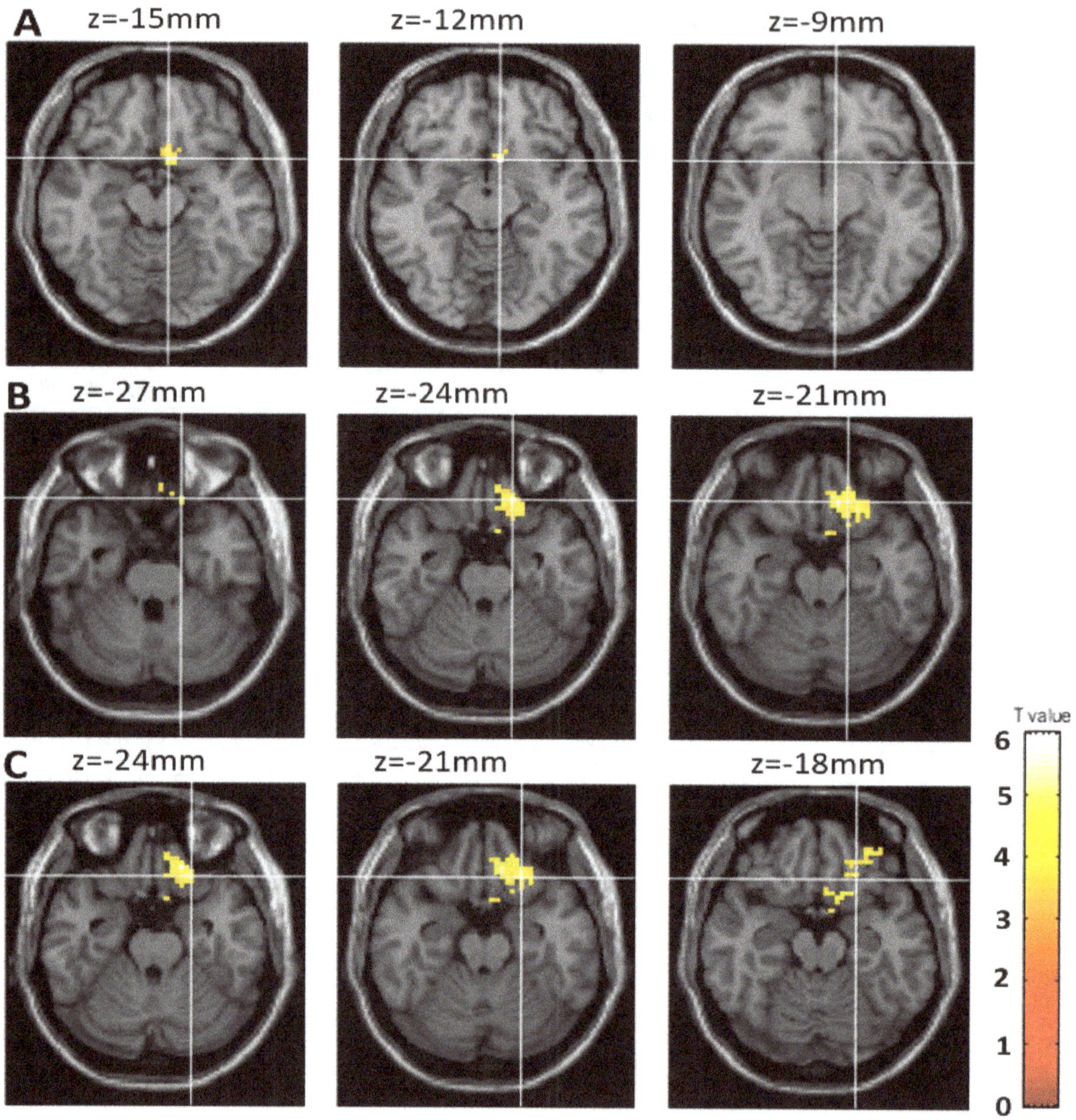

Figure 2. Regions showing differences in the changes of brain activity between the pro-gamer group and IGD adolescent group. (**A**) left subcallosal gyrus (x, y, z, −6, 12, −1), (**B**) left orbital gyrus (x, y, z, −15, 33, −24), (**C**) left inferior frontal gyrus (x, y, z, −21, 27, −21), yellow regions: the IGD adolescent group showed increased brain activity compared to the pro-gamers group.

3.3. Correlation between the fALFF and CBCL Scores in All Adolescents (Student Pro-Gamers and IGD Adolescents)

The fALFF values within the left inferior frontal gyrus were associated with the CBCL-externalizing scores in all adolescents ($r = 0.50$, $p < 0.01$). However, there were no significant correlations between the fALFF values within other areas and the CBCL-total or CBCL-internalizing scores.

4. Discussion

This study compared two groups under the same conditions of excessive internet gaming, one with a support system in place and one with no support system. Even though both groups played internet games for more than seven hours a day, it was assumed that the existence of a support system to keep a regular schedule would lead to different results in terms of behaviors and brain activity. The student pro-gamer group showed improved behavioral scores after a year compared to the baseline. However,

IGD adolescents showed no improvement in behavioral scores and the impulse control network showed dysfunctional brain activity.

4.1. Mproved Problematic Behavioral Scores in Student Pro-Gamers Compared to IGD Adolescents

At baseline, CBCL-internalizing scores in the IGD adolescents were higher than those observed in student pro-gamer group. In addition, the student pro-gamer group showed improved behavioral scores as assessed using the CBCL, compared to IGD adolescent. Moreover, the behavioral score improvements on the CBCL in student pro-gamers included both the CBCL-externalizing and internalizing scores. The CBCL was designed to measure the degree of behavioral and emotional problems in children [43]. The CBCL-externalizing score shows the degree of external problems, including social, thought, and attentional problems, while the CBCL-internalizing score shows the degree of internal problems, including anxiety, depression, and somatic complaints [43]. Additionally, the CBCL-total scores have been suggested as primary screening instruments for ADHD in Korean children [44]. The CBCL-internalizing scores were positively correlated with the Beck Depressive Inventory scores in patients with mood disorders [45]. Altogether, our CBCL results may suggest that the student pro-gamer group showed an improvement in their behavioral and emotional status. With the CBCL results at baseline and follow up, a different interpretation can be suggested. The pro-gamer group was preparing for a pro-gamer career, while the IGD adolescent group had no clear future direction. This situation may have led to the bias of the parental assessment in the CBCL.

Many studies have reported the effects of gaming on adolescent behaviors [46,47]. Greitmeyer et al. [46] suggested that video gaming would affect the social behaviors of gamers, especially when violent and pro-social video games are considered. Shao et al. [47] asserted a positive correlation between the use of violent video games and adolescent aggressiveness. However, our results may indicate that environmental factors and the existence of a support system affects the gamers' behaviors to a greater extent than the game play itself. In a large sample study of adolescents who play violent video games, Przybylski [48] reported that there was no significant correlation between violent video games and aggressive behavior in adolescents. In a survey conducted by the US National Research Council, environmental factors, including family resources and school quality, were seen as crucial factors in preventing mental, emotional, and behavioral disorders in young people [49].

4.2. Increased Brain Activity within the Attention Network (parietal lobe) in Response to One-Year Internet Gameplay in Both Groups

After playing internet games over a year, brain activities within the parietal lobe in both groups increased. The parietal lobe is known as a part of the attention network in the human brain [50]. In previous IGD studies, gaming was seen to affect brain activity within the attention network [25,51,52]. Action video gamers made faster and more precise responses toward targets, using enhanced attention skills [52]. Compared to non-gamers, the frontoparietal network in gamers was used to a greater extent in responding to attention-demanding tasks [51]. Interestingly, repetitive and impulsive internet gaming was thought to be a self-medication for children with ADHD [53,54]. Evren et al. [53] have reported that ADHD was associated with the severity of internet addiction and IGD among university students. Eight weeks of methylphenidate treatment in ADHD children with internet addiction improves ADHD symptoms as well as the severity of internet addiction [55]. Conclusively, increased brain activity within the parietal lobe in both student pro-gamers and the IGD group was associated with internet gaming.

4.3. Increased Brain Activity within the Orbitofrontal Cortex of the IGD Adolescents in Response to a Year of Internet Gaming

Increased brain activity, represented by the fALFF value, within the orbitofrontal cortex was only observed in IGD adolescents in this study. The imbalance between the dorsolateral prefrontal cortex and the orbitofrontal cortex, due to a hyper-activated orbitofrontal cortex, was thought to be related to cognitive control and decision-making dysfunctions, as well as impulsive behaviors in patients with gambling disorders [55]. In the seed base FC analysis, Kim et al. [24] reported the imbalance of FC from the orbitofrontal cortex to the dorsolateral prefrontal cortex in IGD patients. In internet addiction, functional dis-connectivity between the orbitofrontal cortex, dorsolateral prefrontal cortex, and anterior cingulate, due to hyper-activated orbitofrontal cortex, are associated with impulsive and delinquent behaviors [56].

4.4. Association between fALFF Values within the Orbitofrontal and the CBCL-Externalizing Scores

The association between impulsivity, drug seeking behaviors, and dysregulation of the orbitofrontal cortex has been continuously reported in substance use disorder [57,58]. The hyper-activated orbitofrontal cortex might aid to balance the FCs between the dorsolateral prefrontal cortex and the orbitofrontal cortex [11,12].

CBCL-externalizing scores were thought to be associated with impulsive behaviors in children and adolescents [44]. Eisenberg et al. [59] described that problem behaviors in children were related to negative feelings or impulsivity. In other words, difficulty in controlling one's behavior is related to impulsiveness [60].

As the student pro-gamers had a support system in place, this may have helped to promote planning and regular lifestyles. Planning and impulsivity in human behavior have been seen to be closely associated with the functioning of the dorsolateral prefrontal cortex [61,62]. Conclusively, a well-controlled support system that includes planning and a regular life pattern may improve the balance of brain activity between the dorsolateral prefrontal cortex and the orbitofrontal cortex in student pro-gamers.

4.5. Limitations

There were several limitations to our study. First, the number of participants was too small to generalize our results. Because of the small numbers, the brain analysis results have been presented in an uncorrected format. Second, there were few assessment tools used to assess potential environmental factors in our study. Future studies should include a larger number of participants and evaluate the environmental conditions. Third, the assessment tool for excessive internet gaming might be used through objective criteria. Some adolescents may feel that an amount of game playing, that other adolescents feel is not "excessive," can be distressing for them. A subjective perception of "excessive" or "distressing" should be assessed in future studies. Finally, we did not consider different motivations, self-efficacy, and self-worth at the starting point between the pro-gamer students and IGD adolescents. These factors could lead a bias of the results in mental health and brain activity.

5. Conclusions

In response to long term internet game play, increased brain activity within the attention system was found in both groups. However, a well-organized support system, including a regular schedule and a supervisor, would lead to different results in terms of improved behavior scores and suppressing the brain activity within the orbitofrontal cortex.

Author Contributions: Conceptualization, K.H.K., and D.H.H.; methodology, D.H.H.; formal analysis, S.M.K.; investigation, H.C.H.; Writing—Original draft preparation, K.H.K., D.H.H.; Writing—Review and editing, D.H.H.; supervision, D.H.H. All authors have read and agreed to the published version of the manuscript.

Acknowledgments: Thanks A-hyun high school for helping research.

References

1. American Psychiatry Association. *Diagnostic and Statistical Manual of Mental Disorders (DSM-5)*; American Psychiatric Publishing: Arlington, VA, USA, 2013.
2. World Health Organization. *Public Health Implications of Excessive Use of the Internet, Computers, Smartphones and Similar Electronic Devices Meeting Report*; World Health Organization: Tokyo, Japan, 2014.
3. World Health Organization. *The ICD-11 Classification of Mental and Behavioral Disorders: Diagnostic Criteria for Research*; World Health Organization: Geneva, Switzerland, 2018.
4. Gentile, D. Pathological video-game use among youth ages 8 to 18: A national study. *Psychol. Sci.* **2009**, *20*, 594–602. [CrossRef] [PubMed]
5. Stockdale, L.; Coyne, S.M. Video game addiction in emerging adulthood: Cross-sectional evidence of pathology in video game addicts as compared to matched healthy controls. *J. Affect. Disord.* **2018**, *225*, 265–272. [CrossRef] [PubMed]
6. Hull, J.G.; Brunelle, T.J.; Prescott, A.T.; Sargent, J.D. A longitudinal study of risk-glorifying video games and behavioral deviance. *J. Pers. Soc. Psychol.* **2014**, *107*, 300–325. [CrossRef] [PubMed]
7. Weinstein, A.; Lejoyeux, M. New developments on the neurobiological and pharmaco-genetic mechanisms underlying internet and videogame addiction. *Am. J. Addict.* **2015**, *24*, 117–125. [CrossRef] [PubMed]
8. Vaccaro, A.G.; Potenza, M.N. Diagnostic and classification considerations regarding gaming disorder: Neurocognitive and neurobiological features. *Front. Psychiatry* **2019**, *10*, 405. [CrossRef] [PubMed]
9. Kim, J.; Kang, E. Internet game overuse is associated with an alteration of fronto-striatal functional connectivity during reward feedback processing. *Front. Psychiatry* **2018**, *9*, 371. [CrossRef] [PubMed]
10. Wang, Z.; Wu, L.; Yuan, K.; Hu, Y.; Zheng, H.; Du, X.; Dong, G. Cortical thickness and volume abnormalities in internet gaming disorder: Evidence from comparison of recreational internet game users. *Eur. J. Neurosci.* **2018**, *48*, 1654–1666. [CrossRef]
11. Zilverstand, A.; Huang, A.S.; Alia-Klein, N.; Goldstein, R.Z. Neuroimaging Impaired Response Inhibition and Salience Attribution in Human Drug Addiction: A Systematic Review. *Neuron* **2018**, *98*, 886–903. [CrossRef]
12. Koob, G.F.; Volkow, N.D. Neurobiology of addiction: A neurocircuitry analysis. *Lancet Psychiatry* **2016**, *3*, 760–773. [CrossRef]
13. Jeong, E.J.; Ferguson, C.J.; Lee, S.J. Pathological gaming in young adolescents: A longitudinal study focused on academic stress and self-control in South Korea. *J. Youth Adolesc.* **2019**, *48*, 2333–2342. [CrossRef]
14. Pang, S.; Abdin, E.; Chong, S.A.; Chua, B.Y.; Lee, S.P.; Picco, L.; Satghare, P.; Vaingankar, L.; Verma, S.; Subramaniam, M. Correlates of online game play motivations, social anxiety and psychological distress. *Ann. Acad. Med. Singap.* **2017**, *46*, 443–446. [PubMed]
15. Cerniglia, L.; Griffiths, M.D.; Cimino, S.; De Palo, V.; Monacis, L.; Sinatra, M.; Tambelli, R. A latent profile approach for the study of internet gaming disorder, social media addiction, and psychopathology in a normative sample of adolescents. *Psychol. Res. Behav. Manag.* **2019**, *12*, 651–659. [CrossRef] [PubMed]
16. Cerniglia, L.; Zoratto, F.; Cimino, S.; Laviola, G.; Ammaniti, M.; Adriani, W. Internet Addiction in adolescence: Neurobiological, psychosocial and clinical issues. *Neurosci. Biobehav. Rev.* **2017**, *76*, 174–184. [CrossRef] [PubMed]
17. Cerniglia, L.; Guicciardi, M.; Sinatra, M.; Monacis, L.; Simonelli, A.; Cimino, S. The Use of Digital Technologies, Impulsivity and Psychopathological Symptoms in Adolescence. *Behav. Sci.* **2019**, *9*, 82. [CrossRef]
18. Latham, A.J.; Patston, L.L.; Tippett, L.J. The virtual brain: 30 years of video-game play and cognitive abilities. *Front. Psychol.* **2013**, *4*, 629. [CrossRef]
19. Mentiplay, B.F.; FitzGerald, T.L.; Clark, R.A.; Bower, K.J.; Denehy, L.; Spittle, A.J. Do video game interventions improve motor outcomes in children with developmental coordination disorder? A systematic review using the ICF framework. *BMC Pediatr.* **2019**, *19*, 22. [CrossRef]
20. Pallavicini, F.; Ferrari, A.; Mantovani, F. Video games for well-being: A systematic review on the application of computer games for cognitive and emotional training in the adult population. *Front. Psychol.* **2018**, *9*, 2127. [CrossRef]
21. Ballesteros, S.; Mayas, J.; Prieto, A.; Ruiz-Marquez, E.; Toril, P.; Reales, J.M. Effects of video game training on measures of selective attention and working memory in older adults: Results from a randomized controlled trial. *Front. Aging Neurosci.* **2017**, *9*, 354. [CrossRef]

22. Baysak, E.; Yertutanol, F.D.K.; Dalgar, I.; Candansayar, S. How game addiction rates and related psychosocial risk factors change within 2-years: A follow-up study. *Psychiatry Investig.* **2018**, *15*, 984–990. [CrossRef]
23. El-Salhy, M.; Miyazaki, T.; Noda, Y.; Nakajima, S.; Nakayama, H.; Mihara, S.; Kitayuguchi, T.; Higuchi, S.; Muramatsu, T.; Mimura, M. Relationships between internet addiction and clinicodemographic and behavioral factors. *Neuropsychiatr. Dis. Treat.* **2019**, *15*, 739–752. [CrossRef]
24. Kim, J.Y.; Chun, J.W.; Park, C.H.; Cho, H.; Choi, J.; Yang, S.; Ahn, K.J.; Kim, D.J. The correlation between the frontostriatal network and impulsivity in internet gaming disorder. *Sci. Rep.* **2019**, *9*, 1191. [CrossRef] [PubMed]
25. Han, D.H.; Lyoo, I.K.; Renshaw, P.F. Differential regional gray matter volumes in patients with on-line game addiction and professional gamers. *J. Psychiatr. Res.* **2012**, *46*, 507–515. [CrossRef] [PubMed]
26. Wei, X.; Shen, H.; Ren, J.; Li, X.; Xu, X.; Yang, R.; Lai, L.; Chen, L.; Hu, J.; Liu, W.; et al. Altered resting-state connectivity in college students with nonclinical depressive symptoms. *PLoS ONE* **2014**, *9*, e114603. [CrossRef]
27. Lu, H.; Zuo, Y.; Gu, H.; Waltz, J.A.; Zhan, W.; Scholl, C.A.; Rea, W.; Yang, Y.; Stein, E.A. Synchronized delta oscillations correlate with the resting-state functional MRI signal. *Proc. Natl. Acad. Sci. USA* **2007**, *104*, 18265–18269. [CrossRef] [PubMed]
28. Zou, Q.H.; Zhu, C.Z.; Yang, Y.; Zuo, X.N.; Long, X.Y.; Cao, Q.J.; Wang, Y.F.; Zang, Y.F. An improved approach to detection of amplitude of low-frequency fluctuation (ALFF) for resting-state fMRI: Fractional ALFF. *J. Neurosci. Methods* **2008**, *172*, 137–141. [CrossRef] [PubMed]
29. Xu, Y.; Zhuo, C.; Qin, W.; Zhu, J.; Yu, C. Altered spontaneous brain activity in schizophrenia: A meta-analysis and a large-sample study. *Biomed. Res. Int.* **2015**, 204628. [CrossRef] [PubMed]
30. Itahashi, T.; Yamada, T.; Watanabe, H.; Nakamura, M.; Ohta, H.; Kanai, C.; Iwanami, A.; Kato, N.; Hashimoto, R. Alterations of local spontaneous brain activity and connectivity in adults with high-functioning autism spectrum disorder. *Mol. Autism* **2015**, *6*, 30. [CrossRef]
31. Cheng, W.; Ji, X.; Zhang, J.; Feng, J. Individual classification of ADHD patients by integrating multiscale neuroimaging markers and advanced pattern recognition techniques. *Front. Syst. Neurosci.* **2012**, *6*, 58. [CrossRef]
32. Kim, J.I.; Kang, Y.H.; Lee, J.M.; Cha, J.; Park, Y.H.; Kweon, K.J.; Kim, B.N. Resting-state functional magnetic resonance imaging investigation of the neural correlates of cognitive-behavioral therapy for externalizing behavior problems in adolescent bullies. *Prog. Neuro Psychopharmacol. Biol. Psychiatry* **2018**, *86*, 193–202. [CrossRef]
33. Achenbach, T.M. *Manual for the Child Behavior Checklist/4–18 and 1991 Profile*; Burlington: Burlington, NJ, USA, 1991.
34. Lee, S.; Park, J.; Lim, E.; Junh, H. Screening Oppositional Defiant Disorder with the Korean Child Behavior Checklist: The Role of the Subscales of Aggressive and Delinquent Behavior. *J. Korean Acad. Child Adolesc. Psychiatry* **2011**, *22*, 95–102. [CrossRef]
35. Young, K.S. Internet addiction: The emergence of a new clinical disorder. *Cyberpsychol. Behav.* **1998**, *1*, 237–244. [CrossRef]
36. Lee, K.; Lee, H.K.; Gyeong, H.; Yu, B.; Song, Y.M.; Kim, D. Reliability and validity of the Korean version of the internet addiction test among college students. *J. Korean Med. Sci.* **2013**, *28*, 763–768. [CrossRef] [PubMed]
37. Kovacs, M. The Children's Depression, Inventory (CDI). *Psychopharmacol. Bull.* **1985**, *21*, 995–998. [PubMed]
38. Cho, S.C.; Lee, Y.S. Development of the Korean form of the Kovacs' Children's Depression Inventory. *J. Korean Neuropsychiatr. Assoc.* **1990**, *29*, 943–956.
39. Beck, A.T.; Epstein, N.; Brown, G.; Steer, R.A. An inventory for measuring clinical anxiety: Psychometric properties. *J. Consult. Clin. Psychol.* **1998**, *56*, 893. [CrossRef]
40. Kwon, S.M. The assessment of psychopathology in patient with anxiety disorder. *Korean J. Psychopathol.* **1997**, *6*, 37–51.
41. DuPaul, G.J. Parent and teacher ratings of ADHD symptoms: Psychometric properties in a community-based sample. *J. Clin. Child Adolesc. Psychol.* **1991**, *20*, 245–253. [CrossRef]
42. So, Y.K.; Noh, J.S.; Kim, Y.S.; Ko, S.G.; Koh, Y.J. The reliability and validity of Korean parent and teacher ADHD rating scale. *J. Korean Neuropsychiatr. Assoc.* **2002**, *41*, 283–289.
43. Achenbach, T.M.; Ruffle, T.M. The child behavior checklist and related forms for assessing behavioral/emotional problems and competencies. *Pediatr. Rev.* **2000**, *21*, 265–271. [CrossRef]

44. Park, J.I.; Shim, S.H.; Lee, M.; Jung, Y.E.; Park, T.W.; Park, S.H.; Im, Y.J.; Yang, J.C.; Chung, Y.C.; Chung, S.K. The validities and efficiencies of Korean ADHD rating scale and Korean child behavior checklist for screening children with ADHD in the community. *Psychiatry Investig.* **2014**, *11*, 258–265. [CrossRef]
45. Kweon, K.; Lee, H.J.; Park, K.J.; Joo, Y.; Kim, H.W. Child behavior checklist profiles in adolescents with bipolar and depressive disorders. *Compr. Psychiatry* **2016**, *70*, 152–158. [CrossRef] [PubMed]
46. Greitemeyer, T.; Mugge, D.O. Video games do affect social outcomes: A meta-analytic review of the effects of violent and prosocial video game play. *Pers. Soc. Psychol. Bull.* **2014**, *40*, 578–589. [CrossRef] [PubMed]
47. Shao, R.; Wang, Y. The relation of violent video games to adolescent aggression: An examination of moderated mediation effect. *Front. Psychol.* **2019**, *10*, 384. [CrossRef] [PubMed]
48. Przybylski, A.K.; Weinstein, N. Violent video game engagement is not associated with adolescents' aggressive behaviour: Evidence from a registered report. *R. Soc. Open Sci.* **2019**, *6*, 171474. [CrossRef] [PubMed]
49. O'Brien, C. Drug addiction and drug abuse. In *Goodman and Gilman's The Pharmacological Basis of Therapeutics*, 11th ed.; Brunton, L.B., Lazo, J.S., Parker, K.L., Eds.; McGraw-Hill: New York, NY, USA, 2005; pp. 607–629.
50. Ptak, R. The frontoparietal attention network of the human brain: Action, saliency, and a priority map of the environment. *Neuroscientist* **2012**, *18*, 502–515. [CrossRef] [PubMed]
51. Bavelier, D.; Achtman, R.L.; Mani, M.; Focker, J. Neural bases of selective attention in action video game players. *Vis. Res.* **2012**, *61*, 132–143. [CrossRef] [PubMed]
52. Dye, M.W.; Green, C.S.; Bavelier, D. The development of attention skills in action video game players. *Neuropsychologia* **2009**, *47*, 1780–1789. [CrossRef]
53. Evren, C.; Evren, B.; Dalbudak, E.; Topcu, M.; Kutlu, N. Relationships of Internet addiction and Internet gaming disorder symptom severities with probable attention deficit/hyperactivity disorder, aggression and negative affect among university students. *Atten. Defic. Hyperact. Disord.* **2019**, *11*, 413–421. [CrossRef]
54. Han, D.H.; Lee, Y.S.; Na, C.; Ahn, J.Y.; Chung, U.S.; Daniels, M.A.; Haws, C.A.; Renshaw, P.F. The effect of methylphenidate on Internet video game play in children with attention-deficit/hyperactivity disorder. *Compr. Psychiatry* **2009**, *50*, 251–256. [CrossRef]
55. Moccia, L.; Pettorruso, M.; De Crescenzo, F.; De Risio, L.; di Nuzzo, L.; Martinotti, G.; Bifone, A.; Janiri, L.; Di Nicola, M. Neural correlates of cognitive control in gambling disorder: A systematic review of fMRI studies. *Neurosci. Biobehav. Rev.* **2017**, *78*, 104–116. [CrossRef]
56. Park, B.; Han, D.H.; Roh, S. Neurobiological findings related to Internet use disorders. *Psychiatry Clin. Neurosci.* **2017**, *71*, 467–478. [CrossRef] [PubMed]
57. Winstanley, C.A. The orbitofrontal cortex, impulsivity, and addiction: probing orbitofrontal dysfunction at the neural, neurochemical, and molecular level. *Ann. N. Y. Acad. Sci.* **2007**, *1121*, 639–655. [CrossRef] [PubMed]
58. Moorman, D.E. The role of the orbitofrontal cortex in alcohol use, abuse, and dependence. *Prog. Neuropsychopharmacol. Biol. Psychiatry* **2018**, *87*, 85–107. [CrossRef] [PubMed]
59. Eisenberg, N.; Sadovsky, A.; Spinrad, T.L.; Fabes, R.A.; Losoya, S.H.; Valiente, C.; Reiser, M.; Cumberland, A.; Shepard, S.A. The relations of problem behavior status to children's negative emotionality, effortful control, and impulsivity: Concurrent relations and prediction of change. *Dev. Psychol.* **2005**, *41*, 193–211. [CrossRef]
60. Mavrogiorgou, P.; Enzi, B.; Klimm, A.K.; Kohler, E.; Roser, P.; Norra, C.; Juckel, G. Serotonergic modulation of orbitofrontal activity and its relevance for decision making and impulsivity. *Hum. Brain Mapp.* **2017**, *38*, 1507–1517. [CrossRef]
61. Deserno, L.; Wilbertz, T.; Reiter, A.; Horstmann, A.; Neumann, J.; Villringer, A.; Heinze, H.J.; Schlagenhauf, F. Lateral prefrontal model-based signatures are reduced in healthy individuals with high trait impulsivity. *Transl. Psychiatry* **2015**, *5*, e659. [CrossRef]
62. Huang, S.; Zhu, Z.; Zhang, W.; Chen, Y.; Zhen, S. Trait impulsivity components correlate differently with proactive and reactive control. *PLoS ONE* **2017**, *12*, e0176102. [CrossRef]

12

Effects of Internet and Smartphone Addictions on Depression and Anxiety Based on Propensity Score Matching Analysis

Yeon-Jin Kim [1], Hye Min Jang [2], Youngjo Lee [3], Donghwan Lee [2,*,†] and Dai-Jin Kim [4,*,†]

1 Department of Psychiatry, SMG-SNU Boramae Medical Center, Seoul 07061, Korea; loveaj1220@gmail.com
2 Department of Statistics, Ewha Womans University, Seoul 03760, Korea; janghyemin23@naver.com
3 Department of Statistics, Seoul National University, Seoul 08826, Korea; youngjo@snu.ac.kr
4 Department of Psychiatry, Seoul St. Mary's Hospital, The Catholic University of Korea College of Medicine, Seoul 06591, Korea
* Correspondence: donghwan.lee@ewha.ac.kr (D.L.); Kdj922@catholic.ac.kr (D.-J.K.)

† These authors contributed equally to this work.

Abstract: The associations of Internet addiction (IA) and smartphone addiction (SA) with mental health problems have been widely studied. We investigated the effects of IA and SA on depression and anxiety while adjusting for sociodemographic variables. In this study, 4854 participants completed a cross-sectional web-based survey including socio-demographic items, the Korean Scale for Internet Addiction, the Smartphone Addiction Proneness Scale, and the subscales of the Symptom Checklist 90 Items-Revised. The participants were classified into IA, SA, and normal use (NU) groups. To reduce sampling bias, we applied the propensity score matching method based on genetics matching. The IA group showed an increased risk of depression (relative risk 1.207; $p < 0.001$) and anxiety (relative risk 1.264; $p < 0.001$) compared to NUs. The SA group also showed an increased risk of depression (relative risk 1.337; $p < 0.001$) and anxiety (relative risk 1.402; $p < 0.001$) compared to NCs. These findings show that both, IA and SA, exerted significant effects on depression and anxiety. Moreover, our findings showed that SA has a stronger relationship with depression and anxiety, stronger than IA, and emphasized the need for prevention and management policy of the excessive smartphone use.

Keywords: anxiety; depression; Internet addiction; smartphone addiction; propensity score

---

1. Introduction

With the increasing use and convenience of the Internet and smartphones in daily life, the accumulated research has shown the negative effects of the excessive Internet and smartphone use in the realm of mental health [1].

The smartphone user rate in South Korean population is approximately 85%, the highest worldwide [2]. However, the excessive smartphone use is strongly associated with a number of mental health issues, including stress and an increased risk of abnormal anxiety [3,4]. Smartphone addiction (SA) has emerged as a new form of addiction along with Internet addictions (IA), and the clinical characteristic of the SA have received attention in recent years [5]. For example, there are some differences regarding the nature of the devices, such as the easy portability, real-time Internet access and direct communication features of smartphones [6]. Similarities and differences between IA and SA have been reported with respect to demographic variables and the motivational aspects of media use [1,6].

From the environmental aspect, a lack of alternative activities is associated with IA [7]. Additionally, being single has been reported to be strongly associated with both a social network and online gaming [8]. As to the educational level and monthly income dimensions, a recent study in people with SA found significant differences in the health dimension in favor of those who had a lower income and a lower degree of education [9]. Consistent with this finding, a systematic review reported significant correlation between academic performance and severity of IA [10]. With regard to age, a recent review found that problematic Internet use is most relevant to both adolescent and emerging adults (19 years and older) [10], while smartphone addiction is more prevalent in younger adolescents compared with emerging adults (19 years and older) [11]. A recent study showed that women tend to have a higher average of daily usage times and dependency scores for smartphones, compared to men [4]. Choi et al. (2015) reported that the male gender has a relevant risk factor for IA, and the female gender for SA [1]. Regarding the purpose of use, social networking showed to be more strongly related to a high smartphone dependence, compared to other mobile telephone-related functions [11]. In individuals with IA, Anderson et al. (2016) reported that male gender was significantly associated with online PC gaming [10].

With regard to psychological aspects, the positive associations of IA and SA with depression and anxiety have been widely reported [12,13]. Recent studies have suggested that addiction to the Internet and smartphones may arise by user's individual cognitive-emotional and behavioral profile rather than the medium itself [14–16]. A recent study observed the role of empathy and life satisfaction in both IA and SA [17]. With regard to psychopathology, several studies reported a positive correlation between IA, depression, and anxiety [18–20], while a recent study reported a relationship between smartphone use and severity, depression, and anxiety [13]. Therefore, the interrelationship between IA, SA, and mental health problems needs to be precisely delineated. Moreover, given both the overlap and differences between IA and SA [16], then the question that arises is to what extent IA and SA are linked to the increased in the level of depression and anxiety after adjusting the confounding demographic and socioeconomic factors?

It remains unclear whether mental health problems are causes or consequences of excessive reliance on the Internet and smartphones. Cross-sectional studies have employed multiple regression analyses to investigate the relationships between mental health problems, IA, and SA in people [21]. However, in observational studies, which lack randomization, multiple regression analysis has limitations, such as the possibility of overestimation and a poor standard error when numerous covariates are present, in addition to the selection bias [22]. Thus, estimating the effects of addiction by simply examination of a particular outcome, such as depression and anxiety, would be biased by the imbalance of the demographic and socioeconomic factors associated with IA and SA. Moreover, no studies have yet investigated the differential effects according to the characteristics of Internet and smartphone users, including environmental contexts and users' psychological profiles, of IA and SA on depression and anxiety. Propensity score matching (PSM) has become a popular approach to reduce the selection bias in observational studies [23,24]. In this paper, we applied PSM analysis to investigate the effects of IA and SA on depression and anxiety, in order to reduce the selection bias in our data. We chose sex, age, education, marital status, and income as confounding variable, considering the association of these sociodemographic variables with IA and SA in our study [9,25].

The primary aim of this study is to examine the interrelationships between IA, SA, and mood status, that is depression and anxiety, using propensity score matching analysis. Second, we seek to discover how the effects of depression and anxiety differ between IA and SA.

2. Materials and Methods

2.1. Study Participants

The data consisted of the online anonymous self-diagnosis survey responses of 5003 Korean adults (aged 19–49 years), conducted by the Catholic University of Korea, Seoul; and St. Mary's Hospital in December 2014 [26]. The study was conducted in accordance with the Declaration of Helsinki. The institutional review boards of the Catholic University of Korea, Seoul; and St. Mary's Hospital approved this study. All participants were informed about the study and provided written informed consent. The survey participants were recruited by a panel of a research company and self-report questionnaires were administered through Internet without any compensation. Only 149 respondents, who did not use smartphones, were excluded. Finally, we analyzed the data of 4854 participants. In the final sample, the ages were classified into three categories: Below 30 (33.19%), 30–39 (43.94%), and 40–49 (22.87%). There were 2573 males (53.01%) and 2281 females (46.99%). The additional demographic variables of participants considered were education, marital status, and income.

2.2. Measures

2.2.1. Measurement of Internet Addiction

The Korean Scale for Internet Addiction (K-scale) was developed in Korea to assess IA and has been validated in the Korean population with a high reliability of internal consistency [27]. The Cronbach's alpha coefficient for the K-Scale was 0.91 [28]. It has seven subscales and 40 items, measuring daily life disturbance, disturbance of reality testing, automatic addictive thoughts, virtual interpersonal relationships, deviant behavior, withdrawal, and tolerance. This Likert type scale has been set from 1 (not at all) to 4 (always). According to the previous report using this scale, the participants were sorted into three groups: normal, potential risk, and high-risk [29]. The high-risk group was defined as having a standardized score of 70 or higher, in daily life disturbance, automatic addictive thoughts, tolerance factors, or at least 70 in total. The potential risk group was defined as a score of 62 or higher in daily life disturbance, automatic addictive thoughts, tolerance factors, or at least 63 in total. The normal use group contained those scores below these numbers. In this study, IA groups were made up of the potential risk and high-risk groups.

2.2.2. Measurement of Smartphone Addiction

The Smartphone Addiction Proneness Scale (K-SAS) has been validated and widely used to screen for SA [30]. It consists of 15 items rated in a four-point Likert type scale of distress from 1 (not at all) to 4 (always). The questions examined three factors: daily life disturbance, automatic addictive thoughts, and tolerance. The Cronbach's alpha coefficient for the K-SAS was 0.880 [5].

Based on a previous report using this scale, we used the scores to classify the participants into three groups: Normal, potential risk, and high-risk [30]. The high-risk group was defined as having a score of 44 or more in total, or having a subscore of 15 or more in daily life disturbance along with subscores of 13 or more, in both automatic addictive thoughts and tolerance. The potential risk group was defined as having 41 or more in the total score, or 15 or more in the daily life disturbance factor. The normal use group contained those scores below these numbers [30]. In this study, the smartphone-addicted group were made up of high-risk and potential risk groups.

2.2.3. Measurement of Mental Health Problems: Depression and Anxiety

The SCL-90-R is a multidimensional questionnaire developed to screen a range of psychological and psychopathological features of 9 subscales: Somatization, obsessive–compulsive, interpersonal sensitivity, depression, anxiety, hostility, phobic anxiety, paranoid ideation, and psychoticism [31]. The SCL-90 contains 90 items rated in a 5-point scale of distress from 0 (none) to 4 (extreme). The test–retest reliability of the SCL-90-R in the Korean language was 0.76 for depression and 0.77 for anxiety. The internal consistency was 0.89 for depression and 0.86 for anxiety [31]. Depression and anxiety have been reported to be the psychiatric symptoms most strongly associated with IA and SA [12,13]. The specific dimensions of interest to screen in this study included the SCL-90-R subscales for Depression and Anxiety.

2.3. Data Analysis

2.3.1. Statistical Definition

Let Z_i be a binary addiction indicator for the ith subject; that is, $Z_i = 1$ if the ith subject is addicted (IA or SA), and $Z_i = 0$ otherwise. The potential outcome of a mental problem (depression or anxiety) is defined as $Y_i(Z_i)$. Note that only one of the potential outcomes is observed at the same time for each subject, so direct computation of $Y_i(1) - Y_i(0)$ is impossible. Instead of the individual effect, the primary parameter of interest is the expected addiction effect on the addicted population

$$\tau = E(Y_i(1) - Y_i(0)|Z_i = 1) = E(Y_i(1)|Z_i = 1) - E(Y_i(0)|Z_i = 1) \quad (1)$$

However, the estimation of τ still has a problem because $E(Y_i(0)|Z_i = 1)$ cannot be directly estimated. Of course, in randomized experiments, $E(Y_i(0)|Z_i = 1) = E(Y_i(0)|Z_i = 0)$ is satisfied, so τ can easily be estimated. However, in an observation study, the naïve estimation of τ can be biased because $E(Y_i(0)|Z_i = 1) \neq E(Y_i(0)|Z_i = 0)$. To adjust this selection bias, we assume that we can observe the covariates X_i that are not affect by any addiction, and for a given covariates X_i, the potential outcomes $Y_i(1),\ Y_i(0)$ are conditionally independent of addiction indicator Z_i. Furthermore, if potential outcomes are independent of the addiction conditional on covariates X_i, they are also independent of the addiction conditional in the propensity score $P(X_i) = P(Z_i = 1|X_i)$ [19]. The PSM estimator for τ becomes

$$\tau^{PSM} = E_{P(X)|Z=1}[E(Y_i(1)|Z_i = 1,\ P(X_i)) - E(Y_i(0)|Z_i = 0,\ P(X_i))] \quad (2)$$

2.3.2. Estimating the Propensity Score

Propensity scores are calculated using logistic regression, a model used to predict the probability that an addiction occurs

$$\log \frac{P(Z_i = 1|X_i)}{1 - P(Z_i = 1|X_i)} = \alpha + \beta^T X_i \quad (3)$$

In this paper, as the covariates for X_i, we consider five categorical covariates: sex (1 = male and 2 = female), age (1 = 20–29, 2 = 30–39, and 3 = 40–49), education (1 = middle school, 2 = high school, and 3 = university or above), marital status (1 = single, 2 = cohabitation, 3 = married, 4 = divorced, and 5 = bereaved), and income (1 = low, 2 = mid-low, 3 = middle, 4 = mid-high, and 5 = high). In Section 1, these covariates may influence simultaneously the outcomes (depression or anxiety) and addictions. Thus, for each subject, we estimated the propensity scores; that is, the conditional probability of being addicted given the observed covariates [32].

2.3.3. Matching Methods Based on the Estimated Propensity Score

Once the propensity scores are estimated, matching can be used to estimate the treatment effect after adjusting to the differences between the two groups [33]. The goal of matching is to produce a matched sample that balances the distribution of a study's patient and matched the covariates of the control groups observed. This adjusting method allows us to control the confounding variables. In this study, we adopted two widely used matching methods, the optimal and genetic matching [34].

2.3.4. Estimation of the Relative Risks of Addiction on Mental Health Problems after Propensity Score Matching

After propensity score matching by using the observed covariates (age, gender, marriage, income, and education), we have a more balanced dataset. To model the mental health problem (depression or anxiety), we applied generalized linear models (GLMs) to the matched sample. Because the mental health scores are positive and biased, the gamma distribution with log link is fitted. Let Y_i be an outcome of interest (an score of depression or anxiety) with mean μ_i, we can use the Gamma GLM framework with covariates X_i:

$$\log \mu_i = \gamma^T X_i$$

Through modeling, we estimated e^γ as the relative risks (as an expected mean difference between groups) of IA and SA for each covariate.

3. Results

In addition to the 4854 participants, 126 (2.60%) were included in the IA group and 652 (13.43%) were included in the SA group. Table 1 shows the descriptive statistics of the depression and anxiety scores. The mean scores of depression and anxiety of IA and SA groups are larger than those of the normal use (NU) group.

Table 1. Descriptive statistics of Depression and Anxiety scores.

Outcome	Statistics	Total (n = 4854)	Internet: NU (n = 4728)	IA (n = 126)	Smartphone: NU (n = 4202)	SA (n = 652)
Depression	Mean	26.69	26.52	33.01	25.49	34.42
	SD	10.3	10.23	10.7	9.55	11.48
	Min	13	13	13	13	13
	Max	65	65	62	65	65
	Skewness	0.74	0.76	0.29	0.74	0.34
Anxiety	Mean	18.47	18.33	23.75	17.51	24.67
	SD	7.79	7.7	9.21	7.04	9.37
	Min	10	10	10	10	10
	Max	50	50	50	50	50
	Skewness	1.02	1.03	0.56	1	0.47

Abbreviations: SD, standard deviation; NU, normal use; IA, Internet addiction; SA, smartphone addiction.

3.1. Matching Quality of the Propensity Score Matching Method

Although we condition only a few of the covariates in the questionnaires of this study, via the propensity score, we found that the matching procedure was sufficient to balance the distribution of each covariate, Tables 2 and 3. We assessed the distances in the marginal distributions of X_i. For each covariate, we computed the bias; that is, the difference in sample averages of the addicted and normal samples. Before applying the propensity score matching, the biases were not ignored. However, after propensity score matching, the addiction and normal subsamples had a very similar marginal distribution for all covariates.

Table 2. Comparison of the mean percentage of baseline characteristics between IA and normal use groups, in the original sample and the propensity score matched sample, using the genetic and optimal matching.

	Before PSM			After PSM (Genetic)			After PSM (Optimal)		
	Normal (n = 4728)	IA (n = 126)	Bias	Normal (n = 3722)	IA (n = 124)	Bias	Normal (n = 126)	IA (n = 126)	Bias
Sex (male)	53.51	34.13	19.38	33.87	33.87	0	34.92	34.13	0.79
Sex (female)	46.49	65.87	−19.38	66.13	66.13	0	65.08	65.87	−0.79
Age (19–29)	33.1	36.51	−3.41	36.29	36.29	0	32.54	36.51	−3.97
Age (30–39)	43.99	42.06	1.93	42.74	42.74	0	44.44	42.06	2.38
Age (40–49)	22.91	21.43	1.48	20.97	20.97	0	23.02	21.43	1.59
Education (middle school)	0.59	0	0.59	0	0	0	0	0	0
Education (high school)	27.33	30.16	−2.83	30.65	30.65	0	37.3	30.16	7.14
Education (university or above)	72.08	69.84	2.24	69.35	69.35	0	62.7	69.84	−7.14

Table 2. *Cont.*

	Before PSM			After PSM (Genetic)			After PSM (Optimal)		
	Normal (n = 4728)	IA (n = 126)	Bias	Normal (n = 3722)	IA (n = 124)	Bias	Normal (n = 126)	IA (n = 126)	Bias
Marriage (single)	48.1	50	−1.9	50.81	50.81	0	43.65	50	−6.35
Marriage (cohabitation)	0.8	0.79	0.01	0	0	0	0.79	0.79	0
Marriage (married)	49.34	46.03	3.31	46.77	46.77	0	51.59	46.03	5.56
Marriage (divorced)	1.61	3.17	−1.56	2.42	2.42	0	3.97	3.17	0.8
Marriage (bereaved)	0.15	0	0.15	0	0	0	0	0	0
Income (low)	11.84	11.9	−0.06	12.1	12.1	0	14.29	11.9	2.39
Income (mid-low)	31.58	33.33	−1.75	33.06	33.06	0	34.13	33.33	0.8
Income (middle)	44.35	45.24	−0.89	45.97	45.97	0	42.06	45.24	−3.18
Income (mid-high)	10.89	7.14	3.75	6.45	6.45	0	7.14	7.14	0
Income (high)	1.33	2.38	−1.05	2.42	2.42	0	2.38	2.38	0

Abbreviations: PSM, propensity score matching; IA, internet addiction.

Table 3. Comparison of the mean percentage of baseline characteristics between SA and normal groups, in the original sample and the propensity score matched sample, using the genetic and optimal matching.

	Before PSM			After PSM (Genetic)			After PSM (Optimal)		
	Normal (n = 4202)	SA (n = 652)	Bias	Normal (n = 3873)	SA (n = 643)	Bias	Normal (n = 652)	SA (n = 652)	Bias
Sex (male)	55.45	37.27	18.18	36.86	36.86	0	36.5	37.27	−0.77
Sex (female)	44.55	62.73	−18.18	63.14	63.14	0	63.5	62.73	0.77
Age (19–29)	32.2	39.57	−7.37	39.5	39.5	0	39.26	39.57	−0.31
Age (30–39)	43.69	45.55	−1.86	45.72	45.72	0	45.86	45.55	0.31
Age (40–49)	24.11	14.88	9.23	14.77	14.77	0	14.88	14.88	0
Education (middle school)	0.55	0.77	−0.22	0.16	0.16	0	0.92	0.77	0.15
Education (high school)	27.44	27.15	0.29	27.22	27.22	0	28.68	27.15	1.53
Education (university or above)	72.01	72.09	−0.08	72.63	72.63	0	70.4	72.09	−1.69
Marriage (single)	47.52	52.15	−4.63	52.57	52.57	0	52.45	52.15	0.3
Marriage (cohabitation)	0.74	1.23	−0.49	0.93	0.93	0	0.61	1.23	−0.62
Marriage (married)	49.9	45.09	4.81	45.41	45.41	0	45.86	45.09	0.77
Marriage (divorced)	1.67	1.53	0.14	1.09	1.09	0	1.07	1.53	−0.46
Marriage (bereaved)	0.17	0	0.17	0	0	0	0	0	0
Income (low)	11.66	13.04	−1.38	12.75	12.75	0	13.5	13.04	0.46
Income (mid-low)	31.89	29.91	1.98	29.86	29.86	0	28.68	29.91	−1.23
Income (middle)	44.17	45.71	−1.54	46.35	46.35	0	46.01	45.71	0.3
Income (mid-high)	10.97	9.66	1.31	9.64	9.64	0	10.28	9.66	0.62
Income (high)	1.31	1.69	−0.38	1.4	1.4	0	1.53	1.69	−0.16

Abbreviations: PSM, propensity score matching; SA, smartphone addiction.

3.2. *Effects of the Internet Addiction on Depression and Anxiety*

The effects of IA on depression and anxiety obtained using propensity score matching are reported in Table 4. Through genetic matching, 3846 samples were selected. The IA was related to a greater risk of depression (relative risk 1.207, 95% confidence interval 1.128–1.292, and $p < 0.001$) and anxiety (relative risk 1.264, 95% confidence interval 1.173–1.362, and $p < 0.001$). All these relative risk ratios are significant because the confidence interval does not contain the 1. Through optimal matching, 252 samples were selected. The IA was related to a greater depression (relative risk 1.243, 95% confidence interval 1.145–1.348, and $p < 0.001$) and anxiety (relative risk 1.308, 95% confidence interval 1.192–1.435, and $p < 0.001$). Similar to the genetic matching, the relative risk ratios on both, depression and anxiety, are significantly larger than 1.

Table 4. Effects of the internet and smartphone addiction on depression and anxiety, based on propensity score matching.

		Internet Addiction			Smartphone Addiction		
Outcome	**Type of PSM**	*n*	**RR**	**CI**	*n*	**RR**	**CI**
Depression	Optimal	252	1.243	1.145–1.348	1304	1.386	1.334–1.440
	Genetic	3846	1.207	1.128–1.292	4516	1.337	1.296–1.378
Anxiety	Optimal	252	1.308	1.192–1.435	1304	1.44	1.380–1.503
	Genetic	3846	1.264	1.173–1.362	4516	1.402	1.355–1.450

Abbreviations: RR. relative risk; CI, confidence interval.

3.3. Effects of the Smartphone Addiction on Depression and Anxiety

The effects of SA on depression and anxiety using propensity score matching are reported in Table 4. Through genetic matching, 4516 samples were selected. The SA was related to a greater risk of depression (relative risk 1.337, 95% confidence interval 1.296–1.378, and $p < 0.001$) and anxiety (relative risk 1.402, 95% confidence interval 1.355–1.450, and $p < 0.001$). Through optimal matching, 1304 samples were selected. The SA was related to a greater risk of depression (relative risk 1.386, 95% confidence interval 1.334–1.440, and $p < 0.001$) and anxiety (relative risk 1.440, 95% confidence interval 1.380–1.503, and $p < 0.001$). All these relative risk ratios are significant.

3.4. Differences in Effects of the Internet and Smartphone Addiction on Depression and Anxiety

The relative risk ratios for depression and anxiety, from both genetic and optimal matching, were 10% higher for SA than for IA. This means that SA has a greater risk for depression and anxiety than IA. Those confidence intervals do not contain the 1, so we can say that SA is 34–44% more likely to cause a mental disorder.

4. Discussion

Our findings are that both IA and SA exert significant effects on depression and anxiety, even after controlling the confounders using propensity score matching. Epidemiological studies have estimated a higher prevalence of depression in IA [35,36]. A number of cross-sectional studies have reported that individuals with IA or SA showed higher levels of depression and anxiety than normal users [13,37]. In the present study, our results show the roles of IA and SA in developing depression and anxiety. There are some possible explanations for the current findings. First, addictive use of internet and smartphones can increase interpersonal problems, which is related to depression and anxiety, such as family conflicts, lack of off-line relationships, and a heightened need for approval in cyberspace. Second, withdrawal symptoms are proposed as psychopathological patterns in IA and SA, comparable to substance abuse disorders [5]. When they do not have access to a PC or smartphone, the individuals with IA or SA may become anxious, and then desire to use the Internet or a smartphone in to escape such negative feelings [38]. Another possible explanation is that unlike other addictive substances, such as alcohol and nicotine, internet and smartphones over-users may have little insight about their excessive use in daily life because of free and flexible access to the devices [3], making them experience their excessive use as an annoyance rather than as a sign of problematic behavior [39]. Another interesting finding was that SA exerted stronger effects on depression and anxiety than IA. This leads us to speculate that IA and SA have different influences on mental health problems. There could be several possible explanations for this finding. First, considering the media characteristics, it is easier for the excessive smartphone use develops through habit-forming nature of the device, because of its higher accessibility to the wireless network and 24 h of frequent notifications [39]. Second, with regard to environmental factors, this finding may reflect the current radical change of daily life average from PCs to smartphones. People may use the PC internet for complicated work and carry out the other daily tasks with smartphones, leading to a decrease in labor productivity and a higher level of stress [40]. Finally, individuals with SA may use smartphones to maintain relationships and a sense of connectedness with the online social network [41], leading to the fear of missing out and the fear of loss of connection, while triggering a higher smartphone use [42].

This study has several limitations to generalize findings to the entire population, such as the cross-sectional nature of the data limits and the interpretation of causal inference between the Internet and smartphone addiction, depression, and anxiety. Propensity matching also has limitations and requirements. The major limitation is that propensity scores can only control by observed confounders [43]. The possibility of unobserved confounders may remain, limiting the study finding for generalization. Furthermore, because of all observed confounders in this study were collected as categorical variables, there may be information loss when building PSM model. Therefore, our findings should be interpreted with caution. However, to get the robust results of matching, we considered two matching methods, genetic matching and optimal matching. Especially, genetic matching uses a genetic search algorithm, so its process can find a good matching solution with less loss of information [44]. Lastly, assessment of the depression and anxiety symptom was conducted by self-report psychological symptom measure using SCL-90-R. To evaluate mental health problems more accurately and consistently. A structured interview by clinician should be conducted in further studies.

5. Conclusions

In this study, we investigated how IA and SA influence mental health problems, depression and anxiety. To the best of our knowledge, this is the first study to estimate the association between IA, SA and psychopathology using propensity matching score method from cross-sectional data, and to investigate the differential effect in the psychopathology between IA and SA. In conclusion, our findings reveal that both IA and SA increase the risk of depression and anxiety. In addition, SA showed a stronger relationship with depression and anxiety compared to IA.

An implication of these findings is that individuals with a problematic smartphone use should be closely monitored for mental health problems, highlighting the need to establish prevention and management policies aimed at the pre-clinical level of SA. Further prospective studies should investigate the causal directions of the relationships among IA, SA, and mental health problems and should identify the discriminative factors of IA and SA.

Author Contributions: D.-J.K. and D.L. conceived and designed the experiments; H.M.J. analyzed the data; Y.-J.K. wrote the paper. Y.L. supervised the data collection. All authors contributed to the development of the manuscript, revised it critically, and approved the final manuscript.

Acknowledgments: This work was supported by a grant from the National Research Foundation of Korea (Grant No. 2014M3C7A1062894, 2014M3C7A1062896).

References

1. Choi, S.-W.; Kim, D.-J.; Choi, J.-S.; Ahn, H.; Choi, E.-J.; Song, W.-Y.; Kim, S.; Youn, H. Comparison of risk and protective factors associated with smartphone addiction and Internet addiction. *J. Behav. Addict.* **2015**, *4*, 308–314. [CrossRef] [PubMed]
2. *2016 the Survey on Internet Overdependence*; Ministry of Science, ICT and Future Planning: Seoul, Korea, 2017.
3. Lee, Y.-K.; Chang, C.-T.; Lin, Y.; Cheng, Z.-H. The dark side of smartphone usage: Psychological traits, compulsive behavior and technostress. *Comput. Hum. Behav.* **2014**, *31*, 373–383. [CrossRef]
4. Lee, K.E.; Kim, S.-H.; Ha, T.-Y.; Yoo, Y.-M.; Han, J.-J.; Jung, J.-H.; Jang, J.-Y. Dependency on smartphone use and its association with anxiety in Korea. *Public Health Rep.* **2016**, *131*, 411–419. [CrossRef] [PubMed]
5. Kim, D.; Chung, Y.; Lee, J.; Kim, M.; Lee, Y.; Kang, E.; Keum, C.; Nam, J. Development of smartphone addiction proneness scale for adults: Self-report. *Korean J. Couns.* **2012**, *13*, 629–644.
6. Kwon, M.; Lee, J.-Y.; Won, W.-Y.; Park, J.-W.; Min, J.-A.; Hahn, C.; Gu, X.; Choi, J.-H.; Kim, D.-J. Development and validation of a smartphone addiction scale (SAS). *PLoS ONE* **2013**, *8*, e56936. [CrossRef] [PubMed]

7. Kuss, D.J.; Griffiths, M.D.; Karila, L.; Billieux, J. Internet addiction: A systematic review of epidemiological research for the last decade. *Curr. Pharm. Des.* **2014**, *20*, 4026–4052. [CrossRef] [PubMed]
8. Andreassen, C.S.; Billieux, J.; Griffiths, M.D.; Kuss, D.J.; Demetrovics, Z.; Mazzoni, E.; Pallesen, S. The relationship between addictive use of social media and video games and symptoms of psychiatric disorders: A large-scale cross-sectional study. *Psychol. Addict. Behav.* **2016**, *30*, 252. [CrossRef] [PubMed]
9. Aljomaa, S.S.; Qudah, M.F.A.; Albursan, I.S.; Bakhiet, S.F.; Abduljabbar, A.S. Smartphone addiction among university students in the light of some variables. *Comput. Hum. Behav.* **2016**, *61*, 155–164. [CrossRef]
10. Anderson, E.L.; Steen, E.; Stavropoulos, V. Internet use and Problematic Internet Use: A systematic review of longitudinal research trends in adolescence and emergent adulthood. *Int. J. Adolesc. Youth* **2017**, *22*, 430–454. [CrossRef]
11. Haug, S.; Castro, R.P.; Kwon, M.; Filler, A.; Kowatsch, T.; Schaub, M.P. Smartphone use and smartphone addiction among young people in Switzerland. *J. Behav. Addict.* **2015**, *4*, 299–307. [CrossRef] [PubMed]
12. Ko, C.-H.; Yen, J.-Y.; Yen, C.-F.; Chen, C.-S.; Chen, C.-C. The association between Internet addiction and psychiatric disorder: A review of the literature. *Eur. Psychiatry* **2012**, *27*, 1–8. [CrossRef] [PubMed]
13. Demirci, K.; Akgönül, M.; Akpinar, A. Relationship of smartphone use severity with sleep quality, depression, and anxiety in university students. *J. Behav. Addict.* **2015**, *4*, 85–92. [CrossRef] [PubMed]
14. Brand, M.; Young, K.S.; Laier, C.; Wölfling, K.; Potenza, M.N. Integrating psychological and neurobiological considerations regarding the development and maintenance of specific Internet-use disorders: An Interaction of Person-Affect-Cognition-Execution (I-PACE) model. *Neurosci. Biobehav. Rev.* **2016**, *71*, 252–266. [CrossRef] [PubMed]
15. Kim, Y.-J.; Kim, D.-J.; Choi, J. The cognitive dysregulation of Internet addiction and its neurobiological correlates. *Front. Biosci (Elite ed.)* **2017**, *9*, 307–320.
16. Lachmann, B.; Duke, É.; Sariyska, R.; Montag, C. Who's Addicted to the Smartphone and/or the Internet? *Psychol. Pop. Media Cult.* **2017**. [CrossRef]
17. Lachmann, B.; Sindermann, C.; Sariyska, R.Y.; Luo, R.; Melchers, M.C.; Becker, B.; Cooper, A.J.; Montag, C. The Role of Empathy and Life Satisfaction in Internet and Smartphone Use Disorder. *Front. Psychol.* **2018**, *9*, 398. [CrossRef] [PubMed]
18. Banjanin, N.; Banjanin, N.; Dimitrijevic, I.; Pantic, I. Relationship between internet use and depression: Focus on physiological mood oscillations, social networking and online addictive behavior. *Comput. Hum. Behav.* **2015**, *43*, 308–312. [CrossRef]
19. Akin, A.; Iskender, M. Internet addiction and depression, anxiety and stress. *Int. Online J. Educ. Sci.* **2011**, *3*, 138–148.
20. Ostovar, S.; Allahyar, N.; Aminpoor, H.; Moafian, F.; Nor, M.B.M.; Griffiths, M.D. Internet addiction and its psychosocial risks (depression, anxiety, stress and loneliness) among Iranian adolescents and young adults: A structural equation model in a cross-sectional study. *Int. J. Ment. Health Addict.* **2016**, *14*, 257–267. [CrossRef]
21. Cheung, L.M.; Wong, W.S. The effects of insomnia and internet addiction on depression in Hong Kong Chinese adolescents: An exploratory cross-sectional analysis. *J. Sleep Res.* **2011**, *20*, 311–317. [CrossRef] [PubMed]
22. Cepeda, M.S.; Boston, R.; Farrar, J.T.; Strom, B.L. Comparison of logistic regression versus propensity score when the number of events is low and there are multiple confounders. *Am. J. Epidemiol.* **2003**, *158*, 280–287. [CrossRef] [PubMed]
23. Austin, P.C. A critical appraisal of propensity-score matching in the medical literature between 1996 and 2003. *Stat. Med.* **2008**, *27*, 2037–2049. [CrossRef] [PubMed]
24. Austin, P.C.; Grootendorst, P.; Anderson, G.M. A comparison of the ability of different propensity score models to balance measured variables between treated and untreated subjects: A Monte Carlo study. *Stat. Med.* **2007**, *26*, 734–753. [CrossRef] [PubMed]
25. Müller, K.W.; Glaesmer, H.; Brähler, E.; Woelfling, K.; Beutel, M.E. Prevalence of internet addiction in the general population: Results from a German population-based survey. *Behav. Inf. Technol.* **2014**, *33*, 757–766. [CrossRef]
26. Rho, M.J.; Lee, H.; Lee, T.-H.; Cho, H.; Jung, D.; Kim, D.-J.; Choi, I.Y. Risk Factors for Internet Gaming Disorder: Psychological Factors and Internet Gaming Characteristics. *Int. J. Environ. Res. Public Health* **2018**, *15*, 40. [CrossRef] [PubMed]

27. National Information Service Agency. *A Study of Internet Addiction Proneness Scale for Adults*; National Information Service Agency: Seoul, Korea, 2005.
28. Kim, D. *The Follow up Study of Internet Addiction Proneness Scale*; Korea Agency for Digital Opportunity and Promotion: Seoul, Korea, 2008; Available online: http://www.nia.or.kr/site/nia_kor/ex/bbs/View.do?cbIdx=39485&bcIdx=277&parentSeq=277 (accessed on 8 May 2008).
29. Kim, D.-I.; Chung, Y.-J.; Lee, E.-A.; Kim, D.-M.; Cho, Y.-M. Development of internet addiction proneness scale-short form (KS scale). *Korean J. Couns.* **2008**, *9*, 1703–1722.
30. National Information Service Agency. *Development of Korean Smartphone Addiction Proness Scale for Youth and Adults*; National Information Service Agency: Seoul, Korea, 2011; pp. 85–86.
31. Kim, K-I.; Kim, J-W. The standardizaion study of symptom checklist-90-R in Korea III. *Ment. Health Res.* **1984**, *2*, 278–311.
32. Heckman, J.; Smith, J. Assessing the Case for Social Experiments. *J. Econ. Perspect.* **1995**, *9*, 85–110. [CrossRef]
33. Caliendo, M.; Kopeinig, S. Some practical guidance for the implementation of propensity score matching. *J. Econ. Surv.* **2008**, *22*, 31–72. [CrossRef]
34. Sekhon, J.S.; Diamond, A. Genetic Matching for Estimating Causal Effects, unpublished Manuscript. Presented at the Annual Meeting of the Political Methodology, Tallahassee, FL, USA, July 2005.
35. Ghassemzadeh, L.; Shahraray, M.; Moradi, A. Prevalence of Internet addiction and comparison of Internet addicts and non-addicts in Iranian high schools. *Cyberpsychol. Behav.* **2008**, *11*, 731–733. [CrossRef] [PubMed]
36. Yen, J.-Y.; Ko, C.-H.; Yen, C.-F.; Wu, H.-Y.; Yang, M.-J. The comorbid psychiatric symptoms of Internet addiction: Attention deficit and hyperactivity disorder (ADHD), depression, social phobia, and hostility. *J. Adolesc. Health* **2007**, *41*, 93–98. [CrossRef] [PubMed]
37. Tonioni, F.; Mazza, M.; Autullo, G.; Cappelluti, R.; Catalano, V.; Marano, G.; Fiumana, V.; Moschetti, C.; Alimonti, F.; Luciani, M. Is Internet addiction a psychopathological condition distinct from pathological gambling? *J. Addict. Behav.* **2014**, *39*, 1052–1056. [CrossRef] [PubMed]
38. Kuss, D.J.; Griffiths, M.D. Online social networking and addiction—A review of the psychological literature. *Int. J. Environ. Res. Public Health* **2011**, *8*, 3528–3552. [CrossRef] [PubMed]
39. Oulasvirta, A.; Rattenbury, T.; Ma, L.; Raita, E. Habits make smartphone use more pervasive. *Pers. Ubiquitous Comput.* **2012**, *16*, 105–114. [CrossRef]
40. Duke, É.; Montag, C. Smartphone addiction, daily interruptions and self-reported productivity. *Addict. Behav. Rep.* **2017**, *6*, 90–95. [CrossRef] [PubMed]
41. Kuss, D.J.; Griffiths, M.D. Social networking sites and addiction: Ten lessons learned. *Int. J. Environ. Res. Public Health* **2017**, *14*, 311. [CrossRef] [PubMed]
42. Oberst, U.; Wegmann, E.; Stodt, B.; Brand, M.; Chamarro, A. Negative consequences from heavy social networking in adolescents: The mediating role of fear of missing out. *J. Adolesc.* **2017**, *55*, 51–60. [CrossRef] [PubMed]
43. Joffe, M.M.; Rosenbaum, P.R. Invited commentary: Propensity scores. *Am. J. Epidemiol.* **1999**, *150*, 327–333. [CrossRef] [PubMed]
44. Diamond, A.; Sekon, J. Genetic matching for estimating causal effects: A new method of achieving balance in observational studies. *Rev. Econ. Stat.* **2013**, *95*, 932–945. [CrossRef]

13

Self-Perception of Dependence as an Indicator of Smartphone Addiction—Establishment of a Cutoff Point in the SPAI–Spain Inventory

María Luisa Ballestar-Tarín [1], Conchín Simó-Sanz [1,2], Elena Chover-Sierra [1,2,*], Carlos Saus-Ortega [1,3], Carmen Casal-Angulo [1,4] and Antonio Martínez-Sabater [1,5]

1 Nursing Department, Facultat d'Infermeria I Podologia, Universitat de València, 46010 Valencia, Spain; M.luisa.ballestar@uv.es (M.L.B.-T.); conchin.simo@uv.es (C.S.-S.); sausor@uv.es (C.S.-O.); m.carmen.casal@uv.es (C.C.-A.); Antonio.Martinez-Sabater@uv.es (A.M.-S.)
2 Hospital General, Universitario de Valencia, 46014 Valencia, Spain
3 Nursing School La Fe, Universitario de Valencia, 46026 Valencia, Spain
4 Emergencies Service, Extra-hospital, 46010 Valencia, Spain
5 Hospital Clínico, Universitario de Valencia, 46010 Valencia, Spain
* Correspondence: elena.chover@uv.es

Abstract: Background: In recent years, the abusive use of the smartphone has reached a situation that could be considered pathological. In this sense, different instruments to assess this problematic use or addiction to the smartphone are used. One of these instruments is the Smartphone Addition Inventory (SPAI), which has been validated in the Spanish language (SPAI-Spain). The main difficulty of these scales is to establish a cut-off point that determines such mobile addiction. On the other hand, self-perception was used in different addictions as a predictor of the problem. Aim: The objective of this study was to establish the cut-off point in the scores of the SPAI-Spain, using as a reference the self-perception of addiction values. Methods: A receiver operating characteristics (ROC) analysis was carried out, establishing as the cut-off point the one that presented a higher value of Youden J, indicative of its sensitivity and specificity. Results: 2958 participants from the university community completed the SPAI–Spain questionnaire. Differences in SPAI–Spain scores were found among age groups and gender, even though not all of them were statistically significant. When using the self-perception of smartphone addiction as the benchmark value, a score of 44 was established as the cutting point of the SPAI-Spain questionnaire, with a Youden J corresponding to 0.416. Conclusions: The implementation of a cut-off point of the SPAI-Spain questionnaire makes it an instrument that allows early identification of those individuals at risk of addiction, as well as the establishment of preventive and/or intervention measures.

Keywords: smartphones; addiction; self-perceived addiction; ROC analysis; cutoff point; SPAI–Spain

1. Introduction

In the Diagnostic and Statistical Manual of Mental Disorders (DSM–V), the term behavioral addiction is introduced, with the gaming disorder as the only category [1]. It is admitted, therefore, that the "pathological gambling" is an addictive disorder and not a disorder of impulse control, as it was previously classified [2,3]. The World Health Organization (WHO) included gambling and gaming disorder in the International Classification of Diseases (ICD) 11, suggesting that behavioral addictions share some common ground with substance use disorders [4]. Besides, the American Psychiatric Association (APA) recognizes that reward systems are activated in behavioral addictions, and similar behavioral symptoms occur in clinical conditions caused by substance use [1]. This is an open door to other behavioral addictions such as sex, shopping, food, work, physical exercise, mobile, or technologies [5]. However, the DSM–V only points out a small reference to the existence of these excessive behaviors, calling them behavioral syndromes. They are supposed not to have a solid base to be considered as mental disorders [1]. Despite this, many researchers suggest the addictive nature of these behaviors, although they do not share some features with substances' addiction [4,6,7].

This study focuses on the use of the smartphone, to which authors such as Flores et al. [7] catalog it as the consequence of the new "society of autism." The increase in connectivity in different areas of life has led to a behavioral change in people. Moreover, the excessive use of network technology can lead to physical, mental, and social problems [8]. This symptomatology is assimilated to substances addiction, giving rise to the lack of control of impulses, dependence, craving, anxiety, interferences in daily life, in the dream, and/or in personal relationships, among other symptoms [9]. Hence, currently, the problematic use of technologies is considered a social issue, with adolescents and young adults constituting the largest risk group [10–13].

It must be said that adolescence is a period when it is more likely to create dependence on the mobile phone due to the device's almost irresistible characteristics, for instance: autonomy, freedom, identity, social prestige, and entertainment [14]. Although it is true, authors such as Lu et al. [15] suggest that the psychological dependence and abuse created with some of its functionalities are not something exclusive to adolescents. Nevertheless, some other studies indicate that this dependence could affect the adult population [16–19].

Some authors such as De-Sola et al. [20] and Lin [21] have already echoed the need for more studies in other population groups and higher age ranges because there is a lack of awareness about how this device works in them.

On top of that, the difference in use based on gender is another aspect that was analyzed regarding the use of the smartphone. Most studies identify that women use the smartphone much more, and they even have higher levels of addiction [19,22]. Besides, some authors speak of different patterns of use according to gender. Women use the smartphone as an instrument to communicate with others; in contrast, men use it as an instrument for accessing the Internet or gaming [22,23].

Additionally, authors such as Billieux consider the "problematic mobile phones' use" (PMPU) as an inability to regulate the use of mobile phones, which eventually leads to negative consequences in daily life [24]. Studies carried out in Spain find percentages of people with PMPU that vary between 7.99% and 12.5% using different scales [25]. To this end, three different ways were established to define the problematic use of the mobile with its three respective behavior patterns: addictive pattern, antisocial pattern, and risk use pattern. It is necessary to know through validated instruments and semi-structured interviews three aspects of the individual to be catalogued as a user with a real problem: the user profile, the actual use of the device, and the type of problematic use [26]. To achieve the objective of establishing diagnostic criteria for behavioral addictions, it is also necessary to develop reliable and valid measures of these behaviors and regularly assess their psychometric properties, especially because the technological and social trends related to these behaviors change rapidly [8]. Diverse authors designed several instruments to evaluate this problematic use of the mobile phone [25], and even different diagnostic criteria were established for smartphone addiction [27].

Aside from these criteria, self-perception plays an important role in this work. Various authors defined this perception as the process by which people infer their attitudes from their behavior and which refers to the set of evaluations that a person has regarding their abilities [28]. In other words, it is the mental image of oneself. Each person creates it from his or her experiences and needs, and this self-perception is mediated by the circumstances that surround the individual. Escamilla, Córdoba, and Campos [29] consider it a dynamic reality that changes with experience, integrating new data and information, and develops according to social experiences.

In several studies, validated scales asking participants to express their perception regarding the risk indicated or perceived by them are used [30,31]. It is important to emphasize that the degree of problem recognition that anyone has can be related to the valence of the content of their scheme related to consumption [32]. Therefore, self-perception is widely used in different studies as an indicator of disease. In this sense, some factors for it were evaluated, such as the association of self-perception with the dependence on text messages [8], the use/addiction to pornography and personality factors [33], the reasons and barriers in the search for help in gambling problems [34], risk of committing violence [31], alcohol dependence [32,35], and predictors of change in alcohol consumption habits [36]. Even the self-perception of physical health is related as a predictive factor in the use of health services [37] or the degree of participation in endurance sports and self-reported data on self-image, physical and psychological health, and style of life in general [30]. Going further, in other studies, the variable self-perception of health status proves to be a criterion that is strongly related to the presence of chronic diseases [38].

Consequently, this study was performed to establish the cut-off point in the scores of the SPAI–Spain scale [39] related to the self-perceived addiction score indicated by the participants. Besides, the intention is to verify that this criterion variable is better than other measures of dependence, such as the mobile's dedication time.

It is worth highlighting that SPAI is a smartphone addiction screening tool for the adult population, which is already proven to be valid and reliable by research carried out in different countries (China, Italy, Turkey, and Brazil) [40–43]. Its main advantage is its ability to assess aspects as important in other addictions such as compulsive behavior, functional impairment, withdrawal, and tolerance. The authors selected this instrument for its validation in Spanish [39] after carrying out a review of different instruments used to assess mobile addiction [25].

An exploratory study was thereby carried out to establish a cutoff point that allows discrimination between addicted and nonaddicted individuals. Our starting hypothesis is that dependency self-perception is a good indicator of the level of mobile addiction. Therefore, it will be an appropriate criterion to establish this cut-off point.

2. Materials and Methods

2.1. Design

It is a cross-sectional observational study. The data collection instrument (in online format) was distributed among university students by using mailing lists from the University of Valencia's central services as a mean of dissemination after obtaining the permission of the University Rector's office. Data were collected from 5 to 28 April 2017.

The University of Valencia postgraduate studies ethics committee reviewed and approved this study. All the participants gave their written consent to their voluntary and anonymous involvement before completing the inventory.

The inclusion criteria were as follows: age over 17 years old, having a smartphone, and being a student of any discipline at the University of Valencia. The participants were selected using nonprobabilistic convenience sampling. Although the selection of the participants was made by convenience sampling, it must be said that it reflected the reality of the university population.

2.2. Data Collection Instrument

The instrument designed allowed us to collect information about the sociodemographic characteristics of the population, patterns of mobile phone use, and the subjective perception of smartphone dependence, by using a numerical scale (1–10); the SPAI–Spain inventory used for the analysis of smartphone addiction was also included.

The SPAI–Spain instrument [39] shows adequate indices of internal consistency ($\alpha = 0.94$) and consists of 22 items, four less than its original version [41]. Each item is answered by a Likert scale ranging from 1 (strongly agree) to 4 (strongly disagree), obtaining a global score between 22 and 88. The higher the score obtained, the higher the degree of addiction. The original SPAI scale [41] obtained a global Cronbach's alpha of 0.949. Each of its corresponding factors, compulsive behavior, functional impairment, abstinence, and tolerance, obtained the following Cronbach's alpha indexes = 0.856, 0.888, 0.855, and 0.712, respectively. The overall Cronbach's alpha indexes of the SPAI–Spain version [39] were 0.95 for the global scale and 0.87, 0.88, 0.81, and 0.72 for each of its factors.

2.3. *Data Analysis*

Receiver operating characteristics (ROC) analysis was conducted to examine the diagnostic efficacy of the SPAI–Spain for smartphone addiction by using the area under the ROC curve (AUC). Through this analysis, the probability of correctly classifying a subject as an "achiever" of a specific characteristic (sensitivity of the test) was compared with the probability of classifying as "achiever" somebody who was not (1-specificity). This analysis leads to obtaining an optimal cutoff point, from which it was possible to correctly classify the most significant number of subjects [44].

Thus, to obtain a cut-off score of the SPAI–Spain, two variables that measure dependence on the smartphone, self-perception of the dependency and hours of dedication, were used as criterion variables. These two variables were chosen because both obtained high correlations with the final score of the SPAI–Spain, Spearman's r 0.595, and 0.447, respectively.

Self-perception of dependency was evaluated using a Visual Analogical Scale (VAS). The subject was asked to rate their level of dependence from 0 to 10, with 0 being "I do not consider myself dependent on the smartphone at all" and 10 "I consider myself totally dependent on the smartphone." We decided to use a VAS scale to evaluate dependence, in a similar way as this type of scales are used for assess pain levels, thereby being able to evaluate dependence objectively.

The phone usage time was evaluated by asking the subject the number of hours he or she spent using the smartphone daily (less than two hours, between two and four hours, or more than four hours).

Both criterion variables were dichotomized to conduct ROC analysis, considering as "dependent" those subjects who indicated scores between 8 and 10 in the smartphone's dependence self-perception or those who used their phone 4 h or more a day. "Not dependent" subjects were those with scores lower than 8 in the variable smartphone's dependence self-perception or those who used it less than 4 h a day.

The sensitivity, specificity, and Youden's J were calculated for each SPAI–Spain score. The cutoff point for the SPAI–Spain was optimal for smartphone dependence diagnosis when the score was accompanied by the higher Youden's J.

Youden's J is the maximum vertical distance from the ROC curve to the line between (0, 0) and (1, 1). When sensitivity and specificity are equally weighted, the optimal cutoff point is the point with the highest value of J, calculated according to the formula (sensitivity + specificity – 1) [45].

Subsequently, the percentage of false negatives and true positives was assessed using a cross-tabulated table to determine the best criterion variable. Diagnostic accuracy achieved at each score was also calculated.

Analyses were carried out using SPSS Version 24.0. Armonk, NY: IBM Corp. and Microsoft Excel 2010 spreadsheets for Windows.

3. Results

3.1. *Characteristics of the Studied Population*

The SPAI–Spain questionnaire was completed by 2,958 participants whose sociodemographic characteristics, as well as the profile of use of the smartphone, are shown in Table 1.

Table 1. Characteristics of the studied population.

	Mean	SD	*n*	%
Age	27.96	12.13		
18–25			1944	65.7
26–35			408	13.8
36–45			253	8.6
Over 46			353	11.9
Gender				
Men			1025	34.7
Women			1933	65.3
Age When Started Using A Smartphone	17.11	9.27		
Smartphone's Dedication Hours				
<4 (Nondependent)			2062	69.7
≥4 (Dependent)			896	30.3
Smartphone's Dependence Perception				
<8 (Nondependent)			2005	67.8
≥8 (Dependent)			953	32.2

SD: Standard Deviation; *n*: number of participants with this characteristic; %: percentage of participants with this characteristic.

3.2. ROC Analysis Results

The area under the curves is 0.78 [0.763–0.798] by using as a criterion variable the perception of dependence, and 0.699 [0.679–0.719] with the variable dedication time (in hours), as shown in Figures 1 and 2, respectively.

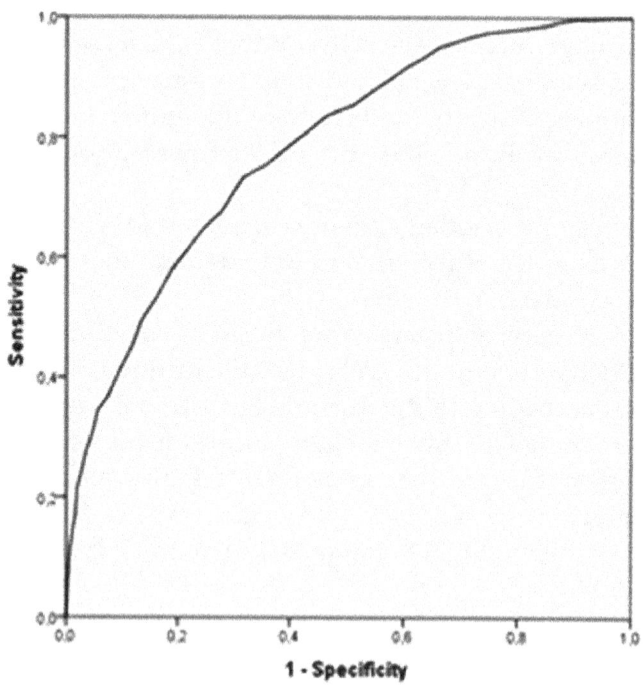

Figure 1. Receiver operating characteristics (ROC) curve. Criterion variable: self-dependence perception.

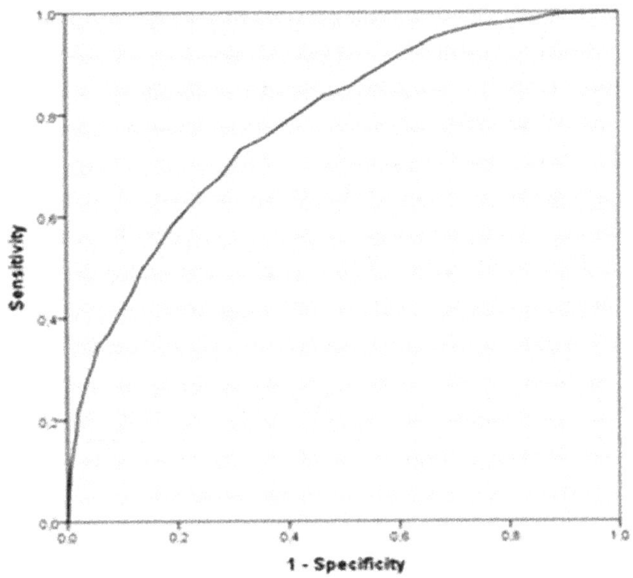

Figure 2. ROC curve. Criterion variable: hours of dedication.

3.3. *SPAI–Spain Cutoff Score Determination*

In order to identify the most suitable cutoff point, the sensitivity and specificity corresponding to each of the scores of the questionnaire for the variable dependence perception and dedication hours, as well as the Youden index, were calculated. It was established that the cutoff point would be the SPAI–Spain score corresponding to the highest value of the Youden index. In the case of dependence self-perception, it was established at score 44 (corresponding to a Youden's J of 0.416). In contrast, in the case of the variable hours of dedication, the cut-off point was established at the value 42 (which corresponds to a Youden's J value of 0.278).

In the supplementary files, we included detailed tables with sensitivity, specificity, positive and negative predictive values, diagnostic accuracy, and Youden's J values for each SPAI–Spain score, according to both external criteria (dependence self-perception and dedication hours).

From these cut-off points identified according to the two established criteria, the percentage of subjects who would be adequately classified with each of said cutoff points was calculated. These results are shown in Table 2.

Table 2. Participant's classification according to their addiction level for the cutoff point for each criterion variable.

		SPAI–Spain: Cut-off point = 44			
		Nondependent		Dependent	
		n	%	*n*	%
Dependence Self-Perception	Nondependent	1371	68.4	632	31.6
	Dependent	255	26.8	698	73.2
		SPAI–Spain: Cut-off point = 42			
		Nondependent		Dependent	
		n	%	*n*	%
Hours of Dedication	Nondependent	1154	56.0	906	44.0
	Dependent	254	28.2	643	71.8

SPAI-Spain: SmartPhone Addiction Inventory Spanish Version; *n*: number of participants with this characteristic.

Although the cutoff point is stricter using the hours of dedication as a criterion variable, the percentage of true positives (dependent–addicts) is higher in the case of the variable self-perception of dependence (73.2% versus 71.8%). Likewise, the percentage of false negatives is higher by using as the variable self-perception of dependence rather than hours of dedication (68.4% versus 56.0%). Subsequently, the score 44 in SPAI–Spain is considered as its cutoff point. It is the one obtained when considering the subjective self-perception of dependence as a criterion since it allows us to classify better both the nondependent subjects and the dependent subjects.

Once the score of 44 (as the cutoff point of the questionnaire) was determined, the percentages of subjects that would be considered as dependent were analyzed, based on characteristics such as the participants' gender and age. These results are shown in Tables 3 and 4.

Table 3. Participant's smartphone dependence according to the variable gender.

		Nondependent		Dependent	
		N	%	*N*	%
Gender	Female	1041	53.9	891	46.1
	Male	585	57.1	439	42.9

Table 4. Participant's smartphone dependence according to the variable age group.

		Nondependent		Dependent	
		N	%	*N*	%
Age Group	18–25	956	49.2	988	50.8
	26–35	240	59.0	167	41.0
	36–45	157	62.1	96	37.9
	Over 46	273	77.6	79	22.4

This analysis of the differences by using the chi-square test allowed us to conclude that there were no statistically significant differences between men and women (chi-square = 2.85 degrees of freedom (df) = 1; $p = 0.09$). However, some significant differences were perceived between age groups (chi-square = 106.68; df = 2; $p < 0.001$).

4. Discussion

In this research, we set out to establish the cutoff point of the SPAI scale validated in Spanish (SPAI–Spain), establishing self-perceived addiction as an external criterion.

The perceived addiction to the smartphone refers to the propensity of a person to report feelings of deregulation and a compulsive device use. In this situation, the focus is on the subjective assessment instead of the objectively measured behaviors, and the focus is on perception, which can be considered as a relevant clinical construct and predicts levels of psychological distress [33].

For this reason, it is understood that the self-perception of dependence on the smartphone, evaluated with the SPAI–Spain scale, can also be a predictor of this addiction. Thus, we divided subjects into "dependent or not dependent" according to their subjective perception, which we have considered an optimal parameter to establish a cutoff point in the SPAI–Spain instrument that could allow researchers to identify those subjects with smartphone addiction. This self-perception of mobile dependence was also measured in other research, such as is this European study performed in 2017. In the study, it emerged that young people in southern Europe (including the Spanish) showed the highest phone usage time, being a predictor of their dependency levels, measured in this case with the Problematic Mobile Phone Use Questionnaire (PMPUQ) [46].

In the validation study of the SPAI–Spain version from which this work for the determination of a cut-off point arises [46], we set out to analyze a series of variables that would serve as comparison criteria with the results of the questionnaire. Among these collected data, we find a subjective criterion, such as the self-perception of mobile addiction, and an objective criterion, such as the number of hours an individual uses the mobile phone. For this reason, we tried to use both measures to establish the cutoff point, finding later that the subjective perception of dependence is a criterion that allows us to predict addiction better than the time the smartphone is used.

The methodology used to establish this cutoff point was based on the determination of the AUC in the ROC curve. Subsequently, the sensitivity (capability to detect addicted individuals), the specificity (capability to detect nonaddicted individuals), and the Youden index for each of the cut points were analyzed, choosing as cutoff that with a higher Youden index [44,47]. This methodology was used in other works in which the objective was to establish this cutoff point from which to establish a classification of the population based on the presence or absence of a specific characteristic, evaluated through any instrument [47–49].

When the self-perception of dependence on the smartphone was used as an external criterion, better diagnostic accuracy values were obtained than when using the criterion of daily hours of smartphone use. Therefore, it also points out that self-perception of dependence was a better indicator than usage hours. Thus, considering that the cutoff point based on the self-perception criterion was the one which allowed us to classify the participants in the study more adequately, it was decided to establish the value 44, which was the one with the highest Youden index (and therefore greater sensitivity).

Using this cut-off point, 23.67% of the participants in the study were classified as dependents to the smartphone. Furthermore, when considering their perception as a descriptor of this dependency, 32.24% of these participants considered themselves as a dependent. These results show how self-perception would be a good predictor of the level of dependence measured by the SPAI-Spain.

The establishment of this cut-off point allowed the identification of those subjects addicted or not addicted to the smartphone. This analysis was also established based on descriptive characteristics of the population, such as gender and age.

As for the analysis of the differences according to gender, this work found a higher percentage of women (53.88%) presented this addiction (although the differences were not statistically significant). In other studies that analyzed these differences, this trend of higher levels of smartphone addiction (or PMPU) in females continues.

In a study carried out in Madrid (Spain) among 1,328 young people, it was found that the estimated prevalence of cell phone dependency was 20% (26.1% in females, 13% in males) [50]. In addition to this, the study by Machado Kouri et al., developed in Brazil, identified female gender as a predictor of mobile addiction [42].

In a study carried out in Belgium and Finland by Lopez-Fernandez et al. [51], women also obtained higher scores in terms of smartphone dependence. The women who participated in the work carried out by Roberts et al. [52] reported using the mobile for longer hours and obtained higher scores on the instrument used to assess cell phone addiction. Also, Choliz et al. showed in two different studies [14,16] that females usually had a higher degree of dependency on mobile phones than did males.

In the case of the differences according to the age of the participants, this study showed statistically significant differences, by finding a higher percentage of mainly younger people who can be classified as addicts.

Most of the research about the excessive use of mobile phones focuses on young people. However, in studies that extend the age of the study population, this greater use or even dependence on mobile phones is also observed in younger people [18]. Thus, for example, the work of Machado Khouri et al. [53], in which subjects between 18 and 35 years of age participated, shows an inverse relationship between age and score in SPAI-BR, and that age between 18 and 25 is a predictive factor of addiction to the mobile. Smetaniuk, in a study with subjects between 18 and 75 years old [54], found significant differences in the score of the instrument used to assess mobile addiction between the different age groups, and the highest scores, indicators of higher addiction levels, were obtained by the youngest subjects, as observed in this work.

Several studies that allude to addiction to the Internet and mobile devices focused on the younger population (even at school age) and tried to identify factors that intervene in the development of this addiction. Some research showed that the younger a subject begins to use these devices, the more likely he or she is to develop addictive behaviors. This fact would explain the lower scores on the SPAI–Spain scale that were obtained in this work by older people who started using their devices at an older age.

It was not possible to compare the cut-off point established for the SPAI-Spain with the versions of the instrument in other languages since only two studies were found that proposed to establish this cutoff point. One of them is the study to develop the short version of the SPAI, with only ten items, instead of the 26 that compose the original instrument. In this study, some diagnostic criteria for smartphone addiction were defined. The cut-off point of the SPAI-SF as well as its capability to classify subjects as dependent and non-dependent, were established through ROC analysis based on the prior defined criteria [49]. There is another study that establishes a cutoff point that uses the Brazilian version of the instrument. In that study, which pinpoints the prevalence of smartphone addiction as an external benchmark for establishing the cut-off point, the researchers consider the 26 elements as dichotomous (yes/no) and establish the cutoff point in seven positive responses [42].

In the development of the original instrument the establishment of a cut-off point from which to define a subject as a dependent was not considered. Moreover, the two studies in which it has been established, the versions of SPAI (or the criteria to establish the cut-off point) are not similar, and also they have been adapted to different populations. All in all makes it difficult to compare the cut-off point established in this work with the other two cut-off points established for different versions of SPAI.

In other versions of the SPAI, such as the Turkish or the Italian one, the establishment of a cut-off point was not considered [40,43]. The study to validate the Iranian version of SPAI alludes to the need to establish a cut point in the instrument, in order to make it a diagnostic instrument, even this cut-off point was not established [54].

The establishment of a cutoff point in the SPAI–Spain instrument, to determine from what score a person could be considered as addicted, allows it to become a diagnostic instrument. An instrument useful to identify subjects with levels of dependence on smartphones and the establishment of measures to prevent/manage addresses this problem. It implies that in the daily practice of health professionals they can use an easy, simple, and manageable tool in the detection of mobile addiction. At the same time, it allows the screening of the general population in the existence of a disorder such as addiction to mobile phones, and thus it can establish therapeutic interventions. On the other hand, it is essential to assess the feeling of self-perception of people regarding their addiction, which will allow their involvement in these therapeutic interventions.

As other researchers claim, problematic mobile use is an evolving public health concern that requires more study to determine the boundary between helpful and harmful technology use [12]. The determination of a risk score can allow future establishment of mobile dependence prevalence studies, as well as the establishment of early detection programs and adequate treatment of this current public health problem.

The information provided by the SPAI–Spain instrument can be highly relevant as a support for researchers and clinicians in the diagnosis and treatment of problematic/addictive use of the smartphone in the adult population. It could be included among the instruments used for evaluating addictive disorders, as well as other tools such as the Münchner Alkoholismus Test (MALT) for the detection of problematic alcohol consumption or the Fagerström tobacco dependence test. As it is a self-administered tool, brief and simple, it can be used in any field of research as a screening method.

Finally, we must not forget that the present work has a series of limitations that we would like to consider.

Regarding the methodology used to establish the cutoff point, although it is the most used for this purpose, we must not forget that the result will depend on the external criterion chosen as the definition of "dependency" (it has been self-perception in this case). Besides, the selection of another external criterion could lead to a different cut point. It must be considered the diversity of criteria, methodological approaches, and lack of conceptual delimitation (abuse, misuse, dependency, and addiction) that guided the various studies related to the PMPU (problematic mobile phone use).

The delimitation of the sample to a university setting could have influenced the high level of studies of the sample and the high percentage of women. It would be interesting to have randomized samples from other populations. The same number of male and female participants in each of the age groups was not recruited. Even so, the participants in our work show a faithful reflection of the population of students at the University of Valencia, with a higher percentage of women, which decreases as the participants' age increases. Besides, we found a percentage of subjects over 45 years old and even over 60 years old, because in this university there is a study program specifically aimed at people over 65 years old.

The means used for the diffusion of the questionnaire and data collection (Internet and email) imply a self-selection bias of the individuals that must also be taken into account. This bias entails that people who use technology regularly and those who use their smartphone more frequently are more likely to have responded.

5. Conclusions

The statistical analysis performed allows the establishment of a cut-off value for the SPAI–SP scale at 44, based on the self-perception of addiction.

The cut-off point established for the SPAI-Spain presents adequate sensitivity and specificity values, as well as adequate diagnostic accuracy.

The establishment of its cut-off point allows the use of the scale as a diagnostic tool to improve the detection and early treatment of addicted persons.

Author Contributions: Conceptualization, M.L.B.-T., A.M.-S., and C.S.-S.; methodology, M.L.B.-T., C.S.-O., and E.C.-S.; formal analysis, M.L.B.-T., and C.S.-O.; data curation, C.C.-A., A.M.-S., M.L.B.-T., C.S.-O., and C.S.-S.; writing—original draft preparation, M.L.B.-T., A.M.-S., and E.C.-S.; writing—review and editing, E.C.-S. and C.C.-A.; supervision, A.M.-S and M.L.B-T. All authors have read and agreed to the published version of the manuscript.

Acknowledgments: We are grateful for permission from the SPAI's authors for its translation and use as well as for the voluntary participation of the University of Valencia members as respondents in this study.

References

1. American Psychiatric Association. *Diagnostic and Statistical Manual of Mental Disorders*, 5th ed.; American Psychiatric Association: Arlington, VA, USA, 2013.
2. Chóliz, M. Historia De Una Adicción: Del Vicio Al Trastorno Del Juego. Cuadernos de medicina psicosomática y psiquiatría de enlace. *Rev. Iberoam. Psicosom.* **2014**, *111*, 84–88.
3. Muñoz-Rivas, M.; Shih, P.C. Abuso de dispositivos móviles. In *Abuso De Internet: Antesala Para La Adicción Al Juego De Azar Online*; Echeburúa, E., Ed.; Pirámide: Madrid, Spain, 2016.
4. Harris, B.; Regan, T.; Schueler, J.; Fields, S.A. Problematic Mobile Phone and Smartphone use Scales: A Systematic Review. *Front. Psychol.* **2020**, *11*, 672. [CrossRef] [PubMed]
5. Griffiths, M. Gambling on the Internet: A Brief Note. *J. Gambl. Stud.* **1996**, *12*, 471–473. [CrossRef] [PubMed]
6. Echeburúa, E. *Adicciones Sin Drogas? Las Nuevas Adicciones: Juego, Sexo, Comida, Compras, Trabajo, Internet*, 2nd ed.; Editorial Desclée de Brouwer: Bilbao, Spain, 2009.

7. Flores Robaina, N.; Jenaro Río, C.; González Gil, F.; Martín, E.; Poy, R. Adicción Al Móvil En Alumnos De Secundaria: Efectos En La Convivencia. *Eur. J. Investig. Health Psychol. Educ.* **2013**, *3*, 215–225. [CrossRef]
8. Liese, B.S.; Benau, E.M.; Atchley, P.; Reed, D.; Becirevic, A.; Kaplan, B. The Self-Perception of Text-Message Dependency Scale (STDS): Psychometric Update Based on a United States Sample. *Am. J. Drug Alcohol Abus.* **2018**, *45*, 42–50. [CrossRef] [PubMed]
9. Lopez-Fernandez, O.; Kuss, D.J.; Pontes, H.M.; Griffiths, M.D.; Dawes, C.; Justice, L.V.; Männikkö, N.; Kääriäinen, M.; Rumpf, H.; Bischof, A.; et al. Measurement Invariance of the Short Version of the Problematic Mobile Phone use Questionnaire (PMPUQ-SV) Across Eight Languages. *Int. J. Environ. Res. Public Health* **2018**, *15*, 1213. [CrossRef]
10. Sasmaz, T.; Oner, S.; Kurt, A.Ö.; Yapici, G.; Yazici, A.E.; Bugdayci, R.; Sis, M. Prevalence and Risk Factors of Internet Addiction in High School Students. *Eur. J. Public Health* **2014**, *24*, 15–20. [CrossRef]
11. Sohn, S.; Rees, P.; Wildridge, B.; Kalk, N.J.; Carter, B. Prevalence of Problematic Smartphone Usage and Associated Mental Health Outcomes Amongst Children and Young People: A Systematic Review, Meta-Analysis and GRADE of the Evidence. *Bmc Psychiatry* **2019**, *19*, 356.
12. Cimino, S.; Cerniglia, L. A Longitudinal Study for the Empirical Validation of an Etiopathogenetic Model of Internet Addiction in Adolescence Based on Early Emotion Regulation. *Biomed Res. Int.* **2018**, *2018*, 4038541–4038548. [CrossRef]
13. Nakayama, H.; Ueno, F.; Mihara, S.; Kitayuguchi, T.; Higuchi, S. Relationship between Problematic Internet use and Age at Initial Weekly Internet Use. *J. Behave. Addict.* **2020**, *9*, 129–139. [CrossRef]
14. Chóliz Montañés, M.; Villanueva Silvestre, V. *Evaluación De La Adicción Al Móvil En La Adolescencia. Rev. Esp. Drogodep*; Departamento de Psicología Básica. Universidad de Valencia: Valencia, Spain, 2011; pp. 165–183.
15. Lu, X.; Watanabe, J.; Liu, Q.; Uji, M.; Shono, M.; Kitamura, T. Internet and Mobile Phone Text-Messaging Dependency: Factor Structure and Correlation with Dysphoric Mood among Japanese Adults. *Comput. Hum. Behav.* **2011**, *27*, 1702–1709. [CrossRef]
16. Chóliz, M.; Pinto, L.; Phansalkar, S.; Corr, E.; Mujjahid, A.; Flores, C.; Barrientos, P. Development of a Brief Multicultural Version of the Test of Mobile Phone Dependence (TMDbrief) Questionnaire. *Front. Psychol.* **2016**, *7*, 650.
17. Körmendi, A.; Brutóczki, Z.; Petra Végh, B.; Székely, R. Smartphone use can be Addictive? A Case Report. *J. Behav. Addict.* **2016**, *5*, 548–552. [CrossRef] [PubMed]
18. Kwon, M.; Lee, J.; Won, W.; Park, J.; Min, J.; Hahn, C.; Gu, X.; Choi, J.; Kim, D. Development and Validation of a Smartphone Addiction Scale (SAS). *PLoS ONE* **2013**, *8*, e56936. [CrossRef] [PubMed]
19. Long, J.; Liu, T.; Liao, Y.; Qi, C.; He, H.; Chen, S.; Billieux, J. Prevalence and Correlates of Problematic Smartphone use in a Large Random Sample of Chinese Undergraduates. *BMC Psychiatry* **2016**, *16*, 408. [CrossRef] [PubMed]
20. De-Sola Gutiérrez, J.; Rodríguez de Fonseca, F.; Rubio, G. Cell-Phone Addiction: A Review. *Front. Psychiatry* **2016**, *7*, 175. [CrossRef]
21. Lin, J.C. Popularity, Funding for Health-Effect Research and Cell-Phone Addiction. *Ap-M* **2010**, *52*, 164–166. [CrossRef]
22. Ivanova, A.; Gorbaniuk, O.; Błachnio, A.; Przepiórka, A.; Mraka, N.; Polishchuk, V.; Gorbaniuk, J. Mobile Phone Addiction, Phubbing, and Depression among Men and Women: A Moderated Mediation Analysis. *Psychiatr. Q.* **2020**. [CrossRef]
23. Fischer-Grote, L.; Kothgassner, O.D.; Felnhofer, A. Risk Factors for Problematic Smartphone use in Children and Adolescents: A review of Existing Literature. *Neuropsychiatr. Klin. Diagn. Ther. Rehabil. Organ Ges. Osterr. Nervenarzte Psychiater* **2019**, *33*, 179–190. [CrossRef]
24. Billieux, J. Problematic use of the Mobile Phone: A Literature Review and a Pathways Model. *Curr. Psychiatry Rev.* **2012**, *15*, 142. [CrossRef]
25. Simó Sanz, C.; Martinez Sabater, A.; Ballestar Tarín, M.; Domínguez Romero, A. Instrumentos De Evaluación Del Uso Problemático Del Teléfono Móvil/Smartphone. *Health Addict. Salud Y Drog.* **2017**, *17*, 5. [CrossRef]
26. Billieux, J.; Maurage, P.; Lopez-Fernandez, O.; Kuss, D.; Griffiths, M. Can Disordered Mobile Phone use be Considered a Behavioral Addiction? an Update on Current Evidence and a Comprehensive Model for Future Research. *Curr. Addict. Rep.* **2015**, *2*, 156–162. [CrossRef]
27. Lin, Y.; Chiang, C.; Lin, P.; Chang, L.; Ko, C.; Lee, Y.; Lin, S. Proposed Diagnostic Criteria for Smartphone Addiction. *PLoS ONE* **2016**, *11*, e0163010. [CrossRef]

28. Becerra Álvarez, D.R.; Delgado Martínez, A.C.; Villamizar Acevedo, G.A. Autopercepción De Estudiantes De Psicología Sobre Sus Competencias En Los Campos Laboral, Educativo Y Salud. *Rexe Rev. Estud. Exp. Educ.* **2014**, *13*, 151–167.
29. Escamilla Cruz, S.; Campos Castolo, M.; Córdoba Ávila, M.Á. Autopercepción De Competencias Profesionales De Alumnos De La Licenciatura En Enfermería. *Rev. Conamed* **2012**, *17*, 67–75.
30. Kirkcaldy, B.D.; Shephard, R.J.; Siefen, R.G. The Relationship between Physical Activity and Self-Image and Problem Behaviour among Adolescents. *Soc. Psychiatry Psychiatr. Epidemiol.* **2002**, *37*, 544–550. [CrossRef]
31. Lockertsen, Ø.; Procter, N.; Vatnar, S.K.B.; Færden, A.; Eriksen, B.M.S.; Roaldset, J.O.; Varvin, S. Screening for Risk of Violence using Service Users' Self-perceptions: A Prospective Study from an Acute Mental Health Unit. *Int. J. Ment. Health Nurs.* **2018**, *27*, 1055–1065. [CrossRef]
32. Domenico, L.H.; Strobbe, S.; Stein, K.F.; Giordani, B.J.; Hagerty, B.M.; Pressler, S.J. Identifying the Structure and Effect of Drinking-Related Self-Schemas. *West. J. Nurs. Res.* **2017**, *39*, 942–981. [CrossRef]
33. Grubbs, J.B.; Wilt, J.A.; Exline, J.J.; Pargament, K.I.; Kraus, S.W. Moral Disapproval and Perceived Addiction to Internet Pornography: A Longitudinal Examination. *Addiction* **2018**, *113*, 496–506. [CrossRef]
34. Suurvali, H.; Hodgins, D.; Toneatto, T.; Cunningham, J. Motivators for Seeking Gambling-Related Treatment among Ontario Problem Gamblers. *J. Gambl. Stud.* **2012**, *28*, 273–296. [CrossRef]
35. Agrawal, A.; Dick, D.M.; Bucholz, K.K.; Madden, P.A.F.; Cooper, M.L.; Sher, K.J.; Heath, A.C. Drinking Expectancies and Motives: A Genetic Study of Young Adult Women. *Addiction* **2008**, *103*, 194–204. [CrossRef] [PubMed]
36. Zins, M.; Carle, F.; Bugel, I.; Leclerc, A.; Orio, F.D.; Goldberg, M. Predictors of Change in Alcohol Consumption among Frenchmen of the GAZEL Study Cohort. *Addiction* **1999**, *94*, 385–395. [CrossRef] [PubMed]
37. Fleury, M.; Ngui, A.N.; Bamvita, J.; Grenier, G.; Caron, J. Predictors of Healthcare Service Utilization for Mental Health Reasons. *Int. J. Environ. Res. Public Health* **2014**, *11*, 10559–10586. [CrossRef] [PubMed]
38. Acosta, L.D.; Carrizo, E.D.; Pelaez, E. Factores Asociados a La Autopercepción De Salud En Adultos Mayores. *Rev. Cuba. Salud Pública* **2015**, *41*, 638–648.
39. Simó-Sanz, C.; Ballestar-Tarín, M.L.; Martínez-Sabater, A. Smartphone Addiction Inventory (SPAI): Translation, Adaptation and Validation of the Tool in Spanish Adult Population. *PLoS ONE* **2018**, *13*, e0205389. [CrossRef]
40. Arpaci, I.; Esgi, N. Psychometric Properties of the Turkish Version of the Smartphone Addiction Inventory (SPAI). *Curr. Psychol.* **2018**, 1–6. [CrossRef]
41. Lin, Y.; Chang, L.; Lee, Y.; Tseng, H.; Kuo, T.B.J.; Chen, S. Development and Validation of the Smartphone Addiction Inventory (SPAI). *PLoS ONE* **2014**, *9*, e98312. [CrossRef]
42. Machado Khoury, J.; Corrêa de Freitas, A.A.; Valente Roque, M.A.; Rodrigues Albuquerque, M.; Maila de Castro, L.N.; Duarte Garcia, F. Assessment of the Accuracy of a New Tool for the Screening of Smartphone Addiction. *PloS ONE* **2017**, *12*, e0176924. [CrossRef]
43. Pavia, L.; Cavani, P.; Di Blasi, M.; Giordano, C. Smartphone Addiction Inventory (SPAI): Psychometric Properties and Confirmatory Factor Analysis. *Comput. Hum. Behav.* **2016**, *63*, 170–178. [CrossRef]
44. Streiner, D.L.; Cairney, J. What's Under the ROC? an Introduction to Receiver Operating Characteristics Curves. *Can. J. Psychiatry* **2007**, *52*, 121–128. [CrossRef] [PubMed]
45. Perkins, N.J.; Schisterman, E.F. The Inconsistency of "Optimal" Cutpoints obtained using Two Criteria Based on the Receiver Operating Characteristic Curve. *Am. J. Epidemiol.* **2006**, *163*, 670–675. [CrossRef] [PubMed]
46. Lopez-Fernandez, O.; Kuss, D.J.; Romo, L.; Morvan, Y.; Kern, L.; Graziani, P.; Rousseau, A.; Rumpf, H.; Bischof, A.; GÄSSLER, A.; et al. Self-Reported Dependence on Mobile Phones in Young Adults: A European Cross-Cultural Empirical Survey. *J. Behav. Addict.* **2017**, *6*, 168–177. [CrossRef] [PubMed]
47. Cerda, J.; Cifuentes, L. Using ROC Curves in Clinical Investigation: Theoretical and Practical Issues. *Rev. Chil. Infectol. Organo Of. Soc. Chil. Infectol.* **2012**, *29*, 138–141. [CrossRef] [PubMed]
48. Nanishi, K.; Green, J.; Taguri, M.; Jimba, M. Determining a Cut-Off Point for Scores of the Breastfeeding Self-Efficacy Scale–Short Form: Secondary Data Analysis of an Intervention Study in Japan. *PLoS ONE* **2015**, *10*, e0129698. [CrossRef] [PubMed]
49. Lin, Y.; Pan, Y.; Lin, S.; Chen, S. Development of Short-Form and Screening Cutoff Point of the Smartphone Addiction Inventory (SPAI-SF). *Int. J. Methods Psychiatr. Res.* **2017**, *26*, e1525. [CrossRef] [PubMed]
50. Sánchez-Martínez, M.; Otero, A. Factors Associated with Cell Phone use in Adolescents in the Community of Madrid (Spain). *Cyberpsychol. Behav.* **2009**, *12*, 131–137. [CrossRef]

51. Lopez-Fernandez, O.; Männikkö, N.; Kääriäinen, M.; Griffiths, M.D.; Kuss, D.J. Mobile Gaming and Problematic Smartphone use: A Comparative Study between Belgium and Finland. *J. Behave. Addict.* **2018**, *7*, 88–99. [CrossRef]
52. Roberts, J.A.; Yaya, L.H.P.; Manolis, C. The Invisible Addiction: Cell-Phone Activities and Addiction among Male and Female College Students. *J. Behav. Addict.* **2014**, *3*, 254–265. [CrossRef]
53. Machado Khoury, J.; Maila de Castro, L.N.; Valente Roque, M.A.; Correa de Freitas, A.A.; Ralil da Costa, M.; Duarte Garcia, F. Smartphone and Facebook Addictions Share Common Risk and Prognostic Factors in a Sample of Undergraduate Students. *Trends Psychiatry Psychother.* **2019**, *41*, 358–368. [CrossRef]
54. Smetaniuk, P. A Preliminary Investigation into the Prevalence and Prediction of Problematic Cell Phone Use. *J. Behav. Addict.* **2014**, *3*, 41–53. [CrossRef]

14

Parental Monitoring and Adolescent Problematic Mobile Phone Use: The Mediating Role of Escape Motivation and the Moderating Role of Shyness

Xinchen Fu [1], Jingxuan Liu [2], Ru-De Liu [1,*], Yi Ding [3], Jia Wang [4], Rui Zhen [5] and Fangkai Jin [1]

1 Beijing Key Laboratory of Applied Experimental Psychology, National Demonstration Center for Experimental Psychology Education (Beijing Normal University), Faculty of Psychology, Beijing Normal University, Beijing 100875, China; fxc_psy@163.com (X.F.); jfk2016@163.com (F.J.)
2 Department of Psychology and Neuroscience, Duke University, Durham, NC 27708, USA; liujingxuan1503@gmail.com
3 Graduate School of Education, Fordham University, New York, NY 10023, USA; yding4@fordham.edu
4 Teachers' College, Beijing Union University, Beijing 100011, China; wangjia@mail.bnu.edu.cn
5 Institute of Psychological Sciences, College of Education, Hangzhou Normal University, No. 2318 Yuhangtang Road, Hangzhou 311121, China; zhenrui1206@126.com
* Correspondence: rdliu@bnu.edu.cn

Abstract: In an attempt to reduce the negative consequences of adolescent media use, parents often monitor their children's online activities. However, research suggests that parental monitoring often does not reduce children's problematic mobile phone use as expected. Based on the results of a survey of 584 Chinese adolescents, we found that parental monitoring positively predicted children's problematic mobile phone use (PMPU) within a Chinese cultural context. The results also showed that children's escape motivation partially mediated this relationship, while their level of shyness moderated both the mediated path and the direct impact of parental monitoring on children's PMPU. The findings suggested that a higher level of shyness increased the likelihood that parental monitoring would increase the child's escape motivation and PMPU. The study results provide guidelines for parents and educators regarding interventions for adolescents' problematic phone use.

Keywords: parental monitoring; problematic mobile phone use; escape motivation; shyness

1. Introduction

Mobile phones are the most common platform used by adolescents to access the internet. In Europe, adolescents use mobile phones more frequently than they do computers to access online information [1]. In China, 98.6% of internet users, or 817 million people, of whom 18% are adolescents, connect to the internet through mobile phones [2]. Some common internet activities adolescents engage in via mobile phones are socializing [3,4], accessing entertainment [5,6], and obtaining study resources [7].

Because mobile phones offer such a wide range of attractions, some adolescents overuse their mobile phones, which can lead to problematic mobile phone use (PMPU) [8,9]. PMPU, also known as mobile phone dependency [10] and mobile phone addiction [11], can elicit unpleasant withdrawal symptoms when an individual's mobile phone access is restricted. Studies have found that adolescents are more prone to mobile phone addiction than adults [12,13].

Considering the wide range of negative health and psychological consequences of PMPU for adolescents [14–16], parents often mediate their child's mobile phone use in an attempt to reduce PMPU. One type of mediation strategy used frequently by parents, parental monitoring, has drawn wide social attention [17]. Parental monitoring refers to parents' tracking of children's online activities [18] and is often thought by parents to be an effective way to prevent their child's PMPU. However, research has shown that parental monitoring may not reduce adolescent PMPU behaviors as expected [8,19,20]. Therefore, the current study aimed to further explore the impact of parental monitoring on children's problematic mobile phone use and to investigate the mechanism underlying such an impact in the Chinese cultural context.

1.1. *Parental Monitoring and Problematic Mobile Phone Use (PMPU)*

PMPU is a type of behavioral addiction [21,22]. It can produce a series of negative health and psychological consequences, such as sleep problems and physical harm [16,23]; decreased level of physical activity [24,25]; social problems [16]; decreased life satisfaction [26]; academic problems [15,27–29]; anxiety when separated from mobile phones [30,31]; negative emotions including stress, anxiety, and depression [14,32]; alexithymia [33,34]; and decreased empathy [26].

In an attempt to reduce the negative effects of children's media use, parents often adopt different mediation strategies to influence their child's media-use behaviors [35]. Parental mediation is a multi-dimensional concept. It encompasses all types of parental strategies, including mediation, controlling, and providing instruction and interpretation regarding media content, to reduce the negative effect of media use on children [36]. Parental mediation was originally divided into three dimensions: restrictive mediation, active mediation, and co-use [37]. These three dimensions were found to be present in parental mediation of children's TV viewing [38,39], gaming [40], and internet use behaviors [35]. However, as internet use became more prevalent among adolescents, researchers suggested that the traditional three dimensions needed to be expanded to further address parental strategies regarding children's internet use behaviors [17,41,42]. Nikken and Jansz [18] proposed a five-dimensional model, in which the restrictive mediation dimension was divided into time restriction and special content restriction, and supervision (i.e., monitoring) was added as a new dimension. Parental monitoring refers to parents' tracking of their child's online activities and history, such as email interactions and website access [17,18,20].

Parental monitoring is the most common mediation strategy for adolescent internet use [43] and can predict adolescent internet-use behaviors [44]. Yet surprisingly, many studies have found that parental monitoring is ineffective in reducing those problematic behaviors. Livingstone and Helsper [17] found that parental monitoring failed to reduce risky online behaviors (such as porn, violence, and privacy viewing) in children aged 9–16 years; a follow-up study showed that parental monitoring was positively correlated with increased internet-related risk [45]. Studies also found that parental monitoring positively predicted children's internet-use behaviors [44] and adolescent internet addiction [46]. In addition, cross-cultural research conducted by Bayraktar [47] found that whereas parental monitoring was negatively correlated with adolescent risky internet-use behaviors (such as porn, viewing violence and excessive internet use) in Europe, it positively predicted adolescent involvement in such risky behaviors in Turkey. With increased adolescent access to the internet via mobile phones, parental monitoring of internet use has evolved to monitoring of internet-related mobile phone-use behaviors [48]. A study conducted in Germany [19] found the correlation between parental monitoring and adolescent mobile phone dependency to be insignificant: Parental monitoring was inefficient in reducing the negative effects of children's PMPU. Similar results were obtained in Taiwan [8]. These study results suggested that parental monitoring may not reduce children's PMPU. The first goal of our study was to examine whether parental monitoring was related to or positively predicted adolescent PMPU.

1.2. *Mediating Role of Escape Motivation*

Parental monitoring refers to parental supervision of children's internet use behaviors with the aim to reduce the negative impacts of media use [48]. Why would parental monitoring perpetuate children's PMPU behaviors instead of reducing them? The underlying mechanism warrants further investigation. Based on the existing theories and study results, we hypothesized that escape motivation might mediate the path between parental monitoring and children's PMPU.

Within the context of adolescent PMPU, escape motivation refers to the motivation that drives adolescents to escape negative emotions via mobile phone use, leading to PMPU [49]. Escaping reality is one of two major functions of PMPU [50]. In many cases, the underlying motivation of addictive behaviors is to escape reality in an effort to reduce painful and negative emotions [51]. Among all types of motivation, escape motivation is often thought to be the most important predictor of internet addiction; it serves as a strong predictor for a wide range of internet and mobile phone-related addictions, including internet addiction [52–54], video game addiction [55,56], online game addiction [57,58], online video apps overuse (i.e., YouTube) [59], and PMPU [60–62].

Parental monitoring can also induce negative emotions in adolescents. According to the self-determination theory, all humans strive for freedom, and therefore their motivation is optimal when they are void of external influence and interference [63]. Thus, when children's freedom is restricted, they may experience reactance [64]. Some studies have already examined the mediating roles of escape motivation in the relations between negative emotions, addictive behaviors, and PMPU. For example, escape motivation was found to mediate the relation between psychological distress (such as emotional imbalance, depression, and anxiety) and video game addiction [65,66] and the relation between psychiatric disorders (such as somatization and OCD) and video game addiction [67]. Escape motivation was also found to mediate the path from loneliness to PMPU [67]. Accordingly, parental monitoring may result in conflicts between parents and child, and thus cause the child to experience stress and negative emotions. As a result, through escape motivation, the child's mobile phone-use behaviors might increase [68,69], leading to PMPU [62].

1.3. *Moderating Role of Shyness*

When choosing mediation strategies to reduce children's PMPU, parents should take their child's temperament into consideration [70]. Shyness, one of the most stable temperament types, should be given special attention [71].

Shyness is a common social experience that involves timidity, discomfort, embarrassment, and fear of being evaluated. It is often accompanied by a desire to minimize social interactions [72–74]. Research suggests that shyness can induce a series of negative consequences, including loneliness [75], anxiety, and depression [76,77]. To reduce or avoid those negative consequences, shy individuals often view online communication as a means to avoid face-to-face interaction [77]. An individual's degree of shyness can positively predict online social activities [78] and internet addictive behaviors [79,80]. Such a predictive effect was shown to be consistent over time [81]. Similarly, many studies suggest that shy individuals increase their mobile phone use to avoid face-to-face contact, which leads to PMPU [82–84].

Research concerning parenting styles suggests that parents should adopt adaptive parenting that is suitable to their child's temperament [85]. Studies have found that inhibitive temperament (similar to shyness) mediates the relation between maternal authoritative parenting and girls' prosocial behaviors [86]. Zarra-Nezhad et al. [87] discovered that parental emotional support positively predicted prosocial behavior only among shy children, while parental control positively predicted prosocial behaviors only among children who were not shy. Because parental mediation strategies are similar to parenting styles to some degree [88], parental monitoring of children's mobile phone use should be similar to parental control. Thus, it could be inferred that parental monitoring exerts different effects based on the shyness level of a child. Furthermore, a study [89] showed that shyness also predicts an individual's drinking motivation; shy individuals are more inclined to reduce their negative emotions and navigate social contexts via drinking, which can eventually lead to alcohol addiction. This suggests that shyness is related to behavioral motivation. Therefore, we hypothesized that parental monitoring would positively predict more escape motivation for shy adolescents than for those who are not shy.

1.4. *The Present Study*

Based on the above, the present study aimed to investigate the mechanism and impact of parental monitoring on adolescent PMPU through a hypothesized moderated mediation model (Figure 1). We anticipated that (a) parental monitoring would positively predict adolescent PMPU (H1) via the mediation of escape motivation (H2), and (b) adolescent level of shyness would moderate the impact of parental monitoring on adolescent escape motivation (H3) and PMPU (H4).

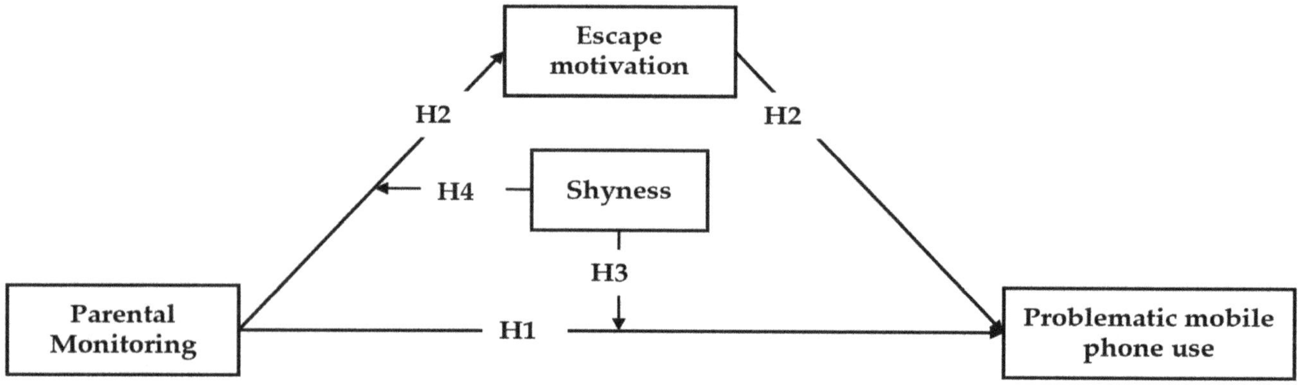

Figure 1. The hypothesized model.

2. Materials and Methods

2.1. *Participants*

In the present study, we contacted an urban middle school in Beijing, China, and informed them of the purpose of our study. All students recruited in grades 7, 8, 10, and 11 were voluntary to participate. A total of 584 students were recruited. The mean age of these participants was 16.13 years (standard deviation (SD) = 2.80) with a range from 13 to 18; 267 (45.7%) were boys, 281 (49.0%) were girls, and 31 (5.3%) did not report gender. Among these students, 23.3% of fathers and 25.8% of mothers received a high-school education or below and 76.7% of fathers and 74.2% of mothers received an undergraduate level of education or above.

2.2. *Procedures*

We obtained the approval to conduct the study from the Research Ethics Committee of a major research university in Beijing and the principals of the participating schools. The students were informed of the voluntary nature of this study and their right to opt out at any time during the course of the study. Then, they were asked to complete a paper-pencil questionnaire that included demographic information, Parental Monitoring, Escape Motivation, Shyness and Problematic mobile phone-use measures.

2.3. *Measures*

2.3.1. Parental Monitoring

Parental monitoring was assessed by the Parental Mediation of Children's Internet Use Scale [18], which was validated in Chinese and exhibited satisfactory reliability and validity [90]. In this study, the word "internet use" was changed to "mobile phone use" to assess parental monitoring of children's mobile phone-use behaviors. The scale included four items (e.g., "My parents check my mobile phone use behaviors; My parents check my mobile phone chatting records; My parents keep an eye on me when I use mobile phone") on a 5-point Likert scale (1 = *never*, 5 = *always*). Higher scores reflected higher levels of parent monitoring of children's mobile phone use. Cronbach's α for the present study was 0.892.

2.3.2. Escape Motivation

Escape motivation was assessed by the Mobile Phone-Use Motivations Scale [49]. It consisted of six items (e.g., I use/play with my smartphone to feel less lonely; to fill uncomfortable silence; to make myself feel better when I feel down) using a 5-point scale ranging from 1 (*strongly disagree*) to 5 (*strongly agree*); higher scores indicated a higher degree of escape motivation. This measure yielded a Cronbach's α of 0.865 in the present study.

2.3.3. Shyness

Shyness was assessed by the Shyness Scale [72], which was validated in Chinese and showed satisfactory reliability and validity [91]. This scale included 13 items (e.g., I have trouble looking someone right in the eye; I feel tense when I'm with people I don't know well; I feel inhibited in social situations.) on a 5-point Likert scale, ranging from 1 (*strongly disagree*) to 5 (*strongly agree*), with higher scores indicating a higher degree of shyness. Cronbach's α for the scale was 0.803 in the present study.

2.3.4. Problematic Mobile Phone Use (PMPU)

Problematic mobile phone use (PMPU) was assessed by the Problematic Mobile Phone-Use Scale [92], which was translated into Chinese and proved to be valid [93]. It consisted of 10 items (e.g., I find it difficult to switch off my mobile phone; I feel anxious if I have not checked for messages or switched on my mobile phone for some time; I find myself engaged on the mobile phone for longer periods of time than intended) on a 5-point scale that ranged from 1 (*strongly disagree*) to 5 (*strongly agree*), with higher scores indicating a higher degree of problematic mobile phone use. Cronbach's α for the present study was 0.821.

2.3.5. Statistical Analysis

We conducted descriptive analyses and Pearson correlations with SPSS 22.0 (IBM, New York, NY, USA). The pattern of missing data was first evaluated. The results showed that 1.25% of the data was missing, and the missing rates on all variables were less than 10%. Therefore, we used the listwise method to handle the missing data in the following structural equation model [94]. Among the 583 participants, 518 provided complete data on all the variables. Next, the moderated mediation model was tested using the SPSS macro PROCESS 3.0 (model 8) (http://www.afhayes.com) recommended by Hayes [95]. We generated 5000 bootstrapped samples to estimate the confidence interval of the model effect. A 95% confidence interval without zero indicates statistical significance.

3. Results

3.1. Preliminary Analyses

The descriptive statistics and correlation matrix are presented in Table 1. Parental monitoring was positively correlated with children's escape motivation, shyness, and PMPU. Children's escape motivation was positively correlated with their shyness level and PMPU. Children's shyness level was positively correlated with PMPU.

Table 1. Means, standard deviations, and correlations between variables.

Variables	M	SD	1	2	3	4	5
1. Age	16.13	2.80	–				
2. Parental monitoring	2.06	1.14	0.114 **	–			
3. Escape motivation	2.86	1.05	−0.023	0.122 **	–		
4. Shyness	2.75	0.70	−0.031	0.135 **	0.147 ***	–	
5. PMPU	2.45	0.76	−0.092 *	0.163 ***	0.607 ***	0.213 ***	–

Note. PMPU = Problematic Mobile Phone Use. * $p < 0.05$. ** $p < 0.01$. *** $p < 0.001$.

3.2. Testing for the Proposed Model

The analysis results of SPSS macro PROCESS are presented in Table 2, which consists of four parts: Model 1, Model 2, conditional indirect effect analysis of Model 1, and conditional direct effect analysis of Model 2. Model 1 was used to test the effects of parental monitoring on children's escape motivation (part of H2), and the interaction between parental monitoring and children's shyness on children's escape motivation (H4), after controlling for age and gender. Model 2 examined the effects of parental monitoring on children's PMPU (H1), children's escape motivation on children's PMPU (part of H2), and the interaction between parental monitoring and children's shyness on children's PMPU (H3).

Table 2. Bootstrap test on moderated mediation effect.

Conditional Process Analysis	β	*SE*	*t*	*p*	*LLCI–ULCI*
Model 1					
Outcome: Escape motivation					
Predictors:					
Age	−0.009	0.014	−0.668	0.505	−0.037–0.018
Gender	0.150	0.079	1.902	0.058	−0.005–0.305
Parental monitoring	0.101 *	0.042	2.392	0.017	0.018–0.183
Shyness	0.129 **	0.041	3.164	0.002	0.050–0.209
Monitoring × Shyness	0.102 *	0.041	2.474	0.014	0.021–0.183
Model 2					
Outcome: PMPU					
Predictors:					
Age	−0.031 **	0.012	−2.672	0.008	−0.054–0.008
Gender	−0.156 *	0.066	−2.352	0.019	−0.287–0.026
Parental monitoring	0.078 *	0.035	2.198	0.028	0.008–0.148
Escape motivation	0.612 ***	0.035	17.571	0.000	0.544–0.681
Shyness	0.124 ***	0.035	3.582	0.000	0.056–0.191
Monitoring × Shyness	0.063 +	0.035	1.806	0.071	−0.005–0.131
Conditional indirect effect analysis of model 1			β	*Boot SE*	*BootLLCI-BootULCI*
M − 1 SD			0.007	0.060	−0.111–0.125
M			0.103 *	0.042	0.021–0.186
M + 1 SD			0.188 ***	0.051	0.087–0.289
Conditional direct effect analysis of model 2			β	*Boot SE*	*BootLLCI-BootULCI*
M − 1 SD			0.020	0.050	−0.079–0.119
M			0.080 *	0.035	0.010–0.149
M + 1 SD			0.132 **	0.044	0.046–0.217

Note. Bootstrap sample size = 5000. SE = standard error, LL = low limit, CI = confidence interval, UL = upper limit. + $p < 0.10$. * $p < 0.05$. ** $p < 0.01$. *** $p < 0.001$.

The conditional indirect effect analysis of Model 1 tested the effects of parental monitoring at its mean, plus one, and minus one standard deviation on children's escape motivation at the mean of shyness. The conditional direct effect analysis of Model 2 tested the effects of parental monitoring at its mean, plus one standard deviation, and minus one standard deviation on children's PMPU at the mean of the shyness. According to Model 1 ($F = 5.96$, $R^2 = 0.05$, $p < 0.001$) and Model 2 ($F = 65.74.45$, $R^2 = 0.41$, $p < 0.001$), after controlling for gender and age, parental monitoring positively predicted children's PMPU ($\beta = 0.078$, $p < 0.05$), supporting H1 (see Figure 2). Parental monitoring positively predicted children's escape motivation ($\beta = 0.101$, $p < 0.05$), and children's escape motivation positively predicted children's PMPU ($\beta = 0.612$, $p < 0.001$), supporting H2.

The interaction of parental monitoring and shyness showed significant effects on children's escape motivation ($\beta = 0.102$, $p < 0.05$). Thus, H4 was supported. This finding suggests that the relation between parental monitoring and children's escape motivation was moderated by children's level of shyness (see Figure 3). In addition, two of the three conditional indirect effects (based on the moderator values at the mean and at plus and minus one standard deviation) were positive and significantly different from zero (see conditional indirect effect analysis of Model 1). That is, according to the interaction of parental monitoring and children's shyness, the indirect effects of parental monitoring on children's escape motivation were stronger when children's shyness level was moderate to high, but lower when children's shyness level was low.

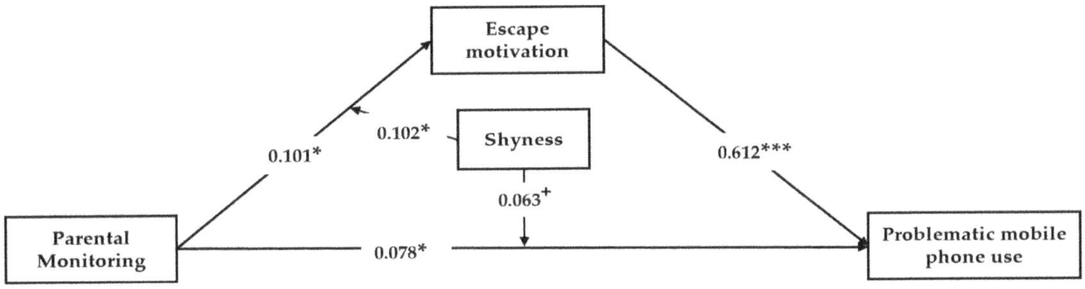

Figure 2. Moderation effects of shyness in the mediation model. All values shown are standardized coefficients. $^{+}$ $p < 0.10$. * $p < 0.05$. *** $p < 0.001$.

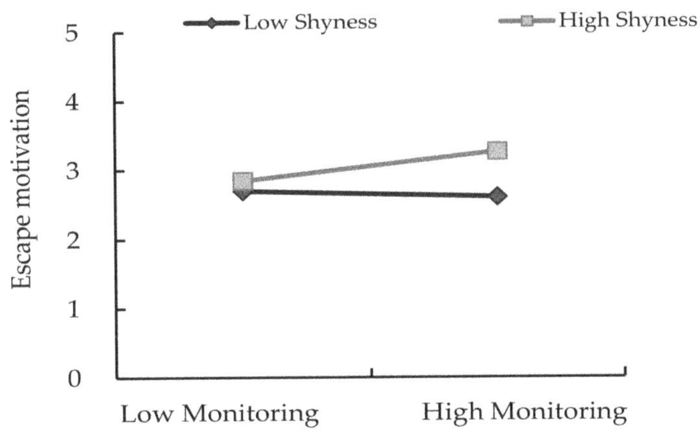

Figure 3. Moderation effect of shyness in the relation between parental monitoring and children's escape motivation.

Furthermore, the interaction of parental monitoring and shyness showed marginally significant effects on children's PMPU ($\beta = 0.063$, $p < 0.10$). Therefore, H3 was supported. Two of the three conditional direct effects (based on the moderator values at the mean and at plus and minus one standard deviation) were positive and significantly different from zero (see conditional direct effect analysis of Model 2). These findings suggest that the relation between parental monitoring and children's PMPU was moderated by children's level of shyness (see Figure 4). The direct effects of parental monitoring on children's PMPU were higher when children's shyness was moderate to high, but lower when children's shyness was low. In conclusion, the above results indicated that parental monitoring affects children's PMPU through a moderated mediation path, with children's escape motivation as the mediator and children's shyness level as the moderator.

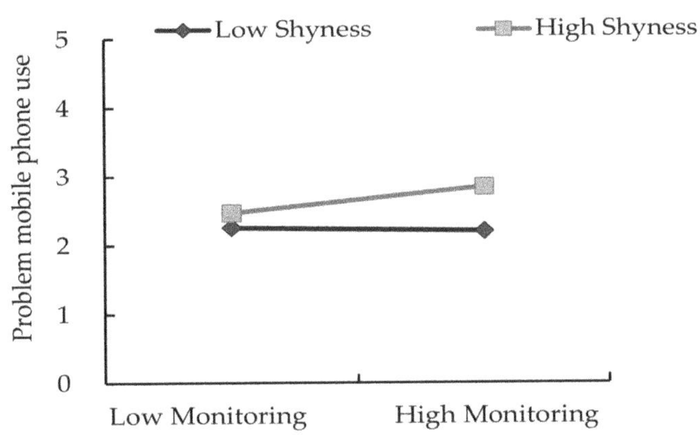

Figure 4. Moderation effect of shyness the relation between parental monitoring and children's PMPU.

4. Discussion

To reduce the negative impact of children's mobile phone use, parental monitoring has not achieved consistent results [45,48]; its underlying mechanism remains unclear. The present study examined a moderated mediation model and found that children's escape motivation partially mediated the association of parental monitoring and their PMPU. In addition, children's degree of shyness moderated the path from parental monitoring to their escape motivation and to PMPU.

4.1. Escape Motivation Partially Mediates the Relation between Parental Monitoring and Adolescent PMPU

Parental monitoring positively correlated with adolescent PMPU, which supports H1. This is consistent with the findings of previous studies regarding internet addiction [46]. Research has shown that adolescents are especially vulnerable to the negative impacts of increased mobile phone use, and parents hope to reduce these negative influences via mediation. Considering that teenage years are a critical period of learning and social development, most parents employ monitoring strategies to mediate their children's mobile phone use. However, research findings suggest that parental monitoring often leads to unexpected results. Because of adolescents' desire for freedom and psychological reactance induced by restriction, they may be subjected to the "Pandora effect" [63,68,96]; as the strength of parental monitoring of mobile phone use increases, adolescents' mobile phone-use behaviors also increase, which can eventually lead to PMPU. Similar results were found in other areas of addiction, including adolescent internet addiction [97], internet dependency [98], and sexual behaviors [99]. From the perspective of the sociology of emotions, emotions serve as an important precursor to effective parental mediation. However, parental monitoring often results in the conflicts between parents and child, causing negative emotions. The model of compensatory internet use suggests that internet use is viewed as a compensatory means to escape the reality. An individual with relatively low overall happiness tends to relieve negative emotions and escape from real-life problems via mobile phone use [100–102]. Moreover, in the family environment, whether the parents' supervision is effective or not partially depends on their own behaviors. According to Bandura's social cognitive theory, children observe the behaviors of others around them and are especially prone to observing, and imitating their parents' behaviors [103]. It has been found that parents' looking down at their own mobile phone (parent phubbing) in the process of communication with their children will not only aggravate children's addiction [104], but also affect children's attitude towards self-control mobile phone use [105]. Therefore, if parents want to achieve efficient monitoring results, they should control their own mobile phone-use behaviors. In general, although parental monitoring aims to improve children's mobile phone-use behaviors, it is often ineffective or leads to undesirable outcomes.

In addition, as we hypothesized, escape motivation mediated the relation between parental monitoring and adolescent PMPU, which supports H2. This result is consistent with similar studies. One study found that escape motivation mediated the predictive effect of negative emotions on PMPU [67]. When individuals face real-life struggles, escape motivation can prompt them to compensate through video games and/or the internet, which can eventually lead to video game or internet addiction [54,106,107]. Furthermore, Erikson [108] proposed that there is a developmental issue in every psychosocial stage of human development; adolescence is a crucial period for identity development, as well as a time when psychological reactance peaks. To adolescents, parental monitoring acts as a restriction of freedom, which could induce their escape motivation. In addition, parental monitoring often creates parent-child conflict, which could cause adolescents to develop negative emotions, thus leading to escape motivation.

4.2. Shyness Moderates Both the Relations of Parental Monitoring with Adolescent Escape Motivation and Adolescent PMPU

The impact of parental monitoring on adolescent PMPU differs across individuals. The present study found that adolescent shyness level moderated the relation between parental monitoring and adolescent escape motivation, and between parental monitoring and adolescent PMPU, which supports

H4 and H3. As children's shyness level increased, increases in parental monitoring strengthened their escape motivation and PMPU. This could be explained by the fact that shy individuals rely more on mobile phones to socialize, and parental monitoring can cause them to generate more negative reactions, such as psychological reactance and feelings of insecurity; this in turn perpetuates their escape motivation and exacerbates PMPU. There are three possible reasons why shy individuals rely more on mobile-phone socialization. First, shyness can be related to social anxiety; to avoid the embarrassment and discomfort elicited by face-to-face interactions, shy individuals tend to socialize via the internet, thus increasing internet use behaviors that can lead to internet and mobile-phone addiction [83,109]. Second, shy individuals often avoid occasions that expose them to evaluation [110]. Internet and mobile phone interactions can disguise their identity and thus protect them from others' evaluations. Third, shyness that originates from social anxiety can expose individuals to psychological challenges [111]. To mitigate and overcome these challenges, shy individuals tend to avoid face-to-face interactions, devote themselves to internet use, and achieve satisfaction through online interactions. Overall, when their parents employ monitoring strategies, shy adolescents might feel insecure and avoid being evaluated, which prompts them to escape reality via mobile phone use.

4.3. Limitation and Implication

The present study has a few limitations. First, our data are cross-sectional, and thus cannot infer strong causational relationships. Experimental or longitudinal designs could be used to further prove the relations between these variables. Second, all of our data came from adolescents' subjective responses. Although our measures have relatively high reliability/validity, the addition of responses from other sources (such as parents) would make our results more persuasive. Data of parental monitoring were obtained from children's self-report, but not from their parents' reports due to the limitation of our research conditions. In future research, obtaining data of parental monitoring from parents will help to reduce potential bias. Third, the findings in this study are in the context of Chinese culture, and its generalization to other culture should be made with caution. In order to avoid the negative effects of mobile phones, many parents in China prohibit children from bringing mobile phones to school. Using mobile phones at home is also often restricted. In comparison to children in other cultural contexts, Chinese children might have less freedom to use mobile phones. Moreover, studies on parental monitoring and children's PMPU have yielded different results under different cultural and national contexts (such as Turkey and Germany) [19,47]. Therefore, future studies can explore the effects of cultural differences and cultural contexts on the effect of parental monitoring on children's PMPU. Finally, future research should involve more schools and students to explore the differences between children in different developmental stages, such as early adolescence (12–13 years) and late adolescence (16–18).

Despite the above limitations, the contributions of the present study are relevant to educators, parents, and adolescents. First, our study results found that parental monitoring positively predicts adolescents' PMPU. However, as the forms of online activities increase and the access to the internet becomes easier, parents are more likely to use monitoring strategies [20]. Moreover, parental monitoring is the most direct mediation method and, therefore, the most convenient for parents [18]. One study points out parents' greater tendency to monitor their child's mobile phone-use behaviors when their use increases [46]. When parental monitoring increases children's mobile phone use, parental monitoring in turn increases, leading to a maladaptive cycle. Parents and educators should be cautious and optimize the use of monitoring strategies to control adolescent mobile phone use. Second, the present study found that parental monitoring positively predicted adolescents' escape motivation, which predicted their PMPU. Third, the effect of parental monitoring on adolescents differed across temperaments. When parents strengthen their monitoring, shy adolescents are more likely to display escape motivation and develop problematic mobile phone-use behaviors. Parents should adopt appropriate mediation strategies according to their child's temperament.

5. Conclusions

Parental monitoring positively predicts children's PMPU, and this predictive effect is partially mediated by children's escape motivation. Children's level of shyness moderates the relation between parental monitoring and children's escape motivation, and the relation between parental monitoring and children's PMPU, Thus, increasing the strength of parental monitoring can lead to an increase in escape motivation and PMPU among shy adolescents.

Author Contributions: Conceptualization, X.F. and J.L.; Formal analysis, X.F. and F.J.; Funding acquisition, R.-D.L.; Investigation, R.Z., F.J. and J.W.; Project administration, R.-D.L.; Supervision, R.-D.L.; Validation, R.-D.L.; Writing—review and editing, X.F., J.L., R.-D.L. and Y.D. All authors have read and agreed to the published version of the manuscript.

References

1. Mascheroni, G.; Ólafsson, K. *Net Children Go Mobile: Risks and Opportunities*, 2nd ed.; Educatt: Milan, Italy, 2014.
2. CNNIC. The 43st China Statistical Report on Internet Development. 2018. Available online: http://www.cnnic.net.cn/hlwfzyj/hlwxzbg/hlwtjbg/201902/P020190318523029756345.pdf (accessed on 20 December 2018).
3. Bolin, G.; Westlund, O. Mobile generations: The role of mobile technology in the shaping of Swedish media generations. *Int. J. Commun.* **2009**, *3*, 108–124.
4. Villanti, A.C.; Johnson, A.L.; Ilakkuvan, V.; Jacobs, M.A.; Graham, A.L.; Rath, J.M. Social media use and access to digital technology in US young adults in 2016. *J. Med. Internet Res.* **2017**, *19*, e196. [CrossRef] [PubMed]
5. Chóliz, M. Mobile-phone addiction in adolescence: The test of mobile phone dependence (TMD). *Prog. Health Sci.* **2012**, *2*, 33–44.
6. Westlund, O. New(s) functions for the mobile: A cross-cultural study. *New Media Soc.* **2010**, *12*, 91–108. [CrossRef]
7. Ott, T.; Magnusson, A.G.; Weilenmann, A.; af Segerstad, Y.H. It must not disturb, it's as simple as that: Students' voices on mobile phones in the infrastructure for learning in Swedish upper secondary school. *Educ. Inf. Technol.* **2018**, *23*, 517–536. [CrossRef]
8. Chang, F.C.; Chiu, C.H.; Chen, P.H.; Chiang, J.T.; Miao, N.F.; Chuang, H.Y.; Liu, S. Children's use of mobile devices, smartphone addiction and parental mediation in Taiwan. *Comput. Hum. Behav.* **2019**, *93*, 25–32. [CrossRef]
9. Nikhita, C.S.; Jadhav, P.R.; Ajinkya, S.A. Prevalence of mobile phone dependence in secondary school adolescents. *J. Clin. Diagn. Res. JCDR* **2015**, *9*, 6–9. [CrossRef]
10. Seo, D.G.; Park, Y.; Kim, M.K.; Park, J. Mobile phone dependency and its impacts on adolescents' social and academic behaviors. *Comput. Hum. Behav.* **2016**, *63*, 282–292. [CrossRef]
11. Kwon, M.; Kim, D.J.; Cho, H.; Yang, S. The smartphone addiction scale: Development and validation of a short version for adolescents. *PLoS ONE* **2013**, *8*, e83558. [CrossRef]
12. Bhise, A.T.; Ghatule, A.A.; Ghatule, A.P. Study of mobile addiction among students wRT Gender and education. *Indian J. Res. Manag. Bus. Soc. Sci.* **2014**, *2*, 17–21.
13. Bianchi, A.; Phillips, J.G. Psychological predictors of problem mobile phone use. *Cyberpsychol. Behav.* **2005**, *8*, 39–51. [CrossRef] [PubMed]
14. Hawi, N.S.; Samaha, M. Relationships among smartphone addiction, anxiety, and family relations. *Behav. Inf. Technol.* **2017**, *36*, 1046–1052. [CrossRef]
15. Kates, A.W.; Wu, H.; Coryn, C.L. The effects of mobile phone use on academic performance: A meta-analysis. *Comput. Educ.* **2018**, *127*, 107–112. [CrossRef]
16. Thomée, S.; Härenstam, A.; Hagberg, M. Mobile phone use and stress, sleep disturbances, and symptoms of depression among young adults-a prospective cohort study. *BMC Public Health* **2011**, *11*, 66. [CrossRef]
17. Livingstone, S.; Helsper, E.J. Parental mediation of children's internet use. *J. Broadcast. Electron. Media* **2008**, *52*, 581–599. [CrossRef]

18. Nikken, P.; Jansz, J. Developing scales to measure parental mediation of young children's internet use. *Learn. Media Technol.* **2014**, *39*, 250–266. [CrossRef]
19. Hefner, D.; Knop, K.; Schmitt, S.; Vorderer, P. Rules? Role model? Relationship? The impact of parents on their children's problematic mobile phone involvement. *Media Psychol.* **2019**, *22*, 82–108. [CrossRef]
20. Sonck, N.; Nikken, P.; de Haan, J. Determinants of Internet mediation: A comparison of the reports by Dutch parents and children. *J. Child. Media* **2013**, *7*, 96–113. [CrossRef]
21. Panova, T.; Carbonell, X. Is smartphone addiction really an addiction? *J. Behav. Addict.* **2018**, *7*, 252–259. [CrossRef]
22. Sunthlia, A.; Ahmad, S.; Singh, S.P. Menace of mobile phone overuse: An emerging public health concern. *Int. J. Commun. Med. Public Health* **2017**, *3*, 153–156. [CrossRef]
23. Randler, C.; Wolfgang, L.; Matt, K.; Demirhan, E.; Horzum, M.B.; Beşoluk, Ş. Smartphone addiction proneness in relation to sleep and morningness–eveningness in German adolescents. *J. Behav. Addict.* **2016**, *5*, 465–473. [CrossRef] [PubMed]
24. Haug, S.; Castro, R.P.; Kwon, M.; Filler, A.; Kowatsch, T.; Schaub, M.P. Smartphone use and smartphone addiction among young people in Switzerland. *J. Behav. Addict.* **2015**, *4*, 299–307. [CrossRef] [PubMed]
25. Rebold, M.J.; Sheehan, T.; Dirlam, M.; Maldonado, T.; O'Donnell, D. The impact of cell phone texting on the amount of time spent exercising at different intensities. *Comput. Hum. Behav.* **2016**, *55*, 167–171. [CrossRef]
26. Lachmann, B.; Sindermann, C.; Sariyska, R.Y.; Luo, R.; Melchers, M.C.; Becker, B.; Montag, C. The role of empathy and life satisfaction in internet and smartphone use disorder. *Front. Psychol.* **2018**, *9*, 398. [CrossRef] [PubMed]
27. Alosaimi, F.D.; Alyahya, H.; Alshahwan, H.; Al Mahyijari, N.; Shaik, S.A. Smartphone addiction among university students in Riyadh, Saudi Arabia. *Saudi Med. J.* **2016**, *37*, 675–683. [CrossRef]
28. Lepp, A.; Barkley, J.E.; Karpinski, A.C. The relationship between cell phone use, academic performance, anxiety, and satisfaction with life in college students. *Comput. Hum. Behav.* **2014**, *31*, 343–350. [CrossRef]
29. Samaha, M.; Hawi, N.S. Relationships among smartphone addiction, stress, academic performance, and satisfaction with life. *Comput. Hum. Behav.* **2016**, *57*, 321–325. [CrossRef]
30. Cheever, N.A.; Rosen, L.D.; Carrier, L.M.; Chavez, A. Out of sight is not out of mind: The impact of restricting wireless mobile device use on anxiety levels among low, moderate and high users. *Comput. Hum. Behav.* **2014**, *37*, 290–297. [CrossRef]
31. Tams, S.; Legoux, R.; Leger, P.M. Smartphone withdrawal creates stress: A moderated mediation model of nomophobia, social threat, and phone withdrawal context. *Comput. Hum. Behav.* **2018**, *81*, 1–9. [CrossRef]
32. Elhai, J.D.; Dvorak, R.D.; Levine, J.C.; Hall, B.J. Problematic smartphone use: A conceptual overview and systematic review of relations with anxiety and depression psychopathology. *J. Affect. Disord.* **2017**, *207*, 251–259. [CrossRef]
33. Hao, Z.; Jin, L.; Li, Y.; Akram, H.R.; Saeed, M.F.; Ma, J.; Huang, J. Alexithymia and mobile phone addiction in Chinese undergraduate students: The roles of mobile phone use patterns. *Comput. Hum. Behav.* **2019**, *97*, 51–59. [CrossRef]
34. Volkmer, S.A.; Lermer, E. Unhappy and addicted to your phone? Higher mobile phone use is associated with lower well-being. *Comput. Hum. Behav.* **2019**, *93*, 210–218. [CrossRef]
35. Warren, R.; Bluma, A. Parental mediation of children's Internet use: The influence of established media. *Commun. Res. Rep.* **2002**, *19*, 8–17. [CrossRef]
36. Nathanson, A.I. Parent and child perspectives on the presence and meaning of parental television mediation. *J. Broadcast. Electron. Media* **2001**, *45*, 201–220. [CrossRef]
37. Bybee, C.R.; Robinson, D.; Turow, J. Determinants of parental guidance of children's television viewing for a special subgroup: Mass media scholars. *J. Broadcast. Electron. Media* **1982**, *26*, 697–710. [CrossRef]
38. Valkenburg, P.M.; Krcmar, M.; Peeters, A.L.; Marseille, N.M. Developing a scale to assess three styles of television mediation: "Instructive mediation," "restrictive mediation," and "social coviewing". *J. Broadcast. Electron. Media* **1999**, *43*, 52–66. [CrossRef]
39. Warren, R.; Gerke, P.; Kelly, M.A. Is there enough time on the clock? Parental involvement and mediation of children's television viewing. *J. Broadcast. Electron. Media* **2002**, *46*, 87–111. [CrossRef]
40. Nikken, P.; Jansz, J. Parental mediation of children's videogame playing: A comparison of the reports by parents and children. *Learn. Media Technol.* **2006**, *31*, 181–202. [CrossRef]

41. Livingstone, S.; Haddon, L.; Görzig, A.; Ólafsson, K. *Risks and Safety on the Internet: The Perspective of European Children: Full Findings and Policy Implications from the EU Kids Online Survey of 9–16 Year Olds and Their Parents in 25 Countries*; EU Kids Online: London, UK, 2011.
42. Mendoza, K. Surveying parental mediation: Connections, challenges and questions for media literacy. *J. Media Lit. Educ.* **2009**, *1*, 28–41.
43. Shin, W.; Li, B. Parental mediation of children's digital technology use in Singapore. *J. Child. Media* **2017**, *11*, 1–19. [CrossRef]
44. Vaala, S.E.; Bleakley, A. Monitoring, mediating, and modeling: Parental influence on adolescent computer and Internet use in the United States. *J. Child. Media* **2015**, *9*, 40–57. [CrossRef]
45. Duerager, A.; Livingstone, S. *How Can Parents Support Children's Internet Safety*; LSE, EU Kids Online: London, UK, 2012.
46. Kalmus, V.; Blinka, L.; Olafsson, K. Does it matter what mama says: Evaluating the role of parental mediation in European adolescents' excessive Internet use. *Child. Soc.* **2015**, *29*, 122–133. [CrossRef]
47. Bayraktar, F. Online Risks and Parental Mediation Strategies Comparison of Turkish Children/Adolescents Who Live in Turkey and Europe. *Educ. Sci. Egit. Ve Bilim* **2017**, *42*, 25–37. [CrossRef]
48. Livingstone, S.; Haddon, L.; Vincent, J.; Mascheroni, G.; Ólafsson, K. *Net Children Go Mobile: The UK Report*; London School of Economics and Political Science: London, UK, 2014.
49. Kim, J.H. Smartphone-mediated communication vs. face-to-face interaction: Two routes to social support and problematic use of smartphone. *Comput. Hum. Behav.* **2017**, *67*, 282–291. [CrossRef]
50. Lowry, P.B.; Gaskin, J.; Moody, G.D. Proposing the multi-motive information systems continuance model (MISC) to better explain end-user system evaluations and continuance intentions. *J. Assoc. Inf. Syst.* **2015**, *16*, 515–579.
51. Peele, S. *The Meaning of Addiction: Compulsive Experience and Its Interpretation*; Lexington Books DC Heath and Com: Lexington, MA, USA, 1985.
52. Parker, B.J.; Plank, R.E. A uses and gratifications perspective on the Internet as a new information source. *Am. Bus. Rev.* **2000**, *18*, 43–49.
53. Song, I.; Larose, R.; Eastin, M.S.; Lin, C.A. Internet gratifications and Internet addiction: On the uses and abuses of new media. *Cyberpsychol. Behav.* **2004**, *7*, 384–394. [CrossRef]
54. Yee, N. Motivations for play in online games. *Cyberpsychol. Behav.* **2006**, *9*, 772–775. [CrossRef]
55. Billieux, J.; Chanal, J.; Khazaal, Y.; Rochat, L.; Gay, P.; Zullino, D.; Van der Linden, M. Psychological predictors of problematic involvement in massively multiplayer online role-playing games: Illustration in a sample of male cybercafé players. *Psychopathology* **2011**, *44*, 165–171. [CrossRef]
56. Dauriat, F.Z.; Zermatten, A.; Billieux, J.; Thorens, G.; Bondolfi, G.; Zullino, D.; Khazaal, Y. Motivations to play specifically predict excessive involvement in massively multiplayer online role-playing games: Evidence from an online survey. *Eur. Addict. Res.* **2011**, *17*, 185–189. [CrossRef]
57. Király, O.; Urbán, R.; Griffiths, M.D.; Ágoston, C.; Nagygyörgy, K.; Kökönyei, G.; Demetrovics, Z. The mediating effect of gaming motivation between psychiatric symptoms and problematic online gaming: An online survey. *J. Med. Internet Res.* **2015**, *17*, e88. [CrossRef] [PubMed]
58. Kuss, D.J.; Griffiths, M.D.; Pontes, H.M. Chaos and confusion in DSM-5 diagnosis of Internet Gaming Disorder: Issues, concerns, and recommendations for clarity in the field. *J. Behav. Addict.* **2017**, *6*, 103–109. [CrossRef] [PubMed]
59. Klobas, J.E.; McGill, T.J.; Moghavvemi, S.; Paramanathan, T. Compulsive YouTube usage: A comparison of use motivation and personality effects. *Comput. Hum. Behav.* **2018**, *87*, 129–139. [CrossRef]
60. Bae, S.M. The relationship between the type of smartphone use and smartphone dependence of Korean adolescents: National survey study. *Child. Youth Serv. Rev.* **2017**, *81*, 207–211. [CrossRef]
61. Khang, H.; Kim, J.K.; Kim, Y. Self-traits and motivations as antecedents of digital media flow and addiction: The Internet, mobile phones, and video games. *Comput. Hum. Behav.* **2013**, *29*, 2416–2424. [CrossRef]
62. Wang, J.L.; Wang, H.Z.; Gaskin, J.; Wang, L.H. The role of stress and motivation in problematic smartphone use among college students. *Comput. Hum. Behav.* **2015**, *53*, 181–188. [CrossRef]
63. Grolnick, W.S.; Deci, E.L.; Ryan, R.M. Internalization within the family: The self-determination theory perspective. In *Parenting and Children's Internalization of Values: A Handbook of Contemporary Theory*; Grusec, J.E., Kuczynski, L., Eds.; John Wiley & Sons Inc.: Hoboken, NJ, USA, 1997; pp. 135–161.

64. White, S.R.; Rasmussen, E.E.; King, A.J. Restrictive mediation and unintended effects: Serial multiple mediation analysis explaining the role of reactance in US adolescents. *J. Child. Media* **2015**, *9*, 510–527. [CrossRef]
65. Maroney, N.; Williams, B.J.; Thomas, A.; Skues, J.; Moulding, R. A stress-coping model of problem online video game use. *Int. J. Ment. Health Addict.* **2019**, *17*, 845–858. [CrossRef]
66. Ballabio, M.; Griffiths, M.D.; Urbán, R.; Quartiroli, A.; Demetrovics, Z.; Király, O. Do gaming motives mediate between psychiatric symptoms and problematic gaming? An empirical survey study. *Addict. Res. Theory* **2017**, *25*, 397–408. [CrossRef]
67. Shen, X.; Wang, J.L. Loneliness and excessive smartphone use among Chinese college students: Moderated mediation effect of perceived stressed and motivation. *Comput. Hum. Behav.* **2019**, *95*, 31–36. [CrossRef]
68. Fikkers, K.M.; Piotrowski, J.T.; Valkenburg, P.M. A matter of style? Exploring the effects of parental mediation styles on early adolescents' media violence exposure and aggression. *Comput. Hum. Behav.* **2017**, *70*, 407–415. [CrossRef]
69. Valkenburg, P.M.; Piotrowski, J.T.; Hermanns, J.; De Leeuw, R. Developing and validating the perceived parental media mediation scale: A self-determination perspective. *Hum. Commun. Res.* **2013**, *39*, 445–469. [CrossRef]
70. Demirhan, E.; Randler, C.; Horzum, M.B. Is problematic mobile phone use explained by chronotype and personality? *Chronobiol. Int.* **2016**, *33*, 821–831. [CrossRef]
71. Rapee, R.M.; Coplan, R.J. Conceptual relations between anxiety disorder and fearful temperament. *New Dir. Child Adolesc. Dev.* **2010**, *127*, 17–31. [CrossRef]
72. Cheek, J.M.; Buss, A.H. Shyness and sociability. *J. Personal. Soc. Psychol.* **1981**, *41*, 330–339. [CrossRef]
73. Henderson, L.; Zimbardo, P.G. Shyness as a clinical condition: The Stanford model. In *International Handbook of Social Anxiety: Concepts, Research and Interventions Relating to the Self and Shyness*; Crozier, W.R., Alden, L.E., Eds.; John Wiley & Sons Ltd.: New York, NY, USA, 2001; pp. 431–447.
74. Rubin, K.H.; Coplan, R.J.; Bowker, J.C. Social withdrawal in childhood. *Annu. Rev. Psychol.* **2009**, *60*, 141–171. [CrossRef] [PubMed]
75. Tan, J.; Ai, Y.; Wen, X.; Wu, Y.; Wang, W. Relationship between shyness and loneliness among Chinese adolescents: Social support as mediator. *Soc. Behav. Personal. Int. J.* **2016**, *44*, 201–208. [CrossRef]
76. Barstead, M.G.; Smith, K.A.; Laursen, B.; Booth-LaForce, C.; King, S.; Rubin, K.H. Shyness, preference for solitude, and adolescent internalizing: The roles of maternal, paternal, and best-friend support. *J. Res. Adolesc.* **2018**, *28*, 488–504. [CrossRef] [PubMed]
77. Laghi, F.; Schneider, B.H.; Vitoroulis, I.; Coplan, R.J.; Baiocco, R.; Amichai-Hamburger, Y.; Flament, M. Knowing when not to use the Internet: Shyness and adolescents' on-line and off-line interactions with friends. *Comput. Hum. Behav.* **2013**, *29*, 51–57. [CrossRef]
78. Appel, M.; Gnambs, T. Shyness and social media use: A meta-analytic summary of moderating and mediating effects. *Comput. Hum. Behav.* **2019**, *98*, 294–301. [CrossRef]
79. Ang, C.S.; Chan, N.N.; Lee, C.S. Shyness, Loneliness Avoidance, and Internet Addiction: What are the Relationships? *J. Psychol.* **2018**, *152*, 25–35. [CrossRef] [PubMed]
80. Chak, K.; Leung, L. Shyness and locus of control as predictors of internet addiction and internet use. *Cyberpsychol. Behav.* **2004**, *7*, 559–570. [CrossRef] [PubMed]
81. Tian, Y.; Bian, Y.; Han, P.; Gao, F.; Wang, P. Associations between psychosocial factors and generalized pathological internet use in Chinese university students: A longitudinal cross-lagged analysis. *Comput. Hum. Behav.* **2017**, *72*, 178–188. [CrossRef]
82. Bian, M.; Leung, L. Linking loneliness, shyness, smartphone addiction symptoms, and patterns of smartphone use to social capital. *Soc. Sci. Comput. Rev.* **2015**, *33*, 61–79. [CrossRef]
83. Han, L.; Geng, J.; Jou, M.; Gao, F.; Yang, H. Relationship between shyness and mobile phone addiction in Chinese young adults: Mediating roles of self-control and attachment anxiety. *Comput. Hum. Behav.* **2017**, *76*, 363–371. [CrossRef]
84. Hong, W.; Liu, R.D.; Oei, T.P.; Zhen, R.; Jiang, S.; Sheng, X. The mediating and moderating roles of social anxiety and relatedness need satisfaction on the relationship between shyness and problematic mobile phone use among adolescents. *Comput. Hum. Behav.* **2019**, *93*, 301–308. [CrossRef]
85. Luke, F.; Chan, C.C.; Au, A.; Lai, S.M. Adaptive parenting for alleviating young children's shyness: A randomized controlled trial of an early intervention program. *Infant Child Dev.* **2017**, *26*, 1–19. [CrossRef]

86. Hastings, P.D.; Rubin, K.H.; DeRose, L. Links among gender, inhibition, and parental socialization in the development of prosocial behavior. *Merrill-Palmer Q.* **2005**, *51*, 467–493. [CrossRef]
87. Zarra-Nezhad, M.; Moazami-Goodarzi, A.; Nurmi, J.E.; Eklund, K.; Ahonen, T.; Aunola, K. Children's Shyness Moderates the Associations between Parenting Behavior and the Development of Children's Pro-Social Behaviors. *J. Child Fam. Stud.* **2018**, *27*, 3008–3018. [CrossRef]
88. Eastin, M.S.; Greenberg, B.S.; Hofschire, L. Parenting the internet. *J. Commun.* **2006**, *56*, 486–504. [CrossRef]
89. Young, C.M.; DiBello, A.M.; Traylor, Z.K.; Zvolensky, M.J.; Neighbors, C. A Longitudinal Examination of the Associations between Shyness, Drinking Motives, Alcohol Use, and Alcohol-Related Problems. *Alcohol. Clin. Exp. Res.* **2015**, *39*, 1749–1755. [CrossRef] [PubMed]
90. Wu, N. The Relationship between Children Internet use with Academic Performance: The Role of Parental Mediation. Ph.D. Thesis, Central China Normal University, Wuhan, China, 2016. (In Chinese).
91. Li, F.F.; Luo, Q.; Zhou, Z.K.; Sun, X.J.; Wei, H. Mediating effect of interpersonal communication disturbances between college students' shyness and dependence of online communication. *J. Clin. Psychol.* **2012**, *20*, 182–184. (In Chinese)
92. Foerster, M.; Roser, K.; Schoeni, A.; Röösli, M. Problematic mobile phone use in adolescents: Derivation of a short scale MPPUS-10. *Int. J. Public Health* **2015**, *60*, 277–286. [CrossRef] [PubMed]
93. Zhuang, H.; Liu, R.-D.; Liu, Y. The impact of peer attachment on problematic mobile phone use among adolescents: Moderated mediation effect of loneliness and self-construa. *Psychol. Sci.* **2017**, *40*, 89–95. (In Chinese)
94. Little, R.J.; Rubin, D.B. *Statistical Analysis with Missing Data*; John Wiley & Sons: Hoboken, NJ, USA, 2019; Volume 793.
95. Hayes, A.F. *Introduction to Mediation, Moderation, and Conditional Process Analysis: A Regression-Based Approach*; The Guilford Press: New York, NY, USA, 2013.
96. Brehm, S.S.; Brehm, J.W. *Psychological Reactance: A Theory of Freedom and Control*; Academic Press: Cambridge, MA, USA, 2013.
97. Yen, J.Y.; Yen, C.F.; Chen, C.C.; Chen, S.H.; Ko, C.H. Family factors of internet addiction and substance use experience in Taiwanese adolescents. *Cyberpsychol. Behav.* **2007**, *10*, 323–329. [CrossRef] [PubMed]
98. Xiuqin, H.; Huimin, Z.; Mengchen, L.; Jinan, W.; Ying, Z.; Ran, T. Mental health, personality, and parental rearing styles of adolescents with Internet addiction disorder. *Cyberpsychol. Behav. Soc. Netw.* **2010**, *13*, 401–406. [CrossRef]
99. Nikken, P.; de Graaf, H. Reciprocal relationships between friends' and parental mediation of adolescents' media use and their sexual attitudes and behavior. *J. Youth Adolesc.* **2013**, *42*, 1696–1707. [CrossRef]
100. Hasan, M.R.; Jha, A.K.; Liu, Y. Excessive use of online video streaming services: Impact of recommender system use, psychological factors, and motives. *Comput. Hum. Behav.* **2018**, *80*, 220–228. [CrossRef]
101. Kardefelt-Winther, D. A conceptual and methodological critique of internet addiction research: Towards a model of compensatory internet use. *Comput. Hum. Behav.* **2014**, *31*, 351–354. [CrossRef]
102. Kardefelt-Winther, D. Conceptualizing Internet use disorders: Addiction or coping process? *Psychiatry Clin. Neurosci.* **2017**, *71*, 459–466. [CrossRef]
103. Bandura, A. Social learning theory of aggression. *J. Commun.* **1978**, *28*, 12–29. [CrossRef] [PubMed]
104. Xie, X.; Chen, W.; Zhu, X.; He, D. Parents' phubbing increases Adolescents' Mobile phone addiction: Roles of parent-child attachment, deviant peers, and gender. *Child. Youth Serv. Rev.* **2019**, *105*, 104426. [CrossRef]
105. Fu, X.; Liu, J.; Liu, R.D.; Ding, Y.; Hong, W.; Jiang, S. The Impact of Parental Active Mediation on Adolescent Mobile Phone Dependency: A Moderated Mediation Model. *Comput. Hum. Behav.* **2020**, *107*, 106280. [CrossRef]
106. Caplan, S.; Williams, D.; Yee, N. Problematic Internet use and psychosocial well-being among MMO players. *Comput. Hum. Behav.* **2009**, *25*, 1312–1319. [CrossRef]
107. Billieux, J.; Van der Linden, M.; Achab, S.; Khazaal, Y.; Paraskevopoulos, L.; Zullino, D.; Thorens, G. Why do you play World of Warcraft? An in-depth exploration of self-reported motivations to play online and in-game behaviours in the virtual world of Azeroth. *Comput. Hum. Behav.* **2013**, *29*, 103–109. [CrossRef]
108. Erikson, E.H. *Identity and the Life Cycle: Selected Papers*; International Universities Press: Oxford, UK, 1959.
109. Odacı, H.; Çelik, Ç.B. Who are problematic internet users? An investigation of the correlations between problematic internet use and shyness, loneliness, narcissism, aggression and self-perception. *Comput. Hum. Behav.* **2013**, *29*, 2382–2387. [CrossRef]

110. Cheek, J.M.; Melchior, L.M. Shyness and anxious self-preoccupation during a social interaction. *J. Soc. Behav. Personal.* **1990**, *5*, 117–130.
111. Jackson, T.; Fritch, A.; Nagasaka, T.; Gunderson, J. Towards explaining the association between shyness and loneliness: A path analysis with American college students. *Soc. Behav. Personal. Int. J.* **2002**, *30*, 263–270. [CrossRef]

15

Relationship between Difficulty in Emotion Regulation and Internet Addiction in College Students: A One-Year Prospective Study

Jui-Kang Tsai [1,2,†], Wei-Hsin Lu [3,4,†], Ray C. Hsiao [5,6], Huei-Fan Hu [7,*] and Cheng-Fang Yen [8,9,*]

1 Department of Psychiatry, Kaohsiung Armed Forces General Hospital, Kaohsiung 80284, Taiwan; regon720@gmail.com
2 Department of Nursing, Meiho University, Pingtung 91202, Taiwan
3 Department of Psychiatry, Ditmanson Medical Foundation Chia-Yi Christian Hospital, Chia-Yi City 60002, Taiwan; wiiseen@gmail.com
4 Department of Senior Citizen Service Management, Chia Nan University of Pharmacy and Science, Tainan 71710, Taiwan
5 Department of Psychiatry and Behavioral Sciences, University of Washington School of Medicine, Seattle, WA 98105, USA; rhsiao@u.washington.edu
6 Department of Psychiatry, Children's Hospital and Regional Medical Center, Seattle, WA 98105, USA
7 Department of Psychiatry, Tainan Municipal Hospital (managed by Show Chwan Medical Care Corporation), Tainan 70173, Taiwan
8 Department of Psychiatry, School of Medicine and Graduate Institute of Medicine, College of Medicine, Kaohsiung Medical University, Kaohsiung 80708, Taiwan
9 Department of Psychiatry, Kaohsiung Medical University Hospital, Kaohsiung 80708, Taiwan
* Correspondence: cych07205@gmail.com (H.-F.H.); chfaye@cc.kmu.edu.tw (C.-F.Y.)

† J.-K.T. and W.-H.L. contributed equally to this study.

Abstract: This prospective study evaluated the predictive effect of difficulty in emotion regulation on the occurrence and remission of Internet addiction (IA) and determined whether IA has a role in changing emotion regulation among college students during a follow-up period of 1 year. A total of 500 college students (262 women and 238 men) were recruited. In baseline and follow-up investigations, the levels of IA and difficulty in emotion regulation were evaluated using the Chen Internet Addiction Scale and the Difficulties in Emotion Regulation Scale (DERS), respectively. The results indicated that the subscale of impulse control difficulties on the DERS predicted the incidence of IA during the follow-up period of 1 year in male participants ($t = -2.875$, $p = 0.005$), whereas no subscale on the DERS predicted the remission of IA. IA did not predict the change in difficulties in emotion regulation. The subscale of impulse control difficulties on the DERS predicted the occurrence of IA in the college students and warrants early intervention.

Keywords: internet addiction; emotion regulation; college student

---

1. Introduction

The Internet has become a key resource in society and everyday life. At social and individual levels, the Internet facilitates interpersonal communication, provides entertainment, and helps individuals create new social networks [1,2]. However, inappropriate or excessive Internet use may result in Internet addiction (IA) and negative life outcomes [3]. People who have IA may have difficulties in controlling their Internet usage and develop problems in occupational or academic performance and in social relationships, as well as psychological and physical problems [4]. Although the Diagnostic and

Statistical Manual of Mental Disorders, Fifth Edition (DSM-5) does not list IA as a formal psychiatric diagnosis, it calls for research to examine Internet gaming disorder, a common type of IA, in terms of its course, symptoms, and underlying mechanisms [5]. Therefore, IA is an issue that warrants further study.

A multinational meta-analysis provided estimates of the global prevalence of IA, which varies across world regions, with the highest prevalence of 10.9% in the Middle East and the lowest prevalence of 2.6% in Northern and Western Europe [6]. The prevalence rate of IA among college students is 3.7% in Japan [7], 8–13% in Taiwan [8], and 13.6% in China [9]. College students may use the Internet for studying, gaming, social networking, gambling, chatting, shopping, and watching pornographic videos [10,11]. However, given that college students have free and unlimited access to the Internet, have flexible schedules, and are free from their parents' interference, they were identified as having a high risk for IA [12].

There have many studies examining the relationship between IA and personality characteristics such as neuroticism [13–15], conscientiousness [13–15], agreeableness [13–15], boredom proneness [16], borderline personality characteristics [17], reinforcement sensitivity [18], and frustration intolerance [18]. Emotion regulation is the attempt to alter emotional experiences via the initiation, maintenance, or modification of frequency, intensity, or duration of emotional experiences [19]. Difficulties with emotion regulation are believed to be risk factors for addiction [20,21]. Gratz and Roemer proposed that emotion regulation involves multiple conceptions, including (a) awareness and understanding of emotions, (b) acceptance of emotions, (c) ability to control impulsive behaviors and behave in accordance with desired goals when experiencing negative emotions, and (d) ability to use situationally appropriate emotion regulation-n strategies flexibly to modulate emotional responses as desired in order to meet individual goals and situational demands [22]. The relative absence of any or all of these abilities would indicate the presence of difficulties in emotion regulation [22].

Research has found that young people with IA had more difficulty in identifying and describing emotions, understanding emotional reactions, and controlling their impulsive behaviors in response to negative emotional experiences, and were less able to use effective emotion regulation strategies than adolescents without IA [23–27]. It is hypothesized that inadequate prefrontal cognitive control to suppress their negative emotions may result in impulsivity and increase the risk of IA [26]. A two-year prospective study also reported that emotional problems, such as depression and social phobia, predict the occurrence of IA in adolescents [28]. However, research also found that Internet use is a common strategy that people use to alleviate emotional distress [29–31]. Based on the principle of functional analysis in behavioral psychology [32], many forms of problematic behaviors and psychopathology can be conceptualized as efforts to escape and avoid emotions, thoughts, memories, and other private experiences [33]. Although IA is generally considered an unhealthy effort to cope with stress and negative emotions [29], whether IA deteriorates or improves the function of emotion regulation warrants survey.

No prospective study has examined the bidirectional relationship between IA and difficulties in emotion regulation. The prospective study design can provide the temporal relationships between IA and difficulties in emotion regulation and infer the causal relationship between them. The aims of this prospective study were to evaluate the predictive effect of difficulty in emotion regulation on the occurrence and remission of IA, and to determine whether IA can predict the change in difficulty in emotion regulation among college students during the follow-up period of 1 year. In particular, given that emotion regulation contains multiple dimensions of conceptions [22], this study aimed to examine whether the relationships between IA and emotion regulation vary according to various dimensions of emotion regulation. Based on the results of previous studies described above, we hypothesized that difficulty in emotion regulation may predict the occurrence of IA and the non-remission of IA during the period of one-year follow-up. Moreover, we also hypothesized that IA may worsen emotion regulation during the period of 1 year.

2. Materials and Methods

2.1. Participants

Participants were recruited using an advertisement posted for college students aged between 20 and 30 years. A total of 500 college students (262 women and 238 men) participated in this study. Regarding the sample size, a previous study found that 8–13% of college students in Taiwan had IA [8]. The sample of 500 participants was determined as adequate based on the estimation with 80% power, 95% confidence interval, and statistically significant level at 5% [34]. The mean age of the participants was 22.1 years (standard deviation (SD): 1.8 years). Informed consent was obtained from all the participants prior to assessment. The study was approved by the Institutional Review Board of Kaohsiung Medical University Hospital (KMUH-IRB-20120249).

2.2. Measures

2.2.1. Chen Internet Addiction Scale (CIAS)

We used the self-administered Chen IA Scale (CIAS) to assess the participants' severity of IA in the month preceding the study [35]. The CIAS contains 26 items rated on a 4-point Likert scale with the minimum and maximum scores of 26 and 104, respectively [35]. A higher total score indicates more severe IA. The internal reliability (Cronbach's α) of the CIAS in the present study was 0.93. According to diagnostic criteria for IA, a score of 68 out of the total CIAS score has the highest diagnostic accuracy and accepted sensitivity and specificity for IA [36]. Accordingly, those with CIAS scores of 68 or more were classified as those with IA.

2.2.2. Difficulties in Emotion Regulation Scale (DERS)

The DERS is a 36-item self-reported measure developed to assess clinically relevant difficulties in emotion regulation [22]. Items are scored on six scales: Nonacceptance of Emotional Responses (6 items), Difficulties Engaging in Goal-Directed Behavior (5 items), Impulse Control Difficulties (6 items), Lack of Emotional Awareness (6 items), Limited Access to Emotion Regulation Strategies (8 items), and Lack of Emotional Clarity (5 items). Participants are asked to indicate how often each of the 36 items applied to them on a 5-point Likert scale ranging from 1 (almost never) to 5 (almost always). Subscale scores are obtained by summating corresponding items. Cronbach's α for the Taiwanese version of the DERS ranged from 0.72 to 0.81. Higher scores on the DERS indicate greater difficulties in emotion regulation.

2.2.3. Demographic Characteristics

The demographic characteristics of participants collected in this study were sex (female or male) and age (years).

2.3. Study Process and Statistical Analysis

In the initial assessment (Stage 1), all the participants were invited to complete the CIAS and DERS. One year later (Stage 2), the participants were invited to complete the CIAS and DERS again. According to the scores of the CIAS at Stage 1 and Stage 2, the participants were classified into one of four groups (Figure 1). The participants deemed not to be addicted at Stage 1 were stratified into the Persistent no IA (PNIA) and New IA (NIA) groups based on subsequent non-addiction and addiction statuses at Stage 2, respectively. The remaining participants, who were initially deemed to be addicted to the Internet at Stage 1, were stratified into the groups of Remitted IA (RIA) and Persistent IA (PIA) based on remission and continuation of the behavior at Stage 2, respectively.

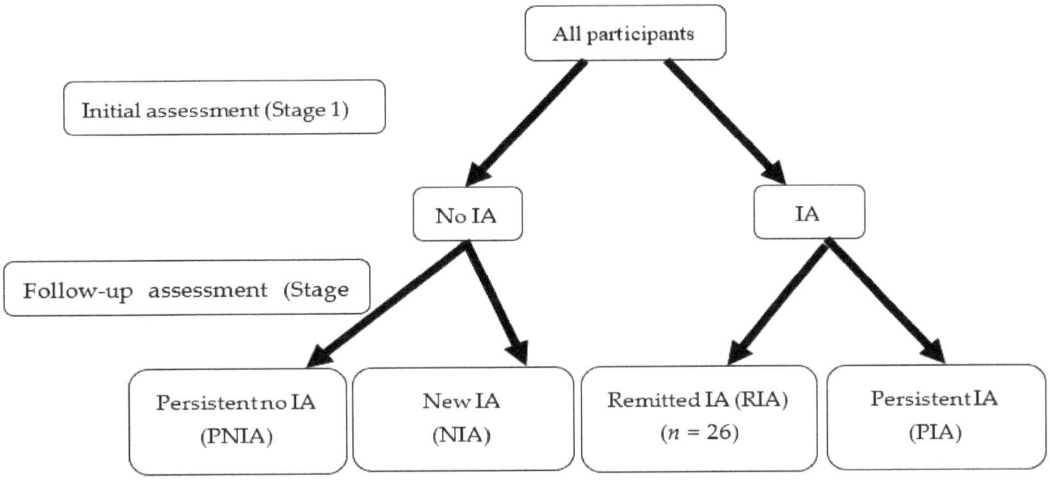

Figure 1. Study participants were assigned to one of four addiction groups. IA: Internet addiction

The incidence rate of IA at Stage 2 and its relationship with difficulty in emotion regulation at Stage 1 were examined in the PNIA and NIA groups. The remission rate of IA at Stage 2 and its relationship with difficulty in emotion regulation at Stage 1 were examined in the RIA and PIA groups. The chi-square test was utilized to evaluate category variables, and Student's t-test was used for continuous variables.

We evaluated whether changes in the difficulty of emotion regulation during the one-year period were different between the college students with and without IA at Stage 1. A repeated-measures two-way analysis of variance (ANOVA) with investigation stages (Stage 1 vs. Stage 2) as a within-subjects factor and the groups (with or without IA at Stage 1) as a between-subjects factor was performed for DERS scores. All statistical analyses were performed using SPSS version 20.0 (SPSS Inc., Chicago, IL, USA). Because of the existence of multiple comparisons, p-values of <0.008 (0.05/6) were considered statistically significant.

3. Results

A total of 324 college students (65.8%, 169 women and 155 men) underwent the follow-up assessment 1 year later. Of the 176 participants (93 women and 83 men) who did not participate in follow-up assessment, 96 (54.5%) could not be contacted, 48 (27.3%) refused to participate in follow-up assessment, and 32 (18.2%) had the desire to participate but were unable to do so due to work or army service. The results of comparing demographic data and the levels of IA on the CIAS and difficulties in emotion regulation on the DERS at initial assessment between participants who participated in and who did not participate in follow-up assessment are shown in Table 1. No differences were found in gender, age, and the levels of IA and difficulties in emotion regulation between these two groups (all $p > 0.008$).

Of the 268 participants in the PNIA and NIA groups who had no IA at Stage 1, 20 were deemed to have IA at Stage 2 (the NIA group), resulting in an incidence rate of 7.5% during the one-year period. Of the 56 individuals in the RIA and PIA groups who had IA at Stage 1, 26 were classified as being without IA at Stage 2 (the RIA group), indicating a one-year remission rate of 46.4%.

Comparisons of demographic characteristics and difficulties in emotion regulation between the PNIA and NIA groups are presented in Table 2. The results revealed that compared with the PNIA group, the NIA group had more severe impulse control difficulties on the DERS at Stage 1, revealing that impulse control difficulties at Stage 1 predicted the incidence of IA at Stage 2 during the follow-up period of 1 year. We further stratified the participants by gender and found that the prediction of impulse control difficulties for the incidence of IA existed in only male ($t = -2.875$, $p = 0.005$) but not in female participants ($t = -1.270$, $p = 0.206$).

Table 1. Comparisons of demographic data and difficulties in emotion regulation between participants who participated in and who did not participate in follow-up assessment.

	No Follow-Up (n =176) n (%) or mean (SD)	Follow-Up (n = 324) n (%) or mean (SD)	χ^2 or t
Gender, n (%)			
Female	93 (52.8)	169 (52.2)	0.884
Male	83 (47.2)	155 (47.8)	
Age (years), mean (SD)	21.9 (1.5)	22.3 (1.9)	0.047
CIAS, mean (SD)	56.6 (13.2)	55.0 (14.2)	1.189
DERS, mean (SD)			
Non-acceptance of emotional responses	12.7 (4.8)	12.6 (3.9)	0.273
Difficulties engaging in goal-directed behavior	12.2 (3.9)	12.0 (3.6)	0.539
Impulse control difficulties	11.2 (4.0)	11.5 (4.2)	−0.802
Lack of emotional awareness	15.3 (4.5)	14.7 (3.9)	1.364
Limited access to emotion regulation strategies	17.1 (5.7)	16.7 (5.3)	0.819
Lack of emotional clarity	9.9 (3.4)	10.0 (2.9)	−0.350

CIAS: Chen Internet Addiction Scale; DERS: Difficulties in Emotion Regulation Scale; SD: Standard deviation.

Table 2. Comparisons of demographic data and difficulties in emotion regulation between the PNIA and NIA groups and the RIA and PIA groups.

	PNIA Group (n = 248) n (%) or mean (SD)	NIA Group (n = 20) n (%) or mean (SD)	χ^2 or t	RIA Group (n = 26) n (%) or mean (SD)	PIA Group (n = 30) n (%) or mean (SD)	χ^2 or t
Gender, n (%)						
Female	129 (50.0)	11 (55)	0.066	15 (57.7)	14 (46.7)	0.678
Male	119 (48.0)	9 (45)		11 (42.3)	16 (53.3)	
Age (years), mean (SD)	22.3 (2.0)	22.4 (1.9)	−0.347	21.6 (1.2)	22.6 (1.9)	−2.421
DERS, mean (SD)						
Non-acceptance of emotional responses	12.2 (3.9)	13.6 (3.2)	−1.532	13.7 (3.6)	14.3 (4.7)	−0.601
Difficulties engaging in goal-directed behavior	11.4 (3.3)	11.9 (3.1)	−0.605	14.8 (3.4)	14.8 (4.3)	−0.029
Impulse control difficulties	10.8 (3.8)	13.4 (4.1)	−2.902 *	14.0 (4.7)	14.2 (5.0)	−0.179
Lack of emotional awareness	14.5 (4.1)	14.0 (2.8)	0.514	16.3 (3.4)	16.0 (3.1)	0.312
Limited access to emotion regulation strategies	15.7 (4.8)	18.5 (4.2)	−2.481	20.1 (6.0)	20.4 (5.6)	−0.229
Lack of emotional clarity	9.7 (2.9)	10.5 (2.9)	−1.168	11.0 (2.1)	11.0 (2.7)	−0.052

* $p < 0.008$. DERS: Difficulties in Emotion Regulation Scale; NIA: No Internet addiction; PIA: Persistent Internet addiction; PNIA: Persistent no Internet addiction; RIA: Remitted Internet addiction; SD: Standard deviation.

Comparisons of demographic characteristics and difficulties in emotion regulation at Stage 1 between the RIA and PIA groups are presented in Table 1. No dimension of difficulty in emotion regulation at Stage 1 was significantly associated with the remission of IA at Stage 2.

The results of the repeated-measures ANOVA for the effect of IA at Stage 1 on changes in DERS scores from Stage 1 to Stage 2 are shown in Table 3. Regarding the results of within-subject analysis, scores for the subscales of lack of emotional awareness (p = 0.017) and limited access to emotion regulation strategies (p = 0.022) tended to decrease more from Stage 1 to Stage 2 in the IA group than in the non-IA group; however, the results did not reach a statistically significant level. Regarding the results of between-subject analysis, there were significant differences in non-acceptance of emotional responses (p = 0.006), difficulties engaging in goal-directed behavior ($p < 0.001$), impulse control difficulties ($p < 0.001$), limited access to emotion regulation strategies ($p < 0.001$), and lack of emotional clarity ($p < 0.001$) between the participants with and without IA at Stage 1.

Table 3. Interactions between Internet addiction and changes in difficulty in emotion regulation analyzed by repeated-measures ANOVA.

	Within-Subject Analysis					Between-Subject Analysis			
	df	Mean Square	F	*p*		df	Mean Square	F	*p*
Non-acceptance of emotional responses									
Cohort	1	0.28	0.03	0.859	Intercept	1	64,390.83	2769.62	<0.001
Cohort × Internet addiction	1	10.75	1.22	0.271	Internet addiction	1	178.02	7.66	0.006
	322	8.84			Error	322	23.25		
Difficulties engaging in goal-directed behavior									
Cohort	1	0.61	0.10	0.755	Intercept	1	63,252.18	3477.03	<0.001
Cohort × Internet addiction	1	12.34	1.96	0.162	Internet addiction	1	831.19	45.69	<0.001
Error	322	6.29			Error	322	18.19		
Impulse control difficulties									
Cohort	1	45.45	5.81	0.016	Intercept	1	55,047.18	2220.87	<0.001
Cohort × Internet addiction	1	24.46	3.13	0.078	Internet addiction	1	655.32	26.44	<0.001
Error	322	7.82			Error	322	24.79		
Lack of emotional awareness									
Cohort	1	331.13	46.49	<0.001	Intercept	1	76,173.83	3796.15	<0.001
Cohort × Internet addiction	1	40.72	5.72	0.017	Internet addiction	1	96.71	4.82	0.029
Error	322	7.12			Error	322	20.07		
Limited access to emotion regulation strategies									
Cohort	1	44.38	3.87	0.050	Intercept	1	116,832.71	3059.68	<0.001
Cohort × Internet addiction	1	60.46	5.28	0.022	Internet addiction	1	1150.13	30.12	<0.001
Error	322	11.46			Error	322	38.19		
Lack of emotional clarity									
Cohort	1	41.63	10.91	0.001	Intercept	1	37,474.75	3280.47	<0.001
Cohort × Internet addiction	1	0.07	0.02	0.892	Internet addiction	1	151.88	13.30	<0.001
Error	322	3.82			Error	322	11.42		

To explore the effects of IA on the changes in difficulties in emotional regulation, the scores on the DERS were further compared between the Stage 1 and Stage 2 investigations using a paired t-test in the participants with and without IA at Stage 1 (Table 4). The results of the paired t-test demonstrated that in the IA group, the scores on the subscale of lack of emotional awareness decreased significantly from Stage 1 to Stage 2. In the non-IA group, the scores on the subscales of lack of emotional awareness and lack of emotional clarity decreased significantly from Stage 1 to Stage 2.

Table 4. Comparisons of difficulties in emotion regulation between the initial (Stage 1) and follow-up (Stage 2) investigations among the participants with and without Internet addiction at Stage 1.

	Stage 1 Mean (SD)	Stage 2 Mean (SD)	Paired t	p
Internet addiction group (n = 56)				
Non-acceptance of emotional responses	14.0 (4.2)	13.7 (4.2)	0.582	0.563
Difficulties engaging in goal-directed behavior	14.8 (3.9)	14.3 (3.8)	0.787	0.435
Impulse control difficulties	14.1 (4.8)	12.9 (4.3)	1.931	0.059
Lack of emotional awareness	16.1 (3.2)	13.6 (3.4)	5.500	<0.001
Limited access to emotion regulation strategies	20.3 (5.7)	18.8 (5.3)	2.084	0.042
Lack of emotional clarity	11.0 (2.4)	10.4 (3.1)	1.520	0.134
Non-Internet addiction group (n = 268)				
Non-acceptance of emotional responses	12.3 (3.8)	12.7 (4.1)	−1.504	0.134
Difficulties engaging in goal-directed behavior	11.4 (3.3)	11.7 (3.6)	−1.372	0.171
Impulse control difficulties	11.0 (3.9)	10.8 (3.9)	0.808	0.420
Lack of emotional awareness	14.4 (4.0)	13.2 (3.5)	5.243	<0.001
Limited access to emotion regulation strategies	16.0 (4.8)	16.1 (4.9)	−0.407	0.684
Lack of emotional clarity	9.8 (2.9)	9.1 (2.6)	4.275	<0.001

4. Discussion

This study revealed that more severe impulse control difficulties predicted a higher incidence of IA during the follow-up period of 1 year in male participants. Related cross-sectional studies have found a significant association between impulsivity and Internet gaming disorder in adolescents and young adults [37,38]. A longitudinal study also indicated that impulsivity is a risk factor for Internet gaming disorders among adolescents [39]. Loss of control of Internet use is an essential criterion for IA [36]; therefore, impulse control difficulties could make individuals more susceptible to the rewarding effects of Internet use and contribute to vulnerability to IA. Impulse control difficulties may also negatively affect young adults' relationships with others and thus increase their desire to seek out friendship and joy from the Internet. Moreover, a Go/NoGo study reported that college students with IA had lower electrophysiological activation in the conflict detection stage than did those without IA [40], indicating that they had lower efficiency in information processing than did their peers without IA. Low efficiency in information processing may limit individuals' ability to access effective emotion regulation strategies. Cognitive-behavioral therapy for IA aims to increase the clients' ability of impulse control by training clients' skills to monitor their inner feelings and control impulse behaviors [41–43]. Research also found that electro-acupuncture had an advantage over psychological intervention in terms of impulsivity control in adolescents with IA [44]. The present study found a gender difference in the prediction of impulse control difficulties for the incidence of IA. Previous studies have also found gender differences in the psychopathology of IA [45,46]. However, the numbers of participants with the incidence of IA during the one-year follow-up period were small. Further study with more participants is warranted to replicate this result.

The one-year remission rate of our study was 46.4%. A previous study on young adolescents in Taiwan found the one-year remission rate of IA was 49.5% [28]. A study on Hong Kong Chinese secondary school students found the one-year remission rate of IA was 59.29/100 person-years [47]. A study on German adolescents found that the one-year remission rate of IA was 71.6% [48]. The results of the present and previous studies indicated that incidence of remission was high without noticeable interventions during adolescence and adulthood. Although the present study did not find a predictive effect of difficulties in emotion regulation on the remission of IA, a previous study found that a lower level of maladaptive emotion regulation strategies significantly predicted for remission one year later [48], indicating that programs enhancing emotion regulation are important for helping people to reduce the severity of IA.

The results of ANOVA examining the changes in difficulties in emotion regulation from Stage 1 to Stage 2 did not show statistically significant differences between the IA and non-IA groups. The results did not support our hypothesis that IA may worsen emotion regulation. The score on the subscale of lack of emotional awareness decreased significantly from Stage 1 to Stage 2 in both IA and non-IA groups, whereas the score on the subscale of lack of emotional clarity decreased significantly in only the non-IA group. However, it is noteworthy that the IA group had higher scores of all subscales of the DERS than the non-IA group at the initial investigation (p-values ranging from <0.001 to 0.003). Research has found that people with negative emotional states, such as depression, anxiety, and feelings of loneliness, were more likely to use the Internet to manage their emotional problems [29–31]. Internet use might be a way for people with negative emotions to experience pleasure and avoid unpleasant experiences [49]. Research found that maladaptive emotion regulation strategies could predict the maintenance of problematic Internet use, whereas a targeted positive development of emotion regulation in childhood and adolescence could promote spontaneous remission of problematic Internet use [48]. Therefore, mental health professionals need to provide intervention programs for people with IA to improve their ability of emotion regulation.

The present study has several limitations that should be addressed. First, the data were exclusively self-reported, and we did not obtain additional information regarding mental health diagnoses or treatment history. Second, although participants recruited from the community are more representative compared with those recruited from clinical units, the volunteers may have had various motivations for participating in the study. Third, we did not assess the content of the Internet activity nor psychiatric diagnoses. Fourth, we did not survey factors that may relate to change in IA in college students, for example, personal traits, socialization process, and enthusiasm devoted to study. Lastly, the four subgroups (PNIA, NIA, RIA, and PIA) were of unequal size; two were comparably small (n = 20 in NIA; n = 30 in PIA). The small sample size might limit the power of statistical analysis.

5. Conclusions

The results of this study indicated that impulse control difficulties predicted the incidence of IA during the follow-up period of 1 year among male college students, whereas IA did not significantly predict the change in difficulties in emotion regulation. Mental health professionals should help college students develop effective strategies for emotion regulation.

Author Contributions: J.-K.T. and C.-F.Y. wrote the report; R.C.H., W.-H.L., H.-F.H., and C.-F.Y. conceived of and performed the study; C.-F.Y. analyzed the data. All authors have read and agreed to the published version of the manuscript.

References

1. Rice, R.E. Influences, usage, and outcomes of Internet health information searching: Multivariate results from the Pew surveys. *Int. J. Med. Inform.* **2006**, *75*, 8–28. [CrossRef] [PubMed]
2. Rodgers, S.; Chen, Q. Internet community group participation: Psychosocial benefits for women with breast cancer. *J. Comput. Mediat. Commun.* **2005**, *10*, 21–26. [CrossRef]
3. Jelenchick, L.A.; Eickhoff, J.; Christakis, D.A.; Brown, R.L.; Zhang, C.; Benson, M.; Moreno, M.A. The Problematic and Risky Internet Use Screening Scale (PRIUSS) for adolescents and young adults: Scale development and refinement. *Comput. Hum. Behav.* **2014**, *35*, 171–178. [CrossRef]

4. Tao, R.; Huang, X.; Wang, J.; Zhang, H.; Zhang, Y.; Li, M. Proposed diagnostic criteria for internet addiction. *Addiction* **2010**, *105*, 556–564. [CrossRef] [PubMed]
5. American Psychiatric Association. *Diagnostic and Statistical Manual of Mental Disorders*, 5th ed.; Arlington American Psychiatric Association: Washington, DC, USA, 2013.
6. Cheng, C.; Li, A.Y. Internet addiction prevalence and quality of (real) life: A meta-analysis of 31 nations across seven world regions. *Cyberpsychol. Behav. Soc. Netw.* **2014**, *17*, 755–760. [CrossRef]
7. Tateno, M.; Teo, A.R.; Shirasaka, T.; Tayama, M.; Watabe, M.; Kato, T.A. Internet addiction and self-evaluated attention-deficit hyperactivity disorder traits among Japanese college students. *Psychiatry Clin. Neurosci.* **2016**, *70*, 567–572. [CrossRef] [PubMed]
8. Ko, C.H.; Hsiao, S.; Liu, G.C.; Yen, J.Y.; Yang, M.J.; Yen, C.F. The characteristics of decision making, potential to take risks, and personality of college students with Internet addiction. *Psychiatry Res.* **2010**, *175*, 121–125. [CrossRef]
9. Yang, T.; Yu, L.; Oliffe, J.L.; Jiang, S.; Si, Q. Regional contextual determinants of internet addiction among college students: A representative nationwide study of China. *Eur. J. Public Health* **2017**, *27*, 1032–1037. [CrossRef]
10. Anderson, K.J. Internet use among college students: An exploratory study. *J. Am. Coll. Health* **2001**, *50*, 21–26. [CrossRef]
11. Balhara, P.S.Y.; Doric, A.; Stevanovic, D.; Knez, R.; Swarndeep ingh, S.; Chowdhury, M.R.R.; Kafali, H.Y.; Sharma, P.; Vally, Z.; Vu, T.V.; et al. Correlates of problematic Internet use among college and university students in eight countries: An international cross-sectional study. *Asian J. Psychiatry* **2019**, *45*, 113–120. [CrossRef]
12. Kuss, D.J.; Griffiths, M.D.; Binder, J.F. Internet addiction in students: Prevalence and risk factors. *Comput. Hum. Behav.* **2013**, *29*, 959–966. [CrossRef]
13. Chang, Y.H.; Lee, Y.T.; Hsieh, S. Internet interpersonal connection mediates the association between personality and Internet addiction. *Int. J. Environ. Res. Public Health* **2019**, *16*, 3537. [CrossRef]
14. Chwaszcz, J.; Lelonek-Kuleta, B.; Wiechetek, M.; Niewiadomska, I.; Palacz-Chrisidis, A. Personality traits, strategies for coping with stress and the level of Internet addiction-A study of Polish secondary-school students. *Int. J. Environ. Res. Public Health* **2018**, *15*, 987. [CrossRef] [PubMed]
15. Shi, M.; Du, T.J. Associations of personality traits with internet addiction in Chinese medical students: The mediating role of attention-deficit/hyperactivity disorder symptoms. *BMC Psychiatry* **2019**, *19*, 183. [CrossRef] [PubMed]
16. Chou, W.J.; Chang, Y.P.; Yen, C.F. Boredom proneness and its correlation with Internet addiction and Internet activities in adolescents with attention-deficit/hyperactivity disorder. *Kaohsiung J. Med. Sci.* **2018**, *34*, 467–474. [CrossRef]
17. Lu, W.H.; Lee, K.H.; Ko, C.H.; Hsiao, R.C.; Hu, H.F.; Yen, C.F. Relationship between borderline personality symptoms and Internet addiction: The mediating effects of mental health problems. *J. Behav. Addict.* **2017**, *6*, 434–441. [CrossRef]
18. Lu, W.H.; Chou, W.J.; Hsiao, R.C.; Hu, H.F.; Yen, C.F. Correlations of Internet addiction severity with reinforcement sensitivity and frustration intolerance in adolescents with attention-deficit/hyperactivity disorder: The moderating effect of medications. *Front. Psychiatry* **2019**, *10*, 268. [CrossRef] [PubMed]
19. Hormes, J.M.; Kearns, B.; Timko, C.A. Craving Facebook? Behavioral addiction to online social networking and its association with emotion regulation deficits. *Addiction* **2014**, *109*, 2079–2088. [CrossRef] [PubMed]
20. Aldao, A.; Nolen-Hoeksema, S.; Schweizer, S. Emotion regulation strategies across psychopathology: A meta-analytic review. *Clin. Psychol. Rev.* **2010**, *30*, 217–237. [CrossRef]
21. Hayes, S.C.; Strosahl, K.D.; Wilson, K.G.; Bissett, R.T.; Pistorello, J.; Toarmino, D.; Polusny, M.A.; Dykstra, T.A.; Batten, S.V.; Bergan, L.; et al. Measuring experiential avoidance: A preliminary test of a working model. *Psychol. Rec.* **2004**, *54*, 553–578. [CrossRef]
22. Gratz, K.L.; Roemer, L. Multidimensional assessment of emotion regulation and dysregulation: Development, factor structure, and initial validation of the difficulties in emotion regulation scale. *J. Psychopathol. Behav. Assess.* **2004**, *26*, 41–54. [CrossRef]
23. Ko, C.H.; Yen, J.Y.; Yen, C.F.; Chen, C.S.; Chen, C.C. The association between Internet addiction and psychiatric disorder: A review of the literature. *Eur. Psychiatry* **2012**, *27*, 1–8. [CrossRef] [PubMed]

24. Estévez, A.; Jáuregui, P.; Sánchez-Marcos, I.; López-González, H.; Griffiths, M.D. Attachment and emotion regulation in substance addictions and behavioral addictions. *J. Behav. Addict.* **2017**, *6*, 534–544. [CrossRef] [PubMed]
25. Karaer, Y.; Akdemir, D. Parenting styles, perceived social support and emotion regulation in adolescents with internet addiction. *Compr. Psychiatry* **2019**, *92*, 22–27. [CrossRef] [PubMed]
26. Lee, J.; Lee, S.; Chun, J.W.; Cho, H.; Kim, D.J.; Jung, Y.C. Compromised prefrontal cognitive control over emotional interference in adolescents with Internet gaming disorder. *Cyberpsychol. Behav. Soc. Netw.* **2015**, *18*, 661–668. [CrossRef] [PubMed]
27. Wang, W.; Li, D.; Li, X.; Wang, Y.; Sun, W.; Zhao, L.; Qiu, L. Parent-adolescent relationship and adolescent internet addiction: A moderated mediation model. *Addict. Behav.* **2018**, *84*, 171–177. [CrossRef]
28. Ko, C.H.; Yen, J.Y.; Chen, C.S.; Yeh, Y.C.; Yen, C.F. Predictive values of psychiatric symptoms for internet addiction in adolescents: A 2-year prospective study. *Arch. Pediatr. Adolesc. Med.* **2009**, *163*, 937–943. [CrossRef]
29. Whang, L.S.; Lee, S.; Chang, G. Internet over-users' psychological profiles: A behavior sampling analysis on internet addiction. *Cyberpsychol. Behav.* **2003**, *6*, 143–150. [CrossRef]
30. Bakken, I.J.; Wenzel, H.G.; Götestam, K.G. Internet addiction among Norwegian adults: A stratified probability sample study. *Scand. J. Psychol.* **2009**, *50*, 121–127. [CrossRef]
31. Van den Eijnden, R.; Vermulst, A.; van Rooij, A.J.; Scholte, R.; van de Mheen, D. The bidirectional relationships between online victimization and psychosocial problems in adolescents: A comparison with real-life victimization. *J. Youth Adolesc.* **2014**, *43*, 790–802. [CrossRef] [PubMed]
32. Kanter, J.W.; Cautilli, J.D.; Busch, A.M.; Baruch, D.E. Toward a comprehensive functional analysis of depressive behavior: Five environmental factors and a possible sixth and seventh. *Behav. Anal. Today* **2005**, *6*, 65–81. [CrossRef]
33. Hayes, S.C.; Wilson, K.G.; Gifford, E.V.; Follette, V.M.; Strosahl, K. Experimental avoidance and behavioral disorders: A functional dimensional approach to diagnosis and treatment. *J. Consult. Clin. Psychol.* **1996**, *64*, 1152–1168. [CrossRef] [PubMed]
34. Hsieh, F.Y. Sample size tables for logistic regression. *Stat. Med.* **1989**, *8*, 795–802. [CrossRef] [PubMed]
35. Chen, S.H.; Weng, L.J.; Su, Y.J.; Wu, H.M.; Yang, P.F. Development of Chinese Internet Addiction Scale and its psychometric study. *Chin. J. Psychol.* **2003**, *45*, 279–294.
36. Ko, C.H.; Yen, J.Y.; Chen, S.H.; Yang, M.J.; Yen, C.F. Proposed diagnostic criteria and the screening and diagnosing tool of Internet addiction in college student. *Compr. Psychiatry* **2009**, *50*, 378–384. [CrossRef]
37. Ding, W.N.; Sun, J.H.; Sun, Y.W.; Chen, X.; Zhou, Y.; Zhuang, Z.G.; Xu, J.R.; Du, Y.S. Trait impulsivity and impaired prefrontal impulse inhibition function in adolescents with Internet gaming addiction revealed by a go/no-go fMRI study. *Behav. Brain. Funct.* **2014**, *10*, 20. [CrossRef]
38. Ko, C.H.; Hsieh, T.J.; Wang, P.W.; Lin, W.C.; Yen, C.F.; Chen, C.S.; Yen, J.Y. Altered gray matter density and disrupted functional connectivity of the amygdala in adults with Internet gaming disorder. *Prog. Neuropsychopharmacol. Biol. Psychiatry* **2015**, *57*, 185–192. [CrossRef] [PubMed]
39. Gentile, D.A.; Choo, H.; Liau, A.; Sim, T.; Li, D.; Fung, D.; Khoo, A. Pathological video game use among youths: A two-year longitudinal study. *Pediatrics* **2011**, *127*, e319–e329. [CrossRef]
40. Dong, G.; Zhou, H.; Zhao, X. Impulse inhibition in people with Internet addiction disorder: Electrophysiological evidence from a Go/NoGo study. *Neurosci. Lett.* **2010**, *485*, 138–142. [CrossRef]
41. Du, Y.S.; Jiang, W.; Vance, A. Longer term effect of randomized, controlled group cognitive behavioural therapy for Internet addiction in adolescent students in Shanghai. *Aust. N. Z. J. Psychiatry* **2010**, *44*, 129–134. [CrossRef]
42. Park, S.Y.; Kim, S.M.; Roh, S.; Soh, M.A.; Lee, S.H.; Kim, H.; Han, D.H. The effects of a virtual reality treatment program for online gaming addiction. *Comput. Methods Programs Biomed.* **2016**, *129*, 99–108. [CrossRef] [PubMed]
43. Torres-Rodríguez, A.; Griffiths, M.D.; Carbonell, X.; Oberst, U. Treatment efficacy of a specialized psychotherapy program for Internet Gaming Disorder. *J. Behav. Addict.* **2018**, *7*, 939–952. [CrossRef] [PubMed]
44. Yang, Y.; Li, H.; Chen, X.X.; Zhang, L.M.; Huang, B.J.; Zhu, T.M. Electro-acupuncture treatment for internet addiction: Evidence of normalization of impulse control disorder in adolescents. *Chin. J. Integr. Med.* **2017**, *23*, 837–844. [CrossRef] [PubMed]

45. Bonnaire, C.; Baptista, D. Internet gaming disorder in male and female young adults: The role of alexithymia, depression, anxiety and gaming type. *Psychiatry Res.* **2019**, *272*, 521–530. [CrossRef] [PubMed]
46. Stockdale, L.; Coyne, S.M. Video game addiction in emerging adulthood: Cross-sectional evidence of pathology in video game addicts as compared to matched healthy controls. *J. Affect. Disord.* **2018**, *225*, 265–272. [CrossRef] [PubMed]
47. Lau, J.T.F.; Wu, A.M.S.; Gross, D.L.; Cheng, K.M.; Lau, M.M.C. Is Internet addiction transitory or persistent? Incidence and prospective predictors of remission of Internet addiction among Chinese secondary school students. *Addict. Behav.* **2017**, *74*, 55–62. [CrossRef]
48. Wartberg, L.; Lindenberg, K. Predictors of spontaneous remission of problematic Internet use in adolescence: A one-year follow-up study. *Int. J. Environ. Res. Public Health* **2020**, *17*, 448. [CrossRef]
49. Chou, W.P.; Lee, K.H.; Ko, C.H.; Liu, T.L.; Hsiao, R.C.; Lin, H.F.; Yen, C.F. Relationship between psychological inflexibility and experiential avoidance and internet addiction: Mediating effects of mental health problems. *Psychiatry Res.* **2017**, *257*, 40–44. [CrossRef]

Problematic Smartphone Use, Deep and Surface Approaches to Learning, and Social Media Use in Lectures

Dmitri Rozgonjuk [1,2,*], Kristiina Saal [1] and Karin Täht [1]

1 Institute of Psychology, University of Tartu, Tartu 50409, Estonia; kristiinasaal@gmail.com (K.S.); karin.taht@ut.ee (K.T.)
2 Department of Psychology, University of Toledo, Toledo, OH 43606, USA
* Correspondence: dmroz@ut.ee
† The preliminary results of this study were presented on the ICBA 2017 Conference on Proneness to Smartphone Addiction, Internet Addiction, and Approaches to Learning, Haifa, Israel, 20–22 February 2017.

Abstract: Several studies have shown that problematic smartphone use (PSU) is related to detrimental outcomes, such as worse psychological well-being, higher cognitive distraction, and poorer academic outcomes. In addition, many studies have shown that PSU is strongly related to social media use. Despite this, the relationships between PSU, as well as the frequency of social media use in lectures, and different approaches to learning have not been previously studied. In our study, we hypothesized that both PSU and the frequency of social media use in lectures are negatively correlated with a deep approach to learning (defined as learning for understanding) and positively correlated with a surface approach to learning (defined as superficial learning). The study participants were 415 Estonian university students aged 19–46 years (78.8% females; age M = 23.37, SD = 4.19); the effective sample comprised 405 participants aged 19–46 years (79.0% females; age M = 23.33, SD = 4.21). In addition to basic socio-demographics, participants were asked about the frequency of their social media use in lectures, and they filled out the Estonian Smartphone Addiction Proneness Scale and the Estonian Revised Study Process Questionnaire. Bivariate correlation analysis showed that PSU and the frequency of social media use in lectures were negatively correlated with a deep approach to learning and positively correlated with a surface approach to learning. Mediation analysis showed that social media use in lectures completely mediates the relationship between PSU and approaches to learning. These results indicate that the frequency of social media use in lectures might explain the relationships between poorer academic outcomes and PSU.

Keywords: problematic smartphone use; smartphone addiction; social media; approaches to learning; deep approach to learning; surface approach to learning

---

1. Introduction

Since their introduction in 2009, smartphones have had a significant impact on daily life across the world. The worldwide ownership of smartphones is around 43% [1], and more than 50% of Estonians own a smartphone [2]. Smartphones have several advantages in educational settings, allowing one to take notes, browse for information, communicate with others, and use specific applications for learning skills [3]. Several studies have shown, however, that there are instances where the excessive use of smartphones leads to the development of "problematic smartphone use" (PSU), a phenomenon characterized by the occurrence of addictive-like symptoms [4]. PSU has been associated with psychopathological symptoms [5] as well as poor academic outcomes [6,7]. Similar findings have been reported with excessive social media use [8]. The aim of this paper is to investigate how

PSU is related to approaches to learning. Specifically, this study addresses the questions of how PSU is related to learning for understanding (known as the deep approach to learning) and learning motivated by external incentives (for example, grades; known as a surface approach to learning) [9]. In addition, the mediating effect of social media use in lectures is analyzed, as it may be the case that the relationship between PSU and approaches to learning is dependent on the frequency of social media use.

Previous works regarding smartphone addiction is often seen as controversial. It has been debated whether or not smartphone "addiction" is a behavioral addiction, and whether or not it may be considered as an actual addiction from the perspective of contemporary addiction theories [10–12]. Nevertheless, one cannot neglect the growing body of evidence that suggests that problematic smartphone usage is related to several psychopathological symptoms, such as depression and anxiety [5,13], poorer health and sleep quality [14], and lower academic achievements [6]. In addition to smartphone addiction, the following terms have been used to describe conceptually the same phenomenon: proneness to smartphone addiction [15,16], smartphone overuse [17,18], excessive smartphone use [19], problematic mobile phone use [20], mobile phone dependence [21], and mobile phone addiction [22,23]. In essence, these terms characterize the excessive use of smartphones accompanied by symptoms resembling those found in contemporary addiction models: dependence, withdrawal, tolerance, and functional impairment [4]; therefore, we conceptualize the phenomenon as problematic smartphone use.

PSU as a maladaptive coping method [24] has received relatively little attention in academic contexts in scientific literature. Although studies have found that the higher levels of PSU are related to poor academic outcomes [6,7], different approaches to learning as potential causal factors for academic outcomes have not yet been researched in the light of problematic technology use.

Empirical findings have led Marton and Säljö [9] to propose a distinction between approaches to learning; these were categorized as surface and deep approaches to learning. Accordingly, one uses a deep approach to learning to fully understand the content studied. In contrast, the surface approach to learning is characterized by instrumental learning which aims to minimally fulfill the requirements of study; with the latter, only the basics of the study material are learned [25]. Biggs [26] defined both of these approaches as motives and strategies. While a deep motive involves intrinsic interest in the content that is learned, and the aim is to develop competence, a surface motive is to meet requirements minimally. In addition, deep strategy is to discover meaning by reading widely, relating one's previous knowledge with learned material, whereas surface strategy is to limit the amount of work one needs to do (through rote learning).

It has been shown that a deep approach to learning facilitates critical thinking, finding causal relationships, creativity, and autonomous thinking. Therefore, this type of approach is an essential ingredient in successful learning, as it leads to a more systematic and thorough comprehension of information [27]. Authors [28] have found that those with a deep approach to learning have better developed organization skills, more spontaneously expressed ideas, and clearer, longer, and more detailed explanations. Those with a deep approach to learning may also make more associations with their work and prior knowledge and experiences [28]. Other works have linked deep learning with a higher need to understand material and a drive to satisfy one's curiosity [29,30]. On the other hand, a surface approach to learning is characterized by incentive-oriented strategy, according to which the student aims to do only as much as is necessary to study, often compulsory, material [25,29]. Those who are prone to this approach tend to focus on learning facts, isolated details, examples and illustrations without connecting the pieces of information to their knowledge to provide a broader perspective [30]. This leads to a focus on understanding simpler principles [27]. Surface learners are rather passive and their attitude towards learning is to regard it as something which inevitably happens. In comparison, a deep approach to learning leads to an increased sense of control over the learning process [9].

As the information suggests, relationships between academic success and learning strategies are well researched. Several studies have shown that surface learners have lower academic outcomes and are less successful in school, whereas those with a deep approach to learning are more successful in school [31–35]. Additionally, the probability of graduating from higher education institutions is lower for students who study superficially [36].

In addition, it has been found that more social media use (on the example of Facebook) is related to worse academic outcomes [37]; also, engaging with social distractors (social media with its functionalities could be considered as one) have shown to be related to poorer concentration and procrastination [38]. Unsurprisingly, one of the main functions of smartphones is social media use [39–42], allowing for almost constant access to continually changing content and engaging with social distractors.

Though some studies have shown that higher levels of PSU and other excessive technology use (e.g., the Internet) are associated with poorer academic outcomes [6,7,43,44], it has not been studied if different levels of PSU are related to deep and surface approach to learning. Furthermore, the role of social media use in lectures is not investigated in the potential relationships between the levels of PSU, and deep and surface approaches to learning.

The aims of this study are (a) to investigate how deep and surface approaches to learning are related to the levels of PSU and social media use in lectures, and (b) to clarify if social media use in lectures mediates the relationship between the levels of PSU and approaches to learning. Based on the empirical findings discussed earlier, we have posed the following hypotheses:

Hypothesis 1 (H1). *The levels of PSU are negatively related to a deep approach to learning and positively related with a surface approach to learning. PSU is a maladaptive coping method [24] that has been found to be associated with several other dysfunctional behaviors or detrimental outcomes, including in academic settings [6,7]. Therefore, we expect the levels of PSU to be correlated negatively to the deep approach to learning (adaptive learning strategy) and positively to the surface approach to learning (maladaptive learning strategy).*

Hypothesis 2 (H2). *The frequency of social media use in lectures is negatively correlated to a deep approach to learning and positively related to a surface approach to learning. Studies have shown that more social media use is related to poorer academic outcomes [37]. Similarly to the previous hypothesis, we expect social media use in lectures to be related to approaches to learning.*

Hypothesis 3 (H3). *The levels of PSU are positively correlated with the frequency of social media use in lectures. The levels of PSU have been shown to be related to the social use of smartphones [39–42]. We expect that is also the case with social media use in lectures, specifically.*

Hypothesis 4 (H4). *Social media use in lectures mediates the relationship between the levels of PSU and approaches to learning. It has been found that levels of PSU are related to social media use and social use in general [15,42,45]. It has also been shown that more social media use is associated with lower academic outcomes [37]. We hypothesize that higher levels of PSU is related to more social media use in lectures, and this is related with a less deep and more surface approach to learning.*

2. Materials and Methods

2.1. Sample and Procedure

Four hundred fifteen Estonian university students (ages ranging from 19 to 46 years, M_{age} = 23.37 ± 4.19 years; 78.8% were female) participated in an online survey in Estonian. Ten participants had missing data in their responses and were, therefore, removed from further analyses. The characteristics of the effective sample are the following: ages ranging from 19 to 46 years, M_{age} = 23.33 ± 4.21 years; 79.0% were female. Therefore, the efficient sample comprised 405 participants (age range from 19 to 46 years, M_{age} = 23.33 ± 4.21 years; 79.0% were female). Three hundred ninety-three (97.04%) participants marked their mother tongue as Estonian, 11 (2.7%) as Russian, and 1 as "other."

The participants were recruited through university mailing lists and via social media. Prior to taking the survey, participants filled out an informed consent form in accordance with the Declaration of Helsinki. The participants were asked to complete a merged questionnaire that consisted of the following parts: (a) general socio-demographics, (b) the Estonian Revised Study Process Questionnaire, (c) questions about social media use in lectures, (d) the Estonian Smartphone Addiction Proneness Scale.

2.2. *Explanations of Measures*

Further details of the measures used are provided.

2.2.1. General Socio-Demographics

These included items about the participants' age (in full years), gender (male/female/other), and mother tongue (Estonian/Russian/other).

2.2.2. The Revised Study Process Questionnaire (Estonian Adaptation)

(R-SPQ-2F; [46]): this is a modified two-dimensional 16-item questionnaire with Likert-type scale (from 1 = "do not agree at all" to 5 = "totally agree") that is inspired by the Revised Study Process Questionnaire developed by Biggs, Kember, and Leung [25]; see [46] for further details about the adaptation process and Table S1 for the items of the scale. The scale measures the extent to which students use a surface (e.g., "I generally restrict my study to what is specifically set as I think it is unnecessary to do anything extra") or deep (e.g., "I find that at times studying gives me a feeling of deep personal satisfaction") approach to learning as their learning strategy. The internal reliability was acceptable for the surface approach to learning subscale (Cronbach's $\alpha = 0.72$), and for the deep approach to learning subscale (Cronbach's $\alpha = 0.75$).

2.2.3. Social Media Use in Lectures

Participants were asked two questions about social media use in lectures, derived from the items and scales used in [47]: firstly, "How frequently do you keep track of social media in lectures?" (1 = "never" ... 5 = "all the time") and, secondly, "How often do you communicate with friends using social networking sites (Facebook, Twitter, etc.) in lectures?" (1 = "never" ... 5 = "all the time"). These items were highly correlated ($r = 0.74$, $p < 0.0001$) and were aggregated into one social media use index.

2.2.4. The Estonian Smartphone Addiction Proneness Scale

(E-SAPS18; [15]: The E-SAPS18 is a five-dimensional questionnaire consisting of 18 items measuring the frequency of smartphone addiction symptoms on a 6-point Likert scale (from 1 = "strongly disagree" to 6 = "strongly agree"). E-SAPS18 consists of five factors (tolerance, positive anticipation, cyberspace-oriented relationships, withdrawal, and physical symptoms), with a higher-order factor of smartphone addiction proneness. The internal reliability of E-SAPS18 is very good (Cronbach's $\alpha = 0.87$), and E-SAPS18 has been validated against other instruments measuring Internet and smartphone addiction proneness.

2.3. *Data Analysis*

RStudio version 3.2.3 (R Core Team, Vienna, Austria) was used for descriptive statistics and correlation analysis. The skewness and kurtosis of distributions of variables were among the acceptable ranges (from −2 to +2) [48,49]. One-tailed Pearson product–moment correlation was used to analyze bivariate relationships between variables, as we expected directional relationships in each correlation. Mplus version 8 was used for mediation analysis.

We used the weighted least squares estimation with a mean- and variance-adjusted chi-square (WLSMV), because it has been shown to be less biased and more accurate than similar estimation methods (e.g., robust maximum likelihood, or MLR) for the data type [50]. Using the WLSMV estimation method, we treated the items of social media use in lectures and E-SAPS18 as categorical/ordinal data, thus involving a polychoric covariance matrix and probit regression coefficients [51]. The summed scale scores for deep and surface approach to learning were treated as observed variables in the models. The cross-products of direct effects to compute mediation effect were used, applying the Delta method for computing indirect effect standard errors, with non-parametric bootstrapping across 1000 samples [52]. Goodness of fit was judged by standard parameters: (a) Comparative Fit Index (CFI) $\geq$ 0.90, (b) Tucker–Lewis Index (TLI) $\geq$ 0.90, and (c) root mean square error of approximation (RMSEA) $\leq$ 0.08.

We used SPSS version 24 to compute Mahalanobis distances to detect the outliers in the multivariate dataset. Altogether, there were 19 cases (4.7%) where $p < 0.05$ (4 cases, or 1% of the sample, with $p < 0.01$). The analyses described above were re-ran in order to detect if these statistical outliers influenced the results cardinally. However, as the results were virtually the same (signs and magnitudes of coefficients, statistical significance of the predictors, and the mediating variable), we retained these multivariate outliers in the sample.

3. Results

3.1. Correlation Analysis

Summary and scale reliability statistics for the study sample are highlighted in Table 1. In order to analyze the relationships between PSU, approaches to learning, and social media use in lectures, Pearson product–moment correlation analyses were carried out. The results are shown in Table 1.

Table 1. Pearson product–moment correlations, means, standard deviations, and internal consistencies of scales and subscales.

	Variable	1	2	3	Min	Max	M	SD	α
1	PSU				18	76	35.52	10.73	0.86
2	SMUL	0.326 ***			2	10	5.92	2.10	0.85
3	DA	−0.109 *	−0.304 ***		11	39	26.80	4.62	0.78
4	SA	0.177 ***	0.297 ***	−0.425 ***	8	34	20.12	4.93	0.75

Notes: $N = 415$. PSU = problematic smartphone use measured by the E-SAPS18; SMUL = Social media use in lectures; DA = deep approach to learning; SA = surface approach to learning. * $p \leq 0.05$, *** $p \leq 0.001$.

It could be observed that all variables are statistically significantly inter-related. Specifically, PSU (as an E-SAPS18 score) is in positive correlation with social media use in lectures and a surface approach to learning; the latter two variables are, in turn, also positively correlated with each other. Additionally, both PSU and social media use in lectures are negatively correlated with a deep approach to learning.

3.2. Mediation Analysis

Confirmatory factor analysis showed that the five-factor E-SAPS18 with one higher-order factor had an acceptable fit: CFI = 0.93; TLI = 0.92; RMSEA = 0.09. The fit indices for two-factor R-SPQ-2F (Estonian adaptation) were CFI = 0.76, TLI = 0.72, and RMSEA = 0.13. Because the latter scale did not show a great fit, we used observed variables (summed scores for deep and surface approach to learning) as outcome variables.

Three mediation models were constructed to investigate if social media use in lectures mediates the relationship between PSU and approaches to learning. In the first model (Model 1), we used only the deep approach to learning as the outcome variable. In the second model (Model 2), we used the surface approach to learning as the outcome model. In both of these models, the mediating variable was controlled for age and gender, as it has been shown that age and gender might impact social media engagement [53]. The third model (Model 3) included both the deep and surface approaches to learning as outcome variables predicted by the levels of PSU and mediated by social media use in lectures. Again, the mediator was controlled for gender; furthermore, deep and surface approaches to learning were specified to covary in that model. As mentioned earlier, measures of PSU and social media use in lectures were modeled as latent (categorical/ordinal), and the summed scores for deep and surface approaches to learning and the covariates (age, gender) were treated as observed variables.

The fit indices for Model 1 were CFI = 0.94, TLI = 0.93, and RMSEA = 0.07; for Model 2, they were CFI = 0.94, TLI = 0.93, and RMSEA = 0.07; and for Model 3: CFI = 0.94, TLI = 0.93, and RMSEA = 0.07. The coefficients of the models are presented in Table 2.

Table 2. The results of mediation models.

Model 1 (Outcome DA)				
Covariates	**Bivariate B (SE)**	***t***	**Multivariate B (SE)**	***t***
PSU	0.001 (0.079)	0.016	0.001 (0.061)	0.016
SMUL	−0.345 (0.060)	−5.751 ***	−0.417 (0.063)	−6.630 ***
PSU -> SMUL	0.547 (0.098)	5.573 ***	0.348 (0.059)	5.874 ***
Age -> SMUL	−0.095 (0.012)	−7.799 ***	−0.440 (0.053)	−8.349 ***
Gender -> SMUL	0.103 (0.139)	0.744	0.046 (0.061)	0.754
PSU -> SMUL -> DA	−0.189 (0.050)	−3.757 ***	−0.145 (0.035)	−4.115 ***
Model 2 (Outcome SA)				
Covariates	**Bivariate B (SE)**	***t***	**Multivariate B (SE)**	***t***
PSU	0.088 (0.061)	1.457	0.093 (0.061)	1.513
SMUL	0.205 (0.050)	4.136 ***	0.336 (0.076)	4.410 ***
PSU -> SMUL	0.548 (0.094)	5.820 ***	0.350 (0.056)	6.247 ***
Age -> SMUL	−0.082 (0.011)	−7.369 ***	−0.382 (0.047)	−8.055 ***
Gender -> SMUL	0.103 (0.124)	0.829	0.046 (0.055)	0.839
PSU -> SMUL -> SA	0.112 (0.035)	3.193 ***	0.118 (0.035)	3.340 ***
Model 3 (Outcomes DA and SA)				
Covariates	**Bivariate B (SE)**	***t***	**Multivariate B (SE)**	***t***
PSU -> DA	0.002 (0.084)	0.024	0.001 (0.060)	0.024
SMUL -> DA	−0.361 (0.060)	−6.008 ***	−0.419 (0.064)	−6.604 ***
PSU -> SA	0.112 (0.071)	1.572	0.097 (0.061)	1.594
SMUL -> SA	0.243 (0.057)	4.261 ***	0.336 (0.074)	4.569 ***
PSU -> SMUL	0.562 (0.102)	5.526 ***	0.353 (0.060)	5.848 ***
Age -> SMUL	−0.097 (0.013)	−7.609 ***	−0.447 (0.053)	−8.364 ***
Gender -> SMUL	0.053 (0.146)	0.365	0.024 (0.064)	0.370
PSU -> SMUL -> DA	−0.203 (0.055)	−3.668 ***	−0.148 (0.037)	−3.969 ***
PSU -> SMUL -> SA	0.137 (0.044)	3.095 **	0.119 (0.037)	3.222 ***
DA <-> SA	−0.228 (0.037)	−6.094 ***	−0.526 (0.051)	−10.365 ***

Notes $N = 415$. PSU = problematic smartphone use measured by the E-SAPS18; SMUL = Social media use in lectures; DA = deep approach to learning; SA = surface approach to learning. ** $p \leq 0.01$, *** $p \leq 0.001$.

It could be observed from all three models that social media use in lectures mediates the relationship between problematic smartphone use and approaches to learning. In Model 1, PSU does not have a direct effect on deep approach to learning; however, social media use in lectures completely mediates the relationship between PSU and deep approach to learning. Furthermore, the indirect effect is negative.

Similarly, social media use in lectures completely mediates the relationship between PSU and surface approach to learning (see Model 2). However, in this case, the indirect effect is positive. Higher PSU leads to higher social media use in lectures which, in turn, is associated with more surface approach to learning.

These effects are present even if both surface and deep approach to learning are included in the same model as outcome variables. Interestingly, gender is not associated with social media use in lectures, whereas in all models, younger people tend to use more social media in lectures.

4. Discussion

According to previous research, PSU and excessive social media use relate to poorer academic outcomes [6]. However, these relationships are often examined in relation to grades or grade point average (GPA), not to deep and surface approaches to learning. As such, in our study, we hypothesized that PSU would be negatively related to a deep approach to learning and positively related to a surface approach to learning. Indeed, the results showed that a higher PSU is associated with less commitment to a deep approach to learning and with greater commitment to a surface approach to learning. We expected, too, that more frequent social media use in lectures would be negatively correlated with a deep approach to learning and positively associated with a surface approach to learning. Our results also confirmed this hypothesis. The relationship between frequent, engaged smartphone use and multitasking [54,55], which may be detrimental to academic achievement [56], may potentially explain these findings. Those with additional access to technology may be more prone to multitasking [57], which may in turn lead to less in-depth or more superficial learning. Future studies should try to take into account multitasking as a potential factor in influencing the relationships reported in this study.

According to our third hypothesis, we expected PSU to be positively associated with the frequency of social media use in lectures. This hypothesis was confirmed by the results. This result is not surprising, as one of the most popular activities on smartphones is social media usage. Therefore, it is natural that those with higher PSU are also more prone to use social media in lectures.

As a second aim of the study, we presented a conceptual mediation model where the relationship between PSU and approaches to learning are mediated by the frequency of social media use in lectures. Our previous results provided the statistical basis for the models [58]. According to the models, social media use in lectures completely mediated the relationship between PSU and approaches to learning. In other words, though PSU and approaches to learning were related in bivariate correlations, these relationships could be explained by the effect of social media use frequency. Indeed, it has been indicated that the most frequent activity carried out on smartphones is social media use [15,45]. Smartphones allow for mobility and availability in terms of online interactions and content consumption from social media platforms.

Several limitations are worth mentioning. Firstly, self-report measures were used, and this might affect the reliability and ecological validity of the findings. It would be interesting to contrast our results with behavioral social media usage data (e.g., the actual measured time of social media usage) and objective academic data (e.g., GPA, test scores, and SAT scores). This kind of approach would allow for more accurate and reliable data, and better generalization. Secondly, the study design was cross-sectional; therefore, one has to be cautious in making causal interpretations. This is especially important to keep in mind while interpreting the results of mediation models. Our hypothesized models are based on the logic that PSU, as a more generic construct, encompasses social media use and that it therefore could be a precondition for more social media consumption. However, it could also be the case that more social media use causes more PSU. Additionally, students' approaches to learning could be influenced by both PSU and social media use; however, it could also be the case that approaches to learning impact how much social media a student consumes in lectures. Finally, we did not ask the participants how much time they spent online (per day or per week) and why the participants engaged in activities involving social media use in lectures. Though studies have shown that self-reported estimated time of technology use is typically inaccurate in comparison to objective use [59–61], knowing learning about the objective usage time and could greatly improve the understanding of these results. Additionally, distinguishing between the activities in which students engage on social media (e.g., learning vs. entertainment that is not related to class content) could specify the potential effects. We encourage the reader to be mindful of these limitations, and we consider experimental and/or longitudinal studies to be helpful in clarifying this issue; we hope the current paper inspires studies of that nature.

This study has both theoretical and practical implications. From a theoretical perspective, this is the first study to investigate the relationships between approaches to learning and PSU. Though it has been shown that a deep approach to learning is positively related to academic outcomes, and a surface approach to learning is found to have negative effects on academic outcomes [31–34], this study provides potential evidence to the findings where PSU has been associated with poor academic outcomes [6]. Specifically, poorer outcomes might be due to a less deep and/or more surface approach to learning. In addition, the findings between PSU and academic outcomes could be explained by students engaging in more social media use.

Among the potential practical implications, this paper suggests that social media use in lectures might be the driver in the relationship between approaches to learning and PSU. Lecturers might consider restricting access to social media use in lectures or to advise their students that engaging in excessive smartphone use and especially social media use in lectures could have detrimental effects on their academic outcomes. However, this idea needs further testing—preferably by implementing experimental and, if possible, longitudinal study design to better understand if this practical suggestion derived from the results of this study have beneficial effects.

5. Conclusions

Recent advances in technology offer many promising advantages in the classroom. However, problematic technology use has been shown to be negatively related to academic outcomes. In the current study, we found that both PSU and social media use in lectures are related to less commitment to a deep approach to learning (learning to fully understand the content studied) in place of a more surface approach to learning (instrumental learning to meet the requirements of one's learning outcomes). Additionally, we proposed hypothetical models where the frequency of social media use in lectures mediates the relationship between PSU and approaches to learning. We found that social media use in lectures completely mediates the aforementioned relationship. Further studies should address the limitations of this study, such as using self-reported measures and cross-sectional study design.

Acknowledgments: This study was not funded. The authors did not receive funds for covering the costs to publish in open access.

Author Contributions: Dmitri Rozgonjuk, Kristiina Saal, and Karin Täht conceived and designed the study; Dmitri Rozgonjuk and Kristiina Saal performed the data collection; Dmitri Rozgonjuk and Karin Täht analyzed the data; Dmitri Rozgonjuk, Kristiina Saal, and Karin Täht wrote the paper.

References

1. Poushter, J. Smartphone Ownership and Internet Usage Continues to Climb in Emerging Economies. 2016. Available online: http://www.pewglobal.org/2016/02/22/smartphone-ownership-and-internet-usage-continues-to-climb-in-emerging-economies/ (accessed on 10 October 2017).
2. Statista. Forecast of the Smartphone User Penetration Rate in Estonia from 2015 to 2022. 2017. Available online: https://www.statista.com/statistics/568089/predicted-smartphone-user-penetration-rate-in-estonia/ (accessed on 11 February 2017).
3. Godwin-Jones, R. Mobile apps for language learning. *Lang. Learn. Technol.* **2011**, *15*, 2–11.
4. Billieux, J.; Maurage, P.; Lopez-Fernandez, O.; Kuss, D.J.; Griffiths, M.D. Can disordered mobile phone use be considered a behavioral addiction? An update on current evidence and a comprehensive model for future research. *Curr. Addict. Rep.* **2015**, *2*, 156–162. [CrossRef]

5. Elhai, J.D.; Dvorak, R.D.; Levine, J.C.; Hall, B.J. Problematic smartphone use: A conceptual overview and systematic review of relations with anxiety and depression psychopathology. *J. Affect. Disord.* **2017**, *207*, 251–259. [CrossRef] [PubMed]
6. Samaha, M.; Hawi, N.S. Relationships among smartphone addiction, stress, academic performance, and satisfaction with life. *Comput. Hum. Behav.* **2016**, *57*, 321–325. [CrossRef]
7. Hawi, N.S.; Samaha, M. To excel or not to excel: Strong evidence on the adverse effect of smartphone addiction on academic performance. *Comput. Educ.* **2016**, *98*, 81–89. [CrossRef]
8. Al-Menayes, J.J. Social Media Use, Engagement and Addiction as Predictors of Academic Performance. *Int. J. Psychol. Stud.* **2015**, *7*, 86–94. [CrossRef]
9. Marton, F.; Säljö, R. On qualitative differences in learning: I—Outcome and process. *Br. J. Educ. Psychol.* **1976**, *46*, 4–11. [CrossRef]
10. Kardefelt-Winther, D.; Heeren, A.; Schimmenti, A.; van Rooij, A.; Maurage, P.; Carras, M.; Edman, J.; Blaszczynski, A.; Khazaal, Y.; Billieux, J. How can we conceptualize behavioural addiction without pathologizing common behaviours? *Addiction* **2017**, *112*, 1709–1715. [CrossRef] [PubMed]
11. Sussman, S.; Rozgonjuk, D.; van den Eijnden, R. Substance and behavioral addictions may share a similar underlying process of dysregulation. *Addiction* **2017**, *112*, 1717–1718. [CrossRef] [PubMed]
12. Griffiths, M.D. Behavioural addiction and substance addiction should be defined by their similarities not their dissimilarities. *Addiction* **2017**, *112*, 1718–1720. [CrossRef] [PubMed]
13. Elhai, J.D.; Levine, J.C.; Dvorak, R.D.; Hallde, B.J. Fear of missing out, need for touch, anxiety and depression are related to problematic smartphone use. *Comput. Hum. Behav.* **2016**, *63*, 509–516. [CrossRef]
14. Demirci, K.; Akgonul, M.; Akpinar, A. Relationship of smartphone use severity with sleep quality, depression, and anxiety in university students. *J. Behav. Addict.* **2015**, *4*, 85–92. [CrossRef] [PubMed]
15. Rozgonjuk, D.; Rosenvald, B.; Janno, S.; Täht, K. Developing a shorter version of the Estonian Smartphone Addiction Proneness Scale (E-SAPS18). *Cyberpsychol. J. Psychosoc. Res. Cyberspace* **2016**, *10*, 4. [CrossRef]
16. Kim, D.; Lee, Y.; Lee, J.; Nam, J.K.; Chung, Y. Development of Korean Smartphone addiction proneness scale for youth. *PLoS ONE* **2014**, *9*, e97920. [CrossRef] [PubMed]
17. Inal, E.E.; Demİrcİ, K.; Çetİntürk, A.; Akgönül, M.; Savaş, S. Effects of smartphone overuse on hand function, pinch strength, and the median nerve. *Muscle Nerve* **2015**, *52*, 183–188. [CrossRef] [PubMed]
18. Lee, H.K.; Kim, J.H.; Fava, M.; Mischoulon, D.; Park, J.H.; Shim, E.J.; Lee, E.H.; Lee, J.H.; Jeon, H.J. Development and validation study of the Smartphone Overuse Screening Questionnaire. *Psychiatry Res.* **2017**, *257*, 352–357. [CrossRef] [PubMed]
19. Chen, J.; Liang, Y.; Mai, C.; Zhong, X.; Qu, C. General Deficit in Inhibitory Control of Excessive Smartphone Users: Evidence from an Event-Related Potential Study. *Front. Psychol.* **2016**, *7*, 511. [CrossRef] [PubMed]
20. Billieux, J.; Van der Linden, M.; d'Acremont, M.; Ceschi, G.; Zermatten, A. Does impulsivity relate to perceived dependence on and actual use of the mobile phone? *Appl. Cogn. Psychol.* **2007**, *21*, 527–537. [CrossRef]
21. Wang, C.; Wang, S.Y.; Li, W.H.; Dong, X.W.; Chi, G.B. Study on the mobile phone dependence syndrome and its distribution among 2213 college students in Guangzhou. *Zhonghua Liu Xing Bing Xue Za Zhi* **2013**, *34*, 949–952. [PubMed]
22. Choliz, M. Mobile phone addiction: A point of issue. *Addiction* **2010**, *105*, 373–374. [PubMed]
23. Pedrero Perez, E.J.; Rodriguez Monje, M.T.; Ruiz Sanchez De Leon, J.M. Mobile phone abuse or addiction. A review of the literature. *Adicciones* **2012**, *24*, 139–152. [PubMed]
24. Elhai, J.D.; Tiamiyu, M.F.; Weeks, J.W. Depression and Social Anxiety in Relation to Problematic Smartphone Use: The Prominent Role of Rumination. *Internet Res.* **2017**, in press.
25. Biggs, J.; Kember, D.; Leung, D.Y. The revised two-factor Study Process Questionnaire: R-SPQ-2F. *Br. J. Educ. Psychol.* **2001**, *71*, 133–149. [CrossRef] [PubMed]
26. Biggs, J. *Study Process Questionnaire Manual. Student Approaches to Learning and Studying*; Australian Council for Educational Research: Hawthorn, Australia, 1987.
27. Warburton, K. Deep learning and education for sustainability. *Int. J. Sustain. High. Educ.* **2003**, *4*, 44–56. [CrossRef]
28. Chin, C.; Brown, D.E. Learning in science: A comparison of deep and surface approaches. *J. Res. Sci. Teach.* **2000**, *37*, 109–138. [CrossRef]

29. Rogaten, J.; Moneta, G.B.; Spada, M.M. Academic performance as a function of approaches to studying and affect in studying. *J. Happiness Stud.* **2013**, *14*, 1751–1763. [CrossRef]
30. Hoeksema, L.H. *Learning Strategy as a Guide to Career Success in Organizations*; DSWO Press, Leiden University: Leiden, The Netherlands, 1995.
31. Arquero, J.L.; Fernández-Polvillo, C.; Hassall, T.; Joyce, J. Vocation, motivation and approaches to learning: A comparative study. *Educ. Train.* **2015**, *57*, 13–30. [CrossRef]
32. Gynnild, V.; Myrhaug, D. Revisiting approaches to learning in science and engineering: A case study. *Eur. J. Eng. Educ.* **2012**, *37*, 458–470. [CrossRef]
33. Heikkilä, A.; Lonka, K. Studying in higher education: Students' approaches to learning, self-regulation, and cognitive strategies. *Stud. High. Educ.* **2006**, *31*, 99–117. [CrossRef]
34. Malie, S.; Akir, O. Bridging the gaps between learning and teaching through recognition of students' learning approaches: A case study. *Res. Educ.* **2012**, *87*, 75–94. [CrossRef]
35. Salamonson, Y.; Weaver, R.; Chang, S.; Koch, J.; Bhathal, R.; Khoo, C.; Wilson, L. Learning approaches as predictors of academic performance in first year health and science students. *Nurse Educ. Today* **2013**, *33*, 729–733. [CrossRef] [PubMed]
36. Rocconi, L.M.; Ribera, A.K.; Laird, T.F.N. College Seniors' Plans for Graduate School: Do Deep Approaches Learning and Holland Academic Environments Matter? *Res. High. Educ.* **2015**, *56*, 178–201. [CrossRef]
37. Kirschner, P.A.; Karpinski, A.C. Facebook® and academic performance. *Comput. Hum. Behav.* **2010**, *26*, 1237–1245. [CrossRef]
38. Dewitte, S.; Schouwenburg, H.C. Procrastination, temptations, and incentives: The struggle between the present and the future in procrastinators and the punctual. *Eur. J. Personal.* **2002**, *16*, 469–489. [CrossRef]
39. Lopez-Fernandez, O.; Kuss, D.J.; Romo, L.; Morvan, Y.; Kern, L.; Graziani, P.; Rousseau, A.; Rumpf, H.J.; Bischof, A.; Gässler, A.K.; et al. Self-reported dependence on mobile phones in young adults: A European cross-cultural empirical survey. *J. Behav. Addict.* **2017**, *6*, 168–177. [CrossRef] [PubMed]
40. Oulasvirta, A.; Rattenbury, T.; Ma, L.; Raita, E. Habits make smartphone use more pervasive. *Pers. Ubiquitous Comput.* **2011**, *16*, 105–114. [CrossRef]
41. Elhai, J.D.; Levine, J.C.; Dvorak, R.D.; Hall, B.J. Non-social features of smartphone use are most related to depression, anxiety and problematic smartphone use. *Comput. Hum. Behav.* **2017**, *69*, 75–82. [CrossRef]
42. Elhai, J.D.; Hall, B.J.; Levine, J.C.; Dvorak, R.D. Types of smartphone usage and relations with problematic smartphone behaviors: The role of content consumption vs. social smartphone use. *Cyberpsychol. J. Psychosoc. Res. Cyberspace* **2017**, *11*, 3. [CrossRef]
43. Rozgonjuk, D.; Täht, K. To what extent does Internet use affect academic performance? Using Evidence from the large-scale PISA study. *Annu. Rev. Cyberther. Telemed.* **2017**, *15*, 39–44.
44. Jiang, Q. Internet addiction among young people in China. *Internet Res.* **2014**, *24*, 2–20. [CrossRef]
45. Kwon, M.; Lee, J.Y.; Won, W.Y.; Park, J.W.; Min, J.A.; Hahn, C.; Gu, X.; Choi, J.H.; Kim, D.J. Development and validation of a smartphone addiction scale (SAS). *PLoS ONE* **2013**, *8*, e56936. [CrossRef] [PubMed]
46. Valk, A.; Marandi, T. How to support deep learning at a university. In Proceedings of the International Conference on Education 2005, Beijing, China, 9–10 April 2015.
47. Junco, R. The relationship between frequency of Facebook use, participation in Facebook activities, and student engagement. *Comput. Educ.* **2012**, *58*, 162–171. [CrossRef]
48. Trochim, W.M.K.; Donnelly, J.P. *The Research Methods Knowledge Base*, 3rd ed.; Atomic Dog: Cincinnati, OH, USA, 2006.
49. Gravetter, F.; Wallnau, L. *Essentials of Statistics for the Behavioral Sciences*, 8th ed.; Wadsworth: Belmont, CA, USA, 2014.
50. Li, C.H. Confirmatory factor analysis with ordinal data: Comparing robust maximum likelihood and diagonally weighted least squares. *Behav. Res. Methods* **2016**, *48*, 936–949. [CrossRef] [PubMed]
51. DiStefano, C.; Morgan, G.B. A Comparison of Diagonal Weighted Least Squares Robust Estimation Techniques for Ordinal Data. *Struct. Equ. Model. Multidiscip. J.* **2014**, *21*, 425–438. [CrossRef]
52. MacKinnon, D.P. *Introduction to Statistical Mediation Analysis*; Routledge Academic: New York, NY, USA, 2008.
53. Kuss, D.J.; Griffiths, M.D. Online social networking and addiction—A review of the psychological literature. *Int. J. Environ. Res. Public Health* **2011**, *8*, 3528–3552. [CrossRef] [PubMed]
54. Grinols, A.B.; Rajesh, R. Multitasking with smartphones in the college classroom. *Bus. Prof. Commun. Q.* **2014**, *77*, 89–95. [CrossRef]

55. Lim, S.; Shim, H. Who Multitasks on Smartphones? Smartphone Multitaskers' Motivations and Personality Traits. *Cyberpsychol. Behav. Soc. Netw.* **2016**, *19*, 223–227. [CrossRef] [PubMed]
56. Walsh, J.L.; Fielder, R.L.; Carey, K.B.; Carey, M.P. Female college students' media use and academic outcomes: Results from a longitudinal cohort study. *Emerg. Adulthood* **2013**, *1*, 219–232. [CrossRef] [PubMed]
57. Kononova, A.; Chiang, Y.H. Why do we multitask with media? Predictors of media multitasking among Internet users in the United States and Taiwan. *Comput. Hum. Behav.* **2015**, *50*, 31–41. [CrossRef]
58. Baron, R.M.; Kenny, D.A. The moderator-mediator variable distinction in social psychological research: Conceptual, strategic, and statistical considerations. *J. Pers. Soc. Psychol.* **1986**, *51*, 1173–1182. [CrossRef] [PubMed]
59. Boase, J.; Ling, R. Measuring Mobile Phone Use: Self-Report versus Log Data. *J. Comput.-Mediat. Commun.* **2013**, *18*, 508–519. [CrossRef]
60. Kobayashi, T.; Boase, J. No Such Effect? The Implications of Measurement Error in Self-Report Measures of Mobile Communication Use. *Commun. Methods Meas.* **2012**, *6*, 126–143. [CrossRef]
61. Elhai, J.D.; Tiamiyu, M.F.; Weeks, J.W.; Levine, J.C.; Picard, K.J.; Hall, B.J. Depression and emotion regulation predict objective smartphone use measured over one week. *Personal. Individ. Differ.* **2017**. [CrossRef]

17

Addictive Features of Social Media/Messenger Platforms and Freemium Games against the Background of Psychological and Economic Theories

Christian Montag [1,*], Bernd Lachmann [1], Marc Herrlich [2] and Katharina Zweig [3]

1 Department of Molecular Psychology, Institute of Psychology and Education, Ulm University, 89081 Ulm, Germany
2 Serious Games Engineering, TU Kaiserslautern, 67663 Kaiserslautern, Germany
3 Algorithm Accountability Lab, TU Kaiserslautern, 67663 Kaiserslautern, Germany
* Correspondence: christian.montag@uni-ulm.de

Abstract: Currently about 2.71 billion humans use a smartphone worldwide. Although smartphone technology has brought many advances, a growing number of scientists discuss potential detrimental effects due to excessive smartphone use. Of importance, the likely culprit to understand over-usage is not the smartphone itself, but the excessive use of applications installed on smartphones. As the current business model of many app-developers foresees an exchange of personal data for allowance to use an app, it is not surprising that many design elements can be found in social media apps and Freemium games prolonging app usage. It is the aim of the present work to analyze several prominent smartphone apps to carve out such elements. As a result of the analysis, a total of six different mechanisms are highlighted to illustrate the prevailing business model in smartphone app development. First, these app-elements are described and second linked to classic psychological/economic theories such as the mere-exposure effect, endowment effect, and Zeigarnik effect, but also to psychological mechanisms triggering social comparison. It is concluded that many of the here presented app-elements on smartphones are able to prolong usage time, but it is very hard to understand such an effect on the level of a single element. A systematic analysis would require insights into app data usually only being available for the app-designers, but not for independent scientists. Nevertheless, the present work supports the notion that it is time to critically reflect on the prevailing business model of 'user data in exchange for app-use allowance'. Instead of using a service in exchange for data, it ultimately might be better to ban or regulate certain design elements in apps to come up with less addictive products. Instead, users could pay a reasonable fee for an app service.

Keywords: social media/messenger apps; Facebook; WhatsApp; Internet addiction; smartphone addiction; Internet use disorder; smartphone use disorder

---

1. Introduction

According to current estimates, about 2.71 billion humans use a smartphone worldwide [1]. Without doubt, one of the major driving forces towards a totally connected world with the Internet available in everyone's pocket was the inception of the iPhone in 2007 [2]. The wide distribution of smartphones led to unprecedented opportunities enabling humans to find their way in unknown territory via services such as Google Maps, to reach out to friends and business partners via a myriad of communication channels, and abundant easy access to knowledge earlier only available via visiting a library and the study of lexicons.

1.1. *Perils of Smartphone Use*

Despite the many advantages of the smartphone, it is heavily discussed among scientists around the globe if problematic usage of the smartphone could have detrimental effects on our mental health [3,4]. Furthermore, associations between anxiety disorder, depression, and problematic use of the smartphone have been observed (underlining the sincerity of this topic), but the causal relationship of effects between the constructs is still unclear [5]. In any case, new research suggests that the many interruptions due to high frequency use and the many daily incoming messages fragmenting everyday life could reduce productivity at work [6–8] and lower a person's well-being [9,10]. Another research group stresses that the availability of smartphones even might lead to "brain drain", when the device is present on the desk while working on a fluid intelligence task or working memory task [11]. In this context, a recent review summarized the literature on cognitive functions [12]. Therefore, this is area of research is not further presented in detail, here.

Beyond the mentioned issues, (excessive use of) smartphones is known to impact on social communication in terms of reducing smiles when interacting with strangers [13], enjoyment of face-to-face interaction [14] or drawing parent's attention away from their children [15]. This might result in a loss of empathy, although so far only correlations between excessive Internet use and lower empathy/social skills could be established [16,17], with only weak associations between excessive smartphone usage and empathy [18]. Again, note that the latter associations base on correlations and so far it is not clear what is cause and what is effect. Moreover, important insights of a study are mentioned which on the one hand observed reduced social skills in excessive Internet users, but on the other hand observed enhanced empathy when the Internet is used in a healthy way [19].

Beyond these observations, a growing number of scientists are focusing on the question of whether excessive smartphone usage could resemble a full-blown addiction [20–22]. Of importance, 'smartphone addiction' is currently not recognized in the official diagnostic manuals such as the International Classification of Diseases-11th Revision (ICD-11) issued by the World Health Organization (WHO) or the Diagnostic and Statistical Manual of Mental Disorders (DSM-5) issued by the American Psychiatric Association (APA). Both ICD-11 and DSM-5 offer practitioners and researchers alike valuable guidance in psycho-diagnostics. With respect to the general debate on the addictive nature of excessive usage of online content, it is noteworthy that Gaming Disorder, as a specific form of 'Internet addiction', has been included in ICD-11 [23]. This means that a first form of 'Internet addiction' is recognized as an official health condition, now.

Given the nomenclature of 'Gaming Disorder' in ICD-11, but also 'Internet Gaming Disorder' in DSM-5 (see Section 3 in the DSM-5's appendix), many researchers currently prefer the term of 'Internet Use Disorder' (IUD) over the classic term 'Internet addiction' [24–26]. With this wording, scientists also stress that a certain kind of online usage and not the Internet per se poses a problem. Therefore, and in line with a prominent model to characterize and understand IUD by Brand et al. [26], the term IUD is also used in the following. Explicitly, it is mentioned that researchers should not over-pathologize everyday life activities [27] and aim at a unification of terms used in the literature in line with the officially suggested nomenclature.

In this context, one currently might prefer the term Smartphone Use Disorder (SUD) over 'smartphone addiction' and understand SUD best as a mobile form of IUD. Of note, many researchers currently use the term problematic smartphone use (PSU), which from our perspective is also 'problematic', because it is not clear if PSU represents a transit zone from healthy towards psychopathological behavior or the end of the spectrum. Correctly, it has been pointed out, that the smartphone does not represent the culprit to understand excessive use of this device [28,29]. Instead one must focus on the manifold installed applications on the smartphones to understand why people are getting 'hooked' to their devices [30]. In this context, it will be of relevance to also distinguish between social and non-social forms of smartphone use to ultimately understand its addictive potential. Interestingly, it has been shown in recent works that higher extraversion (going along with more assertiveness, but also sociality) is not linked to SUD [31,32]. Hence, core social use of social media apps on smartphones (e.g., to stay in touch with friends) might represent the healthy form of smartphone use, reflecting also homo sapiens' urge for social bonding as also outlined in Pankseppian Affective Neuroscience Theory [33]. This all being said, it is understandable that the most prominent categories currently being researched—potentially causing addiction-like symptoms when being overused/or used in the wrong way—are social media/messenger platforms and Freemium games.

As prominent representatives of social media applications, Facebook, Snapchat, Instagram, and Twitter can be named and as a prominent messenger application WhatsApp or Signal. Without doubt, this is the Western view on this topic, whereas in Asia (particularly in China) the application WeChat dominates the market as a hybrid between social media and messenger application plus pay service [34].

The aforementioned term, Freemium, is a hybrid of the English words 'free' and 'premium'. In the realm of Freemium games, this means that the basic version of a game can be downloaded at no monetary cost. However, the person playing a game pays either with his/her data produced while playing, by paying attention to ads, e.g., in exchange for further game-energy, or by paying money to access 'premium' content. Freemium games are very relevant for the present work investigating elements of apps built to prolong usage time, because such games most often run with the business model of 'gaming service in exchange for your data'.

In a work by Montag et al. [35] it has been demonstrated that about 30% of daily smartphone use is accounted for by WhatsApp and Facebook usage in a German sample mainly ranging between ca. 15 and 35 years. Moreover, a recent work by Sha et al. [28] showed that the concepts of SUD and WhatsApp Use Disorder overlap in large parts (correlation of rho = 0.68). A new work underlines the overlap between SUD and excessive social media use, but also links between SUD and (Internet) Gaming Disorder [29]. Once more, this suggests that for the understanding of excessive smartphone use, researchers must also look at the high frequent use of specific applications on the smartphone and not only on the mere use of the total/frequent usage of the smartphone. The focus on social media/messenger applications alone would be a too narrow approach, because according to current numbers also Freemium games play a crucial role when one wants to understand what people are doing on their smartphones. To illustrate this: According to statista.com, "In early 2016 . . . U.S. gamers played an average of 3.6 mobile games per month, and 1.3 games on a daily basis" [36].

1.2. *Main Research Questions in the Available Literature Investigated so Far*

Looking at the growing literature dealing with Internet and Smartphone Use Disorder, it becomes apparent that most studies apply a confirmatory approach to understand IUD/SUD. Since the beginning of this research field with the case study of Kimberly Young [37] scientists tried to test if already existing symptoms in the realm of pathological gambling and/or substance related addictions can be transferred or applied to this potentially new form of a (online) behavioral addiction. It is not surprising that many existing self-report inventories in the field still test if symptoms such as preoccupation with the drug (here the Internet or a certain application), withdrawal symptoms, development of tolerance, loss of control, to name a few, can be associated with excessive Internet usage. Beyond such a confirmatory approach, many studies until this day deal with the important question if and what psychiatric co-morbidities can be observed when dealing with IUD and SUD. Of note, earlier works demonstrated co-morbidities with ADHD and depression [38–40], but also burnout [41] when investigating IUD. Earlier, links between SUD and depression/anxiety disorders have been already mentioned [5]. Of high importance, in the last years the research field has moved forward beyond these questions. Now, researchers also look at the processes explaining how addictive behaviors develop out of habits in the context of IUD and SUD. Up to now, presumably the most promising model to understand this process is the aforementioned I-PACE model by Brand et al. [26]. It argues that a complex interaction between person–affect–cognition and execution variables underlie the development of IUDs. IUDs are explicitly mentioned in plural here because from the introduction it should be clear that distinct forms exist such as Gaming Disorder or Internet Communication Disorder (ICD; or 'social media addiction/use disorder'). This perhaps warrants a more focused research approach—instead of relying too broadly on IUD and SUD (see [31,32] and Montag et al. [42] for overlaps between generalized and specific forms of IUD). Of note, neuroscientific approaches have also been abundantly applied to understand the psycho-biological mechanisms underlying the different forms of IUD/SUD. Due to space restriction, it is referred to a new review study here [43].

Although, the different strains of research presented so far in Section 1 led to valuable insights into the nature of IUDs, only few studies until now aim to understand why specific online applications and their in-built elements are potentially addictive [44,45]. This should be achieved with Section 3 of this work. Of note, in the present work, the term 'application(s)' describes services such as Facebook or Instagram on platform level, whereas the term 'elements/features' refers to certain parts of the applications investigated further in Section 3. Furthermore, it is stated that the terms 'elements' and 'features' are used in an exchangeable way.

2. Methods

In the current work, several features of social media/messenger platforms and Freemium games are presented, which have been developed to grasp a maximum of the online user's attention. The 'classic' app-business model of Silicon Valley asks the user not to pay with money to be able to use a certain application but with his/her personal data. Consequently, app developers have a keen interest in designing their online platforms with the goal to keep users occupied as long as possible [30]. This in turn means that more data per person can be harvested. With an increasing amount of data, revenues tend to rise, due to more effective microtargeting (i.e., sending a person customized ads). This is also shown by Matz et al. [46] demonstrating how clicks and buys can be boosted by the use of personalized ads. In the following, several app mechanisms are presented in alphabetic order. Some of these thoughts have been already covered in a chapter published by the authors in German language [47]. With the present paper, the main points of this earlier work should be made accessible for an international audience. Of importance, the present work is not a systemic review, but rather presents first insights into elements built-in social media and Freemium game apps. These insights have been derived by analysis of prominent and often used apps such as Facebook, WhatsApp, or Candy Crush. What follows is an overview of features built into social media/messenger and Freemium game applications likely prolonging app usage.

3. Results

In this section, we will cover six prominent psychological/economic mechanisms built-in social media apps and/or Freemium games. For an overview, see also Table 1.

3.1. *Endless Scrolling/Streaming and the Concept of Flow*

App and platform technologies are designed to be immersive, hence producing flow while using a certain app. Flow itself is a positive state of mind, which can promote high productivity. An important prerequisite for flow is that the difficulty of a task matches the ability of a person. If there is no fit, the person is either feeling anxious (the task is too difficult) or bored (the task is too easy). Other flow prerequisites are a clear goal set and a sense of personal control over the task. For a detailed introduction into the concept of flow and additional prerequisites, see the seminal work by Csikszentmihalyi [48].

Flow is needed and warranted in different kinds of work processes, however, it can actually be 'fatal' in the case of applications on the smartphone or other 'ubiquitous' devices, when attention should be focused somewhere else: It is well known that flow goes along with a feeling of time distortion and this is exactly what many developers of social media apps and Freemium games aim to achieve—a person being so immersed that he or she is forgetting about time and space while using a platform or app (cf., [30,49,50]). The distracting aspects of many applications on the smartphone are also a well-known danger for every day traffic [51] and in many countries led to the prohibition of smartphone use while driving a car or riding a bike.

One technique used to prolong usage time in this context is the endless scrolling/streaming feature. For example, on the video platform YouTube one can scroll down endlessly with apparently no end. By endlessly scrolling down, the user is getting more and more immersed (perhaps also on a motor level as perceiving the scrolling as a playful activity) while not coming to a natural stop, where he/she might easily reconsider to quit or change the platform. The behavior of endless scrolling is enhanced, because the user finds from time to time something rewarding (e.g., a funny or interesting video), hence intermittent conditioning principles are observed here (see also research on intermittent conditioning principles in the context of slot machine mechanisms by Harrigan & Dixon [52]). The same phenomenon is at work when 'auto play' is the default: e.g., when watching a video on YouTube or the favorite series on Netflix or Amazon Prime. As soon as one video is at the end, the next video begins with either a similar content (on YouTube) or the second episode of a TV show at Netflix and so forth. By this process, viewers get more and more absorbed, which makes it hard to stop watching.

3.2. *Endowment Effect/Mere Exposure Effect*

The endowment and the mere exposure effect play important roles in the areas of social media and games. One very prominent game including a simple variant of both effects is called "Hayday" which was released in 2012. This game is still very popular today but already belonged to the most successful Freemium games in 2013 [53]. In this game, the user aims at building a large farmland, where he/she is entitled to feed cattle, harvest crops and follows other agricultural related activities. As with other games, progress without investing money is very slow, which means that after some fast progress at the beginning of the game (to attract people to the game), rewards in terms of the urgently needed relevant game currency are scarce.

Where do the endowment effect and the mere exposure effect come in? The endowment effect describes that buying or owning a product leads to a higher (emotionally felt) value of the product, often way beyond its actual value [54,55]. In real life, this would explain why after buying a cheap souvenir for 2.99€, this thing starts to rise in the subjectively perceived value: reasons for this could be, that carrying the souvenir home feels like an investment and that fond memories of the holiday are also attached to it. This leads to the effect that the value attached to it, if, e.g., asked to sell the souvenir to someone else, often exceeds the original price. Both ownership and loss aversion are discussed as reasons for the endowment effect.

In the context of smartphone games, this plays out as follows: every time players visit the app platform and invest more time in the construction of the virtual world, it will get harder for them to detach from the game or even delete the app. This is in particular the case, if the progress has been slow and it took the users a very long time to construct the online world. It is their own little world now (resulting in the endowment effect). Also, of importance is the mere exposure effect [56]. The mere exposure effect describes that the more often you are exposed to a certain (neutral) thing or application (here a game), the more you like it. This has even been shown for the initials of your name (for an introduction in the initial preference task, e.g., see Sariyska et al. [57]) and seems to be applicable also for many of the gaming or social media apps.

3.3. *Social Pressure*

A successful way to increase data flow in an application is built into the popular messenger app WhatsApp. WhatsApp represents one of the most successful messenger services used worldwide to exchange text messages and pictures. At the time of writing, WhatsApp has about 1.5 billion users worldwide [58].

Users on WhatsApp are nudged (to encourage someone to do something in a way that is gentle rather than forceful or direct [59]) to communicate fast and often on WhatsApp due to the 'double tick function'. If a user sends a message to a friend, the sender is presented with two gray ticks, which means that the message has successfully arrived at the recipient's phone. If the recipient reads the message, the grey ticks turn blue. As both sides know about these rules, social pressure emerges.

Both parties likely expect a fast answer, above all, if the message apparently has been read. This way, the users of the popular WhatsApp messenger are nudged towards faster communication via social pressure. This process is also known to undermine well-being [60] and might in parts be responsible for rising social concerns when people start to use smartphones [61]. Clearly also a link between features such as the double ticks and the concept of Fear of Missing Out (FoMO) can be established, with FoMO describing the anxiety/fear to miss something in one's own social network [28,62].

Of note, the economic principle of 'nudging' can also be illustrated by the default settings of a fresh WhatsApp installation. The default mode of WhatsApp comes with the 'double tick function' being activated. Most users do not know that they are able to deactivate this app-feature. In general, the 'power of defaults' is a well-known principle applicable to decision making in many different areas and especially in software applications [63,64]. The percentage of users that actually take the time to check or even change the default settings may depend on the specific target group, the importance of the application, and the application design. For instance, there is an anecdotal report by Microsoft that only 5% of Word users change the defaults settings [65].

In sum, system design of apps nudges a person to behave in a certain direction. For person characteristics influencing the perception of these mechanisms, please see Mai et al. [66]. Social pressure plays not only a role on social media platforms to enhance user engagement, but also in computer games. Prominent games such as the massively multiplayer online-role play game (MMORPG) called World of Warcraft (WoW) enable participants to meet in so called 'guilds', hence groups of persons who meet at a certain time online to go on a mission together (in the aforementioned WoW game this could be a 'raid'). As such a guild in particular performs well when being complete, the pressure on the individual of such an online group rises to be at a certain time in the online world to support one's own guild. This goes along with a stronger focus in life on online activities instead on perhaps more pressing issues in the offline world.

3.4. Show Users of an App What They Like

A strong feature for prolonging usage time on social media platforms is the prominent 'Newsfeed' as built-in in the Facebook application. Over the years, Facebook developed machine learning algorithms studying the behavior of their users in detail on the platform. In order to get to know their users better, they do not only record what people 'like' (i.e., give a 'thumbs up') but also how long they hover over a certain post. This could be interpreted as showing a special interest in a certain area. 'Textmining' enables Facebook & Co. to do sentiment analysis and to understand not only what is interesting for their users but also in what mood they are [67–69]. Although, the role of mood for buying decisions/advertising is complex [70,71], such a variable might be of (high) interest to many of the companies behind manifold smartphone/Internet applications. The analysis of the different elements presented in this paragraph technically can all be used to plant the most interesting news in one's own personalized 'Newsfeed'.

The 'Newsfeed' on Facebook is the entry for every user when logging in. Facebook has a great interest in studying the behavior of each person at perfection and in much detail, so that at best only such information is presented in the 'Newsfeed' which is most interesting for the user. Otherwise, people could get bored and close the browser window. For a work dealing with user beliefs considering how the algorithm applied behind the 'Newsfeed' works, please see Rader & Gray [72].

3.5. Social Comparison and Social Reward

Perhaps one of the most prominent features of social reward mechanisms in social media is the iconic 'thumbs up' (giving or getting a 'Like'; (co-)developed by Justin Rosenstein, former worker at Facebook; see also independent.co.uk [73]). Likes demonstrate either positive social feedback on one's own posts or to give another person such a feedback. The power of such feedback has also been proven neuroscientifically, when Instagram users are confronted with their own posted pictures from their account which were manipulated by being presented either with many or few 'Likes' (in this case hearts [74]). Pictures being presented with many Likes elicit stronger activity in the ventral striatum, an area involved of the processing of a rewards [74,75]. It has even been demonstrated that lower gray matter volumes of the nucleus accumbens are associated with longer and higher frequent usage of the Facebook app on smartphones underlining its addictive power [76]. Additionally, several other studies observed that lower gray matter volumes were associated with higher addictive tendencies [77,78].

So far, in this paragraph only social reward via the 'Like' function has been discussed. Beyond that, processes of social comparison also play an important role for revisiting social media platforms because a person gets information on how he/she is perceived by their social network. Without doubt, the social comparison process is not unproblematic, because it might lead to lower self-esteem [79] and the size of one's own real social network to be successfully handled seems to be limited by the so called Dunbar's number (a theoretical limit to the number of people with whom any individual is able to sustain a stable or meaningful social relationship, usually considered to be roughly 150 [80]), likely also valid on social media channels such as Twitter [81]. Social comparison also plays a role in Freemium games, when one thinks of the highscore-boards where you can compare your scores in a game with those from others.

3.6. Zeĭgarnik/Ovsiankina Effect

Classic studies by Zeĭgarnik [82] and Rickers-Ovsiankina [83] made interesting observations concerning memory functions and actions taken after being interrupted while performing a task. In the classic work by Zeĭgarnik, participants of her study got interrupted while solving a puzzle and, in the aftermath, best remembered those tasks where they were interrupted compared to those tasks which they successfully could end. From the same work group, Rickers-Ovsiankina [83] then observed that persons not only seem to be better at remembering the tasks where they got interrupted, but several of the experiment's participants even came back to the unfinished tasks after the experiment ended to ultimately finish the task (and they were not asked to do so).

In sum, these classic works from the field of psychology suggest that individuals involved in the execution of high investment tasks, react with (emotional) strain if interrupted. The final completion of the task will remove this strain. These insights mirror in the design of Freemium games such as Candy Crush Saga. This game has been downloaded an incredible 2.7 billion times in five years [84]. In this game, participants must solve levels in which they follow different missions while playing a Tetris like game (although there are obviously several differences between the games, these cannot be presented in detail here). Of note, when the game has not been played for a while, the gamer is endowed with five lives. Some levels are very hard to solve and in case of Candy Crush Saga it is even mentioned that a "super hard level" is coming up. As some of these levels are "super hard" to solve (rumor has it that it is even impossible at first try), players easily loose several of those free lives ending up with no energy to finish this "super hard level". Being now really attracted by the game, this results in emotional strain which consequently provokes people to spend extra money to buy additional lives/gaming energy, because the next level is only a couple of minutes away.

Table 1. Elements used to prolong usage time of social media apps and/or Freemium games.

Psychological Mechanisms Built-in Social Media/Messenger Apps and/or Freemium Games	Example/Illustration
Endless scrolling/streaming	As soon as one video is at the end on a website such as YouTube, the next video begins with either a similar content or the second episode of a TV show and so forth. By this, viewers get more and more absorbed, which makes it hard to stop watching.
Endowment effect/ mere-exposure effect	Every time players visit the app platform and invest more time in the construction of the virtual world, it will get harder for them to detach from the game or even delete the app. The endowment effect might be both explained by ownership and loss aversion. Also, of importance is the mere exposure effect describing that the more often you are exposed to a certain (neutral) thing or application (here a game), the more you like it.
Social pressure	Illustration from a WhatsApp feature: If a user sends a message to a friend, the sender is presented with two gray ticks, which means that the message has successfully arrived at the recipient's phone. If the recipient reads the message, the grey ticks turn blue. As both sides know about these rules, social pressure emerges. Both parties likely expect a fast answer, above all, if the message apparently has been read.
Show users of an app what they like	Facebook has a great interest in studying the behavior of each person at perfection and in much detail, so that at best only such information is presented in the 'Newsfeed' which is most interesting for the user. Otherwise, people could get bored and close the browser window.
Social comparison and social reward	Perhaps one of the most prominent features of social reward mechanisms in social media is the iconic 'thumbs up'. A 'thumbs up' ('Like') demonstrates either positive social feedback on one's own post or gives another person such a feedback.
Zeĭgarnik effect/ Ovsiankina effect	The Zeigarnik effect refers to better remembering of tasks, where a person has been interrupted. Rickers-Ovsiankina then showed that such interrupted tasks are more likely to be finished later on (even if one is not forced to do this). Illustration: Some levels in Freemium games are very hard to solve and in case of Candy Crush Saga it is even mentioned that a "super hard level" is coming up. As some of these levels are "super hard" to solve (rumor has it that it is even impossible at first try), players easily loose several of those free lives ending up with no energy to finish this "super hard level". Being now really attracted by the game, this results in emotional strain which consequently provokes people to spend extra money to buy additional lives/gaming energy, because the next level is only a couple of minutes away.

4. Discussion

The present article provided its readers with an overview on often observed elements/features of smartphone/Internet applications in-built to prolong the time spent using a certain app. The depicted elements/features embedded in psychological and economic theory underline the notion that these elements indeed have been designed to prolong app usage. Implementing such elements in a smartphone-app will also contribute to a more addictive nature of apps. From our perspective, it is of tremendous importance to further study such in-built elements, because SUD has been associated with loneliness [85]. Although it is not clear what is hen and what is egg in this work (hence the direction of causality), a growing number of studies indeed support such associations with further demonstrating robust links between SUD and negative emotionality [5]. According to the I-PACE model [26] (and its recent update [86]), a history of psychopathology might indeed be a vulnerability factor to develop IUD (and its mobile form of SUD). Nevertheless, it is also imaginable that withdrawal from society and escapism to the online world ultimately might cause loneliness and reduce social connectedness, too [87]. Additional relevant areas discussed in the literature—probably being a result of too much online consumption—are links between IUD and BMI [88] and between IUD and body image avoidance [89]. The latter effect is likely driven by social comparison processes, in particular when a person is confronted with thin models or other (thin) attractive persons [90]. These effects might be in particular strong on platforms such as Instagram and for those users with low self-esteem [91] and being female [92,93]. In this context also the role of selfies [3,94] and the smartphone camera needs to be mentioned [95].

Of importance, apps on smartphones are not in general bad and not always cause negative emotionality or dissatisfaction with one's own body image. In contrast, some applications might even foster physical activity and help persons to improve their diet [96]. However, as mentioned, we focused in the present research on the investigation of social media/messenger and Freemium game applications. Such a focus is warranted because several studies already demonstrated that these applications are important drivers of (excessive) smartphone usage (literature on social media/messenger applications and smartphone usage [28,97,98]; literature on gaming and smartphone usage [29,99,100].

Although it needs to be tested further, the here investigated elements of the apps described against psychological and economic theories all likely prolong usage times. Although literature on each of the elements in the study of SUD is scarce, it has been demonstrated that persons have problems in assessing their smartphone consumption, and this is probably due to time distortions [49,101]. Such time distortions are a well-known companion of flow processes as described in 3.1. Beyond the element of flow, a recent study [102] also found empirical support for the endowment effect indeed playing also a role with online products. The authors of this work observed via an online experiment that "consumers become instantaneously attached to and are reluctant to give up digital services once they have obtained them" ([102], p. 311). This all said, the study of elements in-built in smartphone applications present a rather new research endeavor and many questions are still in need to be answered. One of these questions is highlighted in the next section.

The overview so far presented the features separately. In real-world applications, usually several of the explained elements can be found in one application. To our knowledge, studies are largely lacking aiming at an understanding of how strong each of the aforementioned features of the platforms/games impact upon usage time. Clearly, it will be of high interest to know how the different features interact on usage time. For example, when the design of the 'Newsfeed' according to the idea 'show people what they like' would prolong a person's stay on Facebook by 10 min, and implementation of the 'Like'-function by 5 min, will users stay 15 min longer on Facebook or will these effects interact with each other, resulting in 25 min of online app usage? Indeed, this is hard to study for independent scientists because they usually do not get access to data from platforms such as Facebook or Candy Crush Saga. Therefore, one solution will be ultimately to design independent games/social media apps for research purposes where different features are rolled out in different constellations and in different versions of the same game or services. Of note, tech-companies use this approach often and the literature refers here to 'A/B-testing'. By implementing 'A/B-testing', it can easily be tested if version A compared to version B of an online service prolongs usage time. Ethically, it is of great interest, that most of these tests are unsolicited. This also speaks for that ultimately government regulation might be necessary to force the industry to both open up for scientists from different disciplines to be able to study the impact of the aforementioned elements and to build healthier business models.

5. Limitations and Changes of the Current Business Model in Apps?

The present work is of theoretical nature and carved out relevant mechanisms likely being designed to prolong usage time of app-services dominating everyday life. Clearly, our assumption that these mechanisms have been purely designed to prolong usage time of an app is speculative, but please see also a larger serious scientific area dealing with persuasive design/technologies in the computer sciences [103,104]. It cannot be said for sure what the app developers had in mind when constructing a certain feature, but some developers, such as Justin Rosenstein, confess about the addictive nature of some of the presented elements [73]. Aside from this, it is very likely that the main intention of implementing features as introduced above in an application, represents the prolongation of app usage, because companies such as Facebook and Google earn their money with data.

Nevertheless, it is mentioned that in the last months a movement has been seen in the Silicon Valley aiming to foster "Time Well Spent" on digital platforms [105]. Applications such as "Screentime" on Apple's iPhone or "Time Well Spent" on Facebook should help to reduce online time. How good this actually works has not been investigated and please note that some of the authors (together with computer scientists) presented a similar service for Android users already several years ago, hence years before the app industry launched such a laudable initiative (CM and BL as part of a larger development team with their Menthal application [106,107]). However, it seems that even the tech-industry has learned that detrimental effects for mental health can arise due to their developed addictive app mechanisms. Probably implementation of these new control features also reflects a reaction to pressure from regulating bodies. Results from studies investigating the effect of smartphones and/or social media use on well-being came up with diverse results [28,108–110]. Hence, it also needs to be better understood what kind of use-reduction goes along with the healthiest effects.

Although no one can really predict if this is going to happen soon, the future will see if other healthier business models will be built into applications without the addictive potential currently seen in many of the prominent and often used applications. Apart from these new developments, the recent work by Alutaybi et al. [45] needs to be mentioned, because it came up with ideas on how to reduce FoMO and thereby likely also to reduce addictive tendencies towards social media applications. Before going a bit more in detail concerning some of these ideas, it is noteworthy that the authors presented FoMO eliciting features such as 'temporal events' in their article going beyond what is presented in our work, perhaps also resulting in more addictive tendencies. Of note, a 'temporal event' could be defined by an information being available only for a short time period (this was also one of the most prominent Snapchat functions): Either a person is then fast in consuming the content or simply has not seen what was going on. The authors end their interesting article with thoughts on "FoMO-Aware SNSs Design" [45] (p. 4), in which they basically think about designing social media platforms giving users the ability to make a short note on when they are available. This could help in reducing the urge to constantly check social media, because others are aware of a person being absent (and therefore not being able to reply), but also to set up bilateral or even collective protocols providing persons with rules on when they want to respond to each other. The effects of such an intervention clearly still need to be empirically tested. When comparing the work by Alutaybi et al. [45] and the present one, both of them have merits, as the former has more of a computer science design approach to its analysis (also in carving out 'addictive' or FoMO elements), whereas in the present work it is stronger focused on psychological/economic theories as described above.

Finally, the prominent honeycomb model by Kietzmann et al. [111] is mentioned, because it represents one of the first models to systematically analyze the diverse building blocks of social media. Of importance, this early very influential work addressed business persons in order to help them to recognize the most congruent social media platform for their companies in terms of a social media platform's building blocks called identity, conversation, sharing, presence, relationships, reputation, and groups. When focusing solely on addictive tendencies of social media sites, this framework might be fruitful to be brought together with the present psychological theories in order to empirically tackle the question in which area or areas of the honeycomb model, which of our presented features might have what kind of impact on usage time.

Author Contributions: The present work was carried out and designed by all authors. C.M. wrote the first draft of the manuscript, which was revised by all authors (B.L., M.H., K.Z.). Moreover, all authors approved the final version of this work.

References

1. Statista. Available online: https://www.statista.com/statistics/330695/number-of-smartphone-users-worldwide/ (accessed on 2 April 2019).
2. Maisch, B.; Meckel, M. Innovationskommunikation 2.0—Das Beispiel Apple IPhone. *Mark. Rev. St. Gallen* **2009**, *26*, 42–46. [CrossRef]
3. Montag, C.; Diefenbach, S. Towards Homo Digitalis: Important Research Issues for Psychology and the Neurosciences at the Dawn of the Internet of Things and the Digital Society. *Sustainability* **2018**, *10*, 415. [CrossRef]
4. Scholz, R.; Bartelsman, E.; Diefenbach, S.; Franke, L.; Grunwald, A.; Helbing, D.; Hill, R.; Hilty, L.; Höjer, M.; Klauser, S.; et al. Unintended Side Effects of the Digital Transition: European Scientists' Messages from a Proposition-Based Expert Round Table. *Sustainability* **2018**, *10*, 2001. [CrossRef]
5. Elhai, J.D.; Yang, H.; Montag, C. Cognitive- and Emotion-Related Dysfunctional Coping Processes: Transdiagnostic Mechanisms Explaining Depression and Anxiety's Relations with Problematic Smartphone Use. *Curr. Addict. Rep.* **2019**. [CrossRef]
6. Duke, É.; Montag, C. Smartphone Addiction, Daily Interruptions and Self-Reported Productivity. *Addict. Behav. Rep.* **2017**, *6*, 90–95. [CrossRef] [PubMed]
7. Duke, É.; Montag, C. Smartphone Addiction and Beyond: Initial Insights on an Emerging Research Topic and Its Relationship to Internet Addiction. In *Internet Addiction*; Montag, C., Reuter, M., Eds.; Springer: Cham, Switzerland, 2017; pp. 359–372.
8. Kushlev, K.; Proulx, J.; Dunn, E.W. Silence Your Phones: Smartphone Notifications Increase Inattention and Hyperactivity Symptoms. In Proceedings of the 2016 CHI Conference on Human Factors in Computing Systems, San Jose, CA, USA, 7–12 May 2016; ACM Press: New York, NY, USA, 2016; pp. 1011–1020. [CrossRef]
9. Kushlev, K.; Dunn, E.W. Checking Email Less Frequently Reduces Stress. *Comput. Hum. Behav.* **2015**, *43*, 220–228. [CrossRef]
10. Twenge, J.M.; Martin, G.N.; Campbell, W.K. Decreases in psychological well-being among American adolescents after 2012 and links to screen time during the rise of smartphone technology. *Emotion* **2018**, *18*, 765–780. [CrossRef] [PubMed]
11. Ward, A.F.; Duke, K.; Gneezy, A.; Bos, M.W. Brain drain: The mere presence of one's own smartphone reduces available cognitive capacity. *J. Assoc. Consum. Res.* **2017**, *2*, 140–154. [CrossRef]
12. Wilmer, H.H.; Sherman, L.E.; Chein, J.M. Smartphones and cognition: A review of research exploring the links between mobile technology habits and cognitive functioning. *Front. Psychol.* **2018**, *8*, 605. [CrossRef]
13. Kushlev, K.; Hunter, J.F.; Proulx, J.; Pressman, S.D.; Dunn, E. Smartphones reduce smiles between strangers. *Comput. Hum. Behav.* **2019**, *91*, 12–16. [CrossRef]
14. Dwyer, R.J.; Kushlev, K.; Dunn, E.W. Smartphone use undermines enjoyment of face-to-face social interactions. *J. Exp. Soc. Psychol.* **2018**, *78*, 233–239. [CrossRef]
15. Kushlev, K.; Dunn, E.W. Smartphones distract parents from cultivating feelings of connection when spending time with their children. *J. Soc. Pers. Relatsh.* **2019**, *36*, 1619–1639. [CrossRef]
16. Melchers, M.; Li, M.; Chen, Y.; Zhang, W.; Montag, C. Lower empathy is associated with problematic Internet use: Empirical evidence from Germany and China. *Asian J. Psychiatry* **2015**, *17*, 56–60. [CrossRef] [PubMed]
17. Chou, W.J.; Huang, M.F.; Chang, Y.P.; Chen, Y.M.; Hu, H.F.; Yen, C.F. Social skills deficits and their association with Internet addiction and activities in adolescents with attention-deficit/hyperactivity disorder. *J. Behav. Addict.* **2016**, *6*, 42–50. [CrossRef] [PubMed]
18. Lachmann, B.; Sindermann, C.; Sariyska, R.; Luo, R.; Melchers, M.; Becker, B.; Montag, C. The Role of Empathy and Life Satisfaction in Smartphone Use Disorder. *Front. Psychol.* **2018**, *9*, 398. [CrossRef] [PubMed]
19. Jeon, H.J.; Kim, S.; Chon, W.H.; Ha, J.H. Is Internet overuse associated with impaired empathic ability in Korean college students? *Medicine* **2018**, *97*, e12493. [CrossRef] [PubMed]
20. Lin, Y.-H.; Chang, L.-R.; Lee, Y.-H.; Tseng, H.-W.; Kuo, T.B.J.; Chen, S.-H. Development and Validation of the Smartphone Addiction Inventory (SPAI). *PLoS ONE* **2014**, *9*, e98312. [CrossRef]
21. Kwon, M.; Lee, J.-Y.; Won, W.-Y.; Park, J.-W.; Min, J.-A.; Hahn, C.; Gu, X.; Choi, J.-H.; Kim, D.-J. Development and Validation of a Smartphone Addiction Scale (SAS). *PLoS ONE* **2013**, *8*, e56936. [CrossRef]
22. Samaha, M.; Hawi, N.S. Relationships among smartphone addiction, stress, academic performance, and satisfaction with life. *Comput. Hum. Behav.* **2016**, *57*, 321–325. [CrossRef]

23. Pontes, H.M.; Schivinski, B.; Sindermann, C.; Li, M.; Becker, B.; Zhou, M.; Montag, C. Measurement and conceptualization of Gaming Disorder according to the World Health Organization framework: The development of the Gaming Disorder Test. *Int. J. Ment. Health Addict.* **2019**, 1–21. [CrossRef]
24. Müller, M.; Brand, M.; Mies, J.; Lachmann, B.; Sariyska, R.Y.; Montag, C. The 2D:4D Marker and Different Forms of Internet Use Disorder. *Front. Psychiatry* **2017**, *8*, 213. [CrossRef] [PubMed]
25. Wegmann, E.; Oberst, U.; Stodt, B.; Brand, M. Online-Specific Fear of Missing out and Internet-Use Expectancies Contribute to Symptoms of Internet-Communication Disorder. *Addict. Behav. Rep.* **2017**, *5*, 33–42. [CrossRef] [PubMed]
26. Brand, M.; Young, K.S.; Laier, C.; Wölfling, K.; Potenza, M.N. Integrating Psychological and Neurobiological Considerations Regarding the Development and Maintenance of Specific Internet-Use Disorders: An Interaction of Person-Affect-Cognition-Execution (I-PACE) Model. *Neurosci. Biobehav. Rev.* **2016**, *71*, 252–266. [CrossRef]
27. Billieux, J.; Schimmenti, A.; Khazaal, Y.; Maurage, P.; Heeren, A. Are We Overpathologizing Everyday Life? A Tenable Blueprint for Behavioral Addiction Research. *J. Behav. Addict.* **2015**, *4*, 119–123. [CrossRef] [PubMed]
28. Sha, P.; Sariyska, R.; Riedl, R.; Lachmann, B.; Montag, C. Linking Internet Communication and Smartphone Use Disorder by Taking a Closer Look at the Facebook and WhatsApp Applications. *Addict. Behav. Rep.* **2019**, *9*, 100148. [CrossRef] [PubMed]
29. Leung, H.; Pakpour, A.H.; Strong, C.; Lin, Y.C.; Tsai, M.C.; Griffiths, M.D.; Lin, C.-Y.; Chen, I.H. Measurement invariance across young adults from Hong Kong and Taiwan among three internet-related addiction scales: Bergen Social Media Addiction Scale (BSMAS), Smartphone Application-Based Addiction Scale (SABAS), and Internet Gaming Disorder Scale-Short Form (IGDS-SF9) (Study Part A). *Addict. Behav.* **2019**. [CrossRef]
30. Alter, A. *Irresistible: The Rise of Addictive Technology and the Business of Keeping Us Hooked*; Penguin Press: New York, NY, USA, 2017.
31. Lachmann, B.; Duke, É.; Sariyska, R.; Montag, C. Who's Addicted to the Smartphone and/or the Internet? *Psychol. Pop. Media Cult.* **2019**, *8*, 182–189. [CrossRef]
32. Peterka-Bonetta, J.; Sindermann, C.; Elhai, J.D.; Montag, C. Personality Associations with Smartphone and Internet Use Disorder: A Comparison Study Including Links to Impulsivity and Social Anxiety. *Front. Public Health* **2019**, *7*. [CrossRef]
33. Davis, K.L.; Montag, C. Selected Principles of Pankseppian Affective Neuroscience. *Front. Neurosci.* **2019**, *12*, 1025. [CrossRef]
34. Montag, C.; Becker, B.; Gan, C. The Multipurpose Application WeChat: A Review on Recent Research. *Front. Psychol.* **2018**, *9*, 2247. [CrossRef]
35. Montag, C.; Błaszkiewicz, K.; Sariyska, R.; Lachmann, B.; Andone, I.; Trendafilov, B.; Eibes, M.; Markowetz, A. Smartphone Usage in the 21st Century: Who Is Active on WhatsApp? *BMC Res. Notes* **2015**, *8*, 331. [CrossRef] [PubMed]
36. Statista. Available online: https://www.statista.com/topics/1906/mobile-gaming/ (accessed on 3 April 2019).
37. Young, K.S. Psychology of Computer Use: XL. Addictive Use of the Internet: A Case That Breaks the Stereotype. *Psychol. Rep.* **1996**, *79*, 899–902. [CrossRef] [PubMed]
38. Sariyska, R.; Reuter, M.; Lachmann, B.; Montag, C. Attention Deficit/Hyperactivity Disorder Is a Better Predictor for Problematic Internet Use than Depression: Evidence from Germany. *J. Addict. Res. Ther.* **2015**, *6*, 1–6.
39. Yen, J.-Y.; Ko, C.-H.; Yen, C.-F.; Wu, H.-Y.; Yang, M.-J. The Comorbid Psychiatric Symptoms of Internet Addiction: Attention Deficit and Hyperactivity Disorder (ADHD), Depression, Social Phobia, and Hostility. *J. Adolesc. Health* **2007**, *41*, 93–98. [CrossRef] [PubMed]
40. Yoo, H.J.; Cho, S.C.; Ha, J.; Yune, S.K.; Kim, S.J.; Hwang, J.; Chung, A.; Sung, Y.H.; Lyoo, I.K. Attention Deficit Hyperactivity Symptoms and Internet Addiction. *Psychiatry Clin. Neurosci.* **2004**, *58*, 487–494. [CrossRef] [PubMed]
41. Peterka-Bonetta, J.; Sindermann, C.; Sha, P.; Zhou, M.; Montag, C. The Relationship between Internet Use Disorder, Depression and Burnout among Chinese and German College Students. *Addict. Behav.* **2019**, *89*, 188–199. [CrossRef] [PubMed]

42. Montag, C.; Bey, K.; Sha, P.; Li, M.; Chen, Y.-F.; Liu, W.-Y.; Zhu, Y.-K.; Li, C.-B.; Markett, S.; Keiper, J.; et al. Is It Meaningful to Distinguish between Generalized and Specific Internet Addiction? Evidence from a Cross-Cultural Study from Germany, Sweden, Taiwan and China. *Asia-Pac. Psychiatry* **2015**, *7*, 20–26. [CrossRef] [PubMed]
43. Montag, C.; Becker, M. Psychological and Neuroscientific Advances to Understand Internet Use Disorder. *Neuroforum* **2019**, *25*, 99–107.
44. King, D.L.; Delfabbro, P.H.; Griffiths, M.D. The Role of Structural Characteristics in Problematic Video Game Play: An Empirical Study. *Int. J. Ment. Health Addict.* **2011**, *9*, 320–333. [CrossRef]
45. Alutaybi, A.; Mcalaney, J.; Stefanidis, A.; Phalp, K.; McAlaney, J.; Ali, R. Designing Social Networks to Combat Fear of Missing Out. *Proc. Br. HCI* **2018**, *18*, 1. [CrossRef]
46. Matz, S.C.; Kosinski, M.; Nave, G.; Stillwell, D.J. Psychological Targeting as an Effective Approach to Digital Mass Persuasion. *Proc. Natl. Acad. Sci. USA* **2017**, *114*, 12714–12719. [CrossRef] [PubMed]
47. Zweig, K.A.; Lachmann, B.; Montag, C.; Herrlich, M. Kontinuierliches A/B-Testing Zur Optimierung von Spielerbindung Und Monetarisierung Bei "Freemium"-Spielen. In *Paradoxien des Verbraucherverhaltens*; Springer Fachmedien Wiesbaden: Wiesbaden, Germany, 2019; pp. 43–57.
48. Csikszentmihalyi, M. *Flow: The Classic Work on How to Achieve Happiness*; Random House: London, UK, 2002.
49. Montag, C.; Błaszkiewicz, K.; Lachmann, B.; Sariyska, R.; Andone, I.; Trendafilov, B.; Markowetz, A. Recorded Behavior as a Valuable Resource for Diagnostics in Mobile Phone Addiction: Evidence from Psychoinformatics. *Behav. Sci.* **2015**, *5*, 434–442. [CrossRef] [PubMed]
50. Rau, P.-L.P.; Peng, S.-Y.; Yang, C.-C. Time Distortion for Expert and Novice Online Game Players. *CyberPsychol. Behav.* **2006**, *9*, 396–403. [CrossRef] [PubMed]
51. Kim, H.-J.; Min, J.-Y.; Kim, H.-J.; Min, K.-B. Accident Risk Associated with Smartphone Addiction: A Study on University Students in Korea. *J. Behav. Addict.* **2017**, *6*, 699–707. [CrossRef] [PubMed]
52. Harrigan, K.A.; Dixon, M. PAR Sheets, Probabilities, and Slot Machine Play: Implications for Problem and Non-Problem Gambling. *J. Gambl. Issues* **2009**, 81. [CrossRef]
53. Wikipedia.org. Available online: https://en.wikipedia.org/wiki/Hay_Day (accessed on 2 April 2019).
54. Kahneman, D.; Knetsch, J.L.; Thaler, R.H. Anomalies: The Endowment Effect, Loss Aversion, and Status Quo Bias. *J. Econ. Perspect.* **1991**, *5*, 193–206. [CrossRef]
55. Thaler, R. Toward a Positive Theory of Consumer Choice. *J. Econ. Behav. Organ.* **1980**, *1*, 39–60. [CrossRef]
56. Zajonc, R.B. Mere Exposure: A Gateway to the Subliminal. *Curr. Dir. Psychol. Sci.* **2001**, *10*, 224–228. [CrossRef]
57. Sariyska, R.; Reuter, M.; Bey, K.; Sha, P.; Li, M.; Chen, Y.-F.; Liu, W.-Y.; Zhu, Y.-K.; Li, C.-B.; Suárez-Rivillas, A.; et al. Self-Esteem, Personality and Internet Addiction: A Cross-Cultural Comparison Study. *Personal. Individ. Differ.* **2014**, *61*, 28–33. [CrossRef]
58. Statista. Available online: https://de.statista.com/statistik/daten/studie/285230/umfrage/aktive-nutzer-von-whatsapp-weltweit/ (accessed on 21 July 2019).
59. Thaler, R.; Sunstein, C. *Improving Decisions about Health, Wealth and Happiness*; Penguin Books; Yale University Press: New Haven, CT, USA, 2008.
60. Blabst, N.; Diefenbach, S. WhatsApp and Wellbeing: A Study on WhatsApp Usage, Communication Quality and Stress. In Proceedings of the 31st British Computer Society Human Computer Interaction Conference, Sunderland, UK, 3–6 July 2017; BCS Learning & Development Ltd.: Swindon, UK, 2017; pp. 1–6. [CrossRef]
61. Hadar, A.; Hadas, I.; Lazarovits, A.; Alyagon, U.; Eliraz, D.; Zangen, A. Answering the Missed Call: Initial Exploration of Cognitive and Electrophysiological Changes Associated with Smartphone Use and Abuse. *PLoS ONE* **2017**, *12*. [CrossRef]
62. Przybylski, A.K.; Murayama, K.; DeHaan, C.R.; Gladwell, V. Motivational, Emotional, and Behavioral Correlates of Fear of Missing Out. *Comput. Hum. Behav.* **2013**, *29*, 1841–1848. [CrossRef]
63. Dinner, I.; Johnson, E.J.; Goldstein, D.G.; Liu, K. Partitioning Default Effects: Why People Choose Not to Choose. *J. Exp. Psychol. Appl.* **2011**, *17*, 332–341. [CrossRef] [PubMed]
64. Kesan, J.P.; Shah, R.C. Setting Software Defaults: Perspectives from Law, Computer Science and Behavioral Economics. *Notre Dame Law Rev.* **2006**, *82*, 583–634.
65. Available online: https://archive.uie.com/brainsparks/2011/09/14/do-users-change-their-settings/ (accessed on 17 April 2019).

66. Mai, L.M.; Freudenthaler, R.; Schneider, F.M.; Vorderer, P. "I Know You've Seen It!" Individual and Social Factors for Users' Chatting Behavior on Facebook. *Comput. Hum. Behav.* **2015**, *49*, 296–302. [CrossRef]
67. Eichstaedt, J.C.; Smith, R.J.; Merchant, R.M.; Ungar, L.H.; Crutchley, P.; Preoţiuc-Pietro, D.; Asch, D.A.; Schwartz, H.A. Facebook Language Predicts Depression in Medical Records. *Proc. Natl. Acad. Sci. USA* **2018**, *115*, 11203–11208. [CrossRef] [PubMed]
68. Kramer, A.D.I.; Guillory, J.E.; Hancock, J.T. Experimental Evidence of Massive-Scale Emotional Contagion through Social Networks. *Proc. Natl. Acad. Sci. USA* **2014**, *111*, 8788–8790. [CrossRef] [PubMed]
69. Schwartz, H.A.; Eichstaedt, J.; Kern, M.L.; Park, G.; Sap, M.; Stillwell, D.; Kosinski, M.; Ungar, L. Towards Assessing Changes in Degree of Depression through Facebook. In Proceedings of the Workshop on Computational Linguistics and Clinical Psychology: From Linguistic Signal to Clinical Reality, Baltimore, MD, USA, June 2014; pp. 118–125.
70. Bakamitsos, G.A.; Siomkos, G.J. Context Effects in Marketing Practice: The Case of Mood. *J. Consum. Behav. Int. Res. Rev.* **2004**, *3*, 304–314. [CrossRef]
71. Gardner, M.P. Mood States and Consumer Behavior: A Critical Review. *J. Consum. Res.* **1985**, *12*, 281. [CrossRef]
72. Rader, E.; Gray, R. Understanding User Beliefs about Algorithmic Curation in the Facebook News Feed. In Proceedings of the 33rd Annual ACM Conference on Human Factors in Computing Systems—CHI '15, Seoul, Korea, 8–23 April 2015; ACM Press: New York, NY, USA, 2015; pp. 173–182. [CrossRef]
73. Man Who Invented 'Like' Button Deletes Facebook App over Addiction Fears. Available online: https://www.independent.co.uk/life-style/gadgets-and-tech/facebook-like-inventor-deletes-app-iphone-justin-rosenstein-addiction-fears-a7986566.html (accessed on 3 April 2019).
74. Sherman, L.E.; Payton, A.A.; Hernandez, L.M.; Greenfield, P.M.; Dapretto, M. The Power of the Like in Adolescence: Effects of Peer Influence on Neural and Behavioral Responses to Social Media. *Psychol. Sci.* **2016**, *27*, 1027–1035. [CrossRef]
75. Sherman, L.E.; Greenfield, P.M.; Hernandez, L.M.; Dapretto, M. Peer Influence via Instagram: Effects on Brain and Behavior in Adolescence and Young Adulthood. *Child Dev.* **2018**, *89*, 37–47. [CrossRef]
76. Montag, C.; Markowetz, A.; Blaszkiewicz, K.; Andone, I.; Lachmann, B.; Sariyska, R.; Trendafilov, B.; Eibes, M.; Kolb, J.; Reuter, M.; et al. Facebook Usage on Smartphones and Gray Matter Volume of the Nucleus Accumbens. *Behav. Brain Res.* **2017**, *329*, 221–228. [CrossRef]
77. Makris, N.; Oscar-Berman, M.; Jaffin, S.K.; Hodge, S.M.; Kennedy, D.N.; Caviness, V.S.; Marinkovic, K.; Breiter, H.C.; Gasic, G.P.; Harris, G.J. Decreased Volume of the Brain Reward System in Alcoholism. *Biol. Psychiatry* **2008**, *64*, 192–202. [CrossRef] [PubMed]
78. Seifert, C.L.; Magon, S.; Sprenger, T.; Lang, U.E.; Huber, C.G.; Denier, N.; Vogel, M.; Schmidt, A.; Radue, E.-W.; Borgwardt, S.; et al. Reduced Volume of the Nucleus Accumbens in Heroin Addiction. *Eur. Arch. Psychiatry Clin. Neurosci.* **2015**, *265*, 637–645. [CrossRef] [PubMed]
79. Vogel, E.A.; Rose, J.P.; Roberts, L.R.; Eckles, K. Social Comparison, Social Media, and Self-Esteem. *Psychol. Pop. Media Cult.* **2014**, *3*, 206–222. [CrossRef]
80. Dunbar, R. *How Many Friends Does One Person Need? Dunbar's Number and Other*; Faber & Faber: London, UK, 2010.
81. Gonçalves, B.; Perra, N.; Vespignani, A. Modeling Users' Activity on Twitter Networks: Validation of Dunbar's Number. *PLoS ONE* **2011**, *6*, e22656. [CrossRef] [PubMed]
82. Zeĭgarnik, B.V. *Über das Behalten von Erledigten und Unerledigten Handlungen*; J. Springer: Wiesbaden, Germany, 1927.
83. Rickers-Ovsiankina, M.A. *Die Wiederaufnahme Unterbrochener Handlungen*; Springer: Berlin, Germany, 1928.
84. Candy Crush Saga: 2.73 Billion Downloads in Five Years and still Counting. Available online: https://venturebeat.com/2017/11/17/candy-crush-saga-2-73-billion-downloads-in-five-years-and-still-counting/ (accessed on 2 April 2019).
85. Bian, M.; Leung, L. Linking loneliness, shyness, smartphone addiction symptoms, and patterns of smartphone use to social capital. *Soc. Sci. Comput. Rev.* **2015**, *33*, 61–79. [CrossRef]
86. Brand, M.; Wegmann, E.; Stark, R.; Müller, A.; Wölfling, K.; Robbins, T.W.; Potenza, M.N. The Interaction of Person-Affect-Cognition-Execution (I-PACE) model for addictive behaviors: Update, generalization to addictive behaviors beyond Internet-use disorders, and specification of the process character of addictive behaviors. *Neurosci. Biobehav. Rev.* **2019**, *104*, 1–10. [CrossRef]

87. Savci, M.; Aysan, F. Technological addictions and social connectedness: Predictor effect of internet addiction, social media addiction, digital game addiction and smartphone addiction on social connectedness. *Dusunen Adam J. Psychiatry Neurol. Sci.* **2017**, *30*, 202–216. [CrossRef]
88. Canan, F.; Yildirim, O.; Ustunel, T.Y.; Sinani, G.; Kaleli, A.H.; Gunes, C.; Ataoglu, A. The relationship between internet addiction and body mass index in Turkish adolescents. *Cyberpsychol. Behav. Soc. Netw.* **2014**, *17*, 40–45. [CrossRef]
89. Rodgers, R.F.; Melioli, T.; Laconi, S.; Bui, E.; Chabrol, H. Internet addiction symptoms, disordered eating, and body image avoidance. *Cyberpsychol. Behav. Soc. Netw.* **2013**, *16*, 56–60. [CrossRef]
90. Brown, Z.; Tiggemann, M. Attractive celebrity and peer images on Instagram: Effect on women's mood and body image. *Body Image* **2016**, *19*, 37–43. [CrossRef] [PubMed]
91. Ahadzadeh, A.S.; Sharif, S.P.; Ong, F.S. Self-schema and self-discrepancy mediate the influence of Instagram usage on body image satisfaction among youth. *Comput. Hum. Behav.* **2017**, *68*, 8–16. [CrossRef]
92. Cohen, R.; Newton-John, T.; Slater, A. The relationship between Facebook and Instagram appearance-focused activities and body image concerns in young women. *Body Image* **2017**, *23*, 183–187. [CrossRef] [PubMed]
93. Meier, E.P.; Gray, J. Facebook photo activity associated with body image disturbance in adolescent girls. *Cyberpsychol. Behav. Soc. Netw.* **2014**, *17*, 199–206. [CrossRef] [PubMed]
94. Cohen, R.; Newton-John, T.; Slater, A. 'Selfie'-objectification: The role of selfies in self-objectification and disordered eating in young women. *Comput. Hum. Behav.* **2018**, *79*, 68–74. [CrossRef]
95. Glitsos, L. The camera phone in the concert space: Live music and moving images on the screen. *Music Sound Mov. Image* **2018**, *12*, 33–52, 85. [CrossRef]
96. Schoeppe, S.; Alley, S.; Rebar, A.L.; Hayman, M.; Bray, N.A.; Van Lippevelde, W.; Gnam, J.P.; Bachert, P.; Direito, A.; Vandelanotte, C. Apps to improve diet, physical activity and sedentary behaviour in children and adolescents: A review of quality, features and behaviour change techniques. *Int. J. Behav. Nutr. Phys. Act.* **2017**, *14*, 83. [CrossRef]
97. Haug, S.; Paz Castro, R.; Kwon, M.; Filler, A.; Kowatsch, T.; Schaub, M.P. Smartphone use and smartphone addiction among young people in Switzerland. *J. Behav. Addict.* **2015**, *4*, 299–307. [CrossRef]
98. Zhitomirsky-Geffet, M.; Blau, M. Cross-generational analysis of predictive factors of addictive behavior in smartphone usage. *Comput. Hum. Behav.* **2016**, *64*, 682–693. [CrossRef]
99. Lopez-Fernandez, O.; Männikkö, N.; Kääriäinen, M.; Griffiths, M.D.; Kuss, D.J. Mobile gaming and problematic smartphone use: A comparative study between Belgium and Finland. *J. Behav. Addict.* **2018**, *7*, 88–99. [CrossRef]
100. Lopez-Fernandez, O.; Kuss, D.J.; Romo, L.; Morvan, Y.; Kern, L.; Graziani, P.; Rousseau, A.; Rumpf, H.J.; Bischof, A.; Gässler, A.K.; et al. Self-reported dependence on mobile phones in young adults: A european cross-cultural empirical survey. *J. Behav. Addict.* **2017**, *6*, 168–177. [CrossRef] [PubMed]
101. Lin, Y.H.; Lin, Y.C.; Lee, Y.H.; Lin, P.H.; Lin, S.H.; Chang, L.R.; Tseng, H.W.; Yen, L.Y.; Yang, C.C.; Kuo, T.B. Time distortion associated with smartphone addiction: Identifying smartphone addiction via a mobile application (App). *J. Psychiatr. Res.* **2015**, *65*, 139–145. [CrossRef] [PubMed]
102. Fritze, M.P.; Eisingerich, A.B.; Benkenstein, M. Digital transformation and possession attachment: Examining the endowment effect for consumers' relationships with hedonic and utilitarian digital service technologies. *Electron. Commer. Res.* **2019**, *19*, 311–337. [CrossRef]
103. Hamari, J.; Koivisto, J.; Pakkanen, T. Do persuasive technologies persuade?-a review of empirical studies. In *International Conference on Persuasive Technology*; Springer: Cham, Switzerland, 2014; pp. 118–136.
104. Oinas-Kukkonen, H.; Harjumaa, M. A systematic framework for designing and evaluating persuasive systems. In *International Conference on Persuasive Technology*; Springer: Berlin/Heidelberg, Germany, 2008; pp. 164–176.
105. Facebook. Available online: https://de-de.facebook.com/timewellspent.io/ (accessed on 2 April 2019).
106. Andone, I.; Błaszkiewicz, K.; Eibes, M.; Trendafilov, B.; Montag, C.; Markowetz, A. Menthal: A Framework for Mobile Data Collection and Analysis. In Proceedings of the 2016 ACM International Joint Conference on Pervasive and Ubiquitous Computing Adjunct—UbiComp '16, Heidelberg, Germany, 12–16 September 2016; ACM Press: New York, NY, USA, 2016; pp. 624–629. [CrossRef]
107. Andone, I.; Błaszkiewicz, K.; Trendafilov, B.; Eibes, M.; Montag, C.; Markowetz, A. Menthal—Running a Science Project as a Start-Up. In Proceedings of the Computing in Mental Health, Workshop at CHI 2016, San Jose, CA, USA, 7–12 May 2016.

108. Stieger, S.; Lewetz, D. A week without using social media: Results from an ecological momentary intervention study using smartphones. *Cyberpsychol. Behav. Soc. Netw.* **2018**, *21*, 618–624. [CrossRef] [PubMed]
109. Tromholt, M. The Facebook experiment: Quitting Facebook leads to higher levels of well-being. *Cyberpsychol. Behav. Soc. Netw.* **2016**, *19*, 661–666. [CrossRef] [PubMed]
110. Vanman, E.J.; Baker, R.; Tobin, S.J. The burden of online friends: The effects of giving up Facebook on stress and well-being. *J. Soc. Psychol.* **2018**, *158*, 496–508. [CrossRef] [PubMed]
111. Kietzmann, J.H.; Hermkens, K.; McCarthy, I.P.; Silvestre, B.S. Social Media? Get Serious! Understanding the Functional Building Blocks of Social Media. *Bus. Horiz.* **2011**, *54*, 241–251. [CrossRef]

18

Fear of Missing Out as a Predictor of Problematic Social Media Use and Phubbing Behavior among Flemish Adolescents

Vittoria Franchina [1,*], Mariek Vanden Abeele [2,*], Antonius J. van Rooij [3,4], Gianluca Lo Coco [1] and Lieven De Marez [3]

1 Department of Psychology and Educational Sciences, University of Palermo, 90133 Palermo, Italy; gianluca.lococo@unipa.it
2 Tilburg School of Humanities and Digital Sciences, Tilburg University, 5037AB Tilburg, The Netherlands
3 imec-mict-UGent, Department of Communication Sciences, Ghent University, 9000 Ghent, Belgium; trooij@trimbos.nl (A.J.v.R.); lieven.demarez@ugent.be (L.D.M.)
4 Department of Youth & Risky Behavior, Trimbos Institute, 3521 VS Utrecht, The Netherlands
* Correspondence: vittoria.franchina923005@gmail.com (V.F.); m.m.p.vandenabeele@tilburguniversity.edu (M.V.A.)

Abstract: Fear-of-missing-out (FOMO) refers to feelings of anxiety that arise from the realization that you may be missing out on rewarding experiences that others are having. FOMO can be identified as an intra-personal trait that drives people to stay up to date of what other people are doing, among others on social media platforms. Drawing from the findings of a large-scale survey study among 2663 Flemish teenagers, this study explores the relationships between FOMO, social media use, problematic social media use (PSMU) and phubbing behavior. In line with our expectations, FOMO was a positive predictor of both how frequently teenagers use several social media platforms and of how many platforms they actively use. FOMO was a stronger predictor of the use of social media platforms that are more private (e.g., Facebook, Snapchat) than platforms that are more public in nature (e.g., Twitter, Youtube). FOMO predicted phubbing behavior both directly and indirectly via its relationship with PSMU. These findings support extant research that points towards FOMO as a factor explaining teenagers' social media use.

Keywords: fear of missing out (FOMO); social media; problematic social media use (PSMU); phubbing; teenagers; adolescents; addiction

---

1. Introduction

Behavioral addiction researchers argue that the psychological processes that explain problematic behavior require greater attention [1–5]. Understanding underlying processes is particularly relevant when examining problematic forms of (digital) media use. Digital devices, such as mobile phones, can be used and misused in a variety of different ways. It is likely that the way in which problem use manifests itself depends on the particular underlying psychological mechanism [6,7].

One psychological process that may underlie problematic digital media use is the Fear-Of-Missing-Out (FOMO). FOMO refers to the "pervasive apprehension that others might be having rewarding experiences from which one is absent" [8]. Persons who have a greater FOMO are assumed to have a greater desire to stay continually up-to-date of what others are doing, for example via the use of social media. According to Przybylski et al. [8], FOMO originates from psychological deficits in people's competence and relatedness needs [9]. One way of satisfying these needs, the authors claim, is through the use of social media applications, because the dynamic nature of social media applications provides users with a consistent stream of social and informational rewards [10].

The purpose of the current study is to contribute to the extant body of research on FOMO in relation to social media use. The study has four aims. First, it investigates whether teenagers with higher levels of FOMO have more social media accounts (i.e., the breadth of social media use) and whether they access these accounts more frequently (i.e., the depth of social media use [11]) than teenagers with lower levels of FOMO. Second, assuming that teenagers with higher levels of FOMO are mostly motivated to check up on people in their personal social networks, we examine whether FOMO is a stronger predictor of the use of platforms that connect teenagers to their offline networks (e.g., Facebook, Snapchat) than of the use of platforms that connect to a largely unknown audience (e.g., Youtube, Twitter). Third, the study examines if teenagers with greater FOMO report higher levels of problematic social media use (PSMU) and, four, are more likely to report one particular form of problematic social media use, which is the use of social media during conversations with co-present others (cf. "phubbing"). These research aims are addressed with data from a large-scale cross-sectional survey that was administered to 2663 Flemish adolescents.

2. Theoretical Framework

People have always had a tendency to think about what others are thinking and doing [12]. In the 1970 and 1980 scholars already identified that some people developed anxieties around missing out, contemplating on the rewarding experiences that others might be having (e.g., in the context of romantic relationships) [13]. FOMO is thus not an entirely new concept.

FOMO can be understood as such an anxiety around missing out on rewarding experiences that results from people's desire for interpersonal attachments [12]. This desire, which is grounded in people's need to belong, is an innate and fundamental motivation which humans have [14]. People gratify this need by seeking belongingness to social groups. Social groups nowadays exist in both physical and virtual shapes and people have access to their social groups in both ways, online and offline. Social media, which can be defined as "Internet-based applications that build on the ideological and technological foundations of Web 2.0, and that allow the creation and exchange of User Generated Content" [15,16], offer a place where users can keep in touch with their social circles. Social network sites (SNS) such as Facebook or Instagram, for example, offer users an online connection to persons in their personal networks, facilitating the practice of keeping in touch.

Nowadays the digital world is considered an extension of the Self [17,18]. In addition to the personal mind and physical body, the Self can be thought to include people, places, physical possessions, as well as affiliation groups to which a person feels attached [19]. Social media platforms are a part of this: they are the digital portals to affiliation groups. In contemporary society we thus manage the affiliation network both offline and online; virtual groups are as real and important as the physical ones. Not being able to connect with those affiliation groups on social media may cause feelings of being out of touch with "real" life [17]. After all, losing or missing a person one is attached to, can bring feelings of loss and grieving as much as if a part of the Self was damaged [19].

The fear of being socially excluded plays a role in experiencing a FOMO [12]. Social exclusion produces a loss of belongingness, and therefore causes anxiety. Thus, when people cannot access their social media accounts, they might feel anxiety because of a fear that they are being socially excluded [12].

Social exclusion also elicits feelings of worthlessness [12]. These feelings lead people to the act of comparing themselves to others on social media [20] with the purpose of deciding upon their own personal value [21]. Social networks offer a place where consumers, particularly young generations, can continuously keep up with what peers are doing and checking on what they are missing out on (e.g., social events, life experiences, life opportunities, and so on and so forth). FOMO can thus drive social media use, as checking up on other people may lead to a temporary relief of one's anxiety.

2.1. FOMO and the Use of Different Social Media Platforms

Users may use different media to gratify different needs [22–24]. This can explain differences in the popularity of certain social media platforms. In January 2015, the Global Web Index summary showed that the most popular social media platform was the social network site Facebook, immediately followed by YouTube, Twitter and Instagram. The same year Instagram's popularity outperformed Twitter. According to some, this is because pictures are more effective than words in achieving self-presentational objectives, which are central motivations for social media use [25]. Given that each social media platform is characterized by its own features and affordances, it is relevant to differentiate between social media platforms in research on social media use: Different platforms may connect users to different persons and networks, and give access to different forms of information of which users may wish to stay up-to-date.

Current research findings reveal that FOMO is a predictor of the use of SNS with which users connect to people in their personal networks, such as Instagram [25] and Facebook [26]. Instagram use, for example, is found to be motivated by the desire to keep in touch with others [25] and to "to keep up with or gain knowledge about what others (i.e., friends, family and strangers) are doing" [27]. FOMO has also been found to predict Facebook use [28,29] and Instagram use [30,31]. The above study findings thus indicate that FOMO predicts the use of at least these social network sites, but potentially also the use of other social media platforms.

With respect to social media use, a difference can be made between the "depth" and the "breadth" of one's use, where the depth of use refers to aspects such as the frequency and duration of social media use, and the breadth of use refers to the variety of social media platforms that are actively used. For teens in particular, not only frequent use, but also the use of a broad variety of social media platforms may serve the purpose of relieving anxieties with regard to not knowing what others are thinking and doing, as the differences in the relational affordances of different platforms [32] mean that they may give access to at least partially different networks and contents. Hence, for the current study we expect that not only the depth, operationalized as the frequency of social media use, but also the breadth, operationalized as the number of active social media platforms teenagers use, are predicted by FOMO:

Hypothesis 1. *Teens who experience greater FOMO, use social media more frequently (Hypothesis 1a;* i.e., *the depth of social media use), and use more different social media accounts (Hypothesis 1b;* i.e., *the breadth of social media use).*

2.2. FOMO and the Use of More Private versus More Public Social Media Platforms

As mentioned above, the use of different social media platforms may gratify different underlying needs. For example, a recent study shows that users significantly differ in the gratifications they derive from using Facebook, Instagram, Twitter and Snapchat [33]. One affordance in which platforms may differ is in the extent to which content is restricted to a (sub-)set of contacts, or fully public—in other words, whether content is shared with a mostly known versus a mostly unknown audience. On platforms such as Facebook, Instagram or Snapchat, people's online social network usually overlaps with their offline affiliation group (e.g., Facebook/Snapchat contacts need to know each other's names or phone numbers to see each other's posts and profiles). Platforms such as Twitter or Youtube, on the other hand, usually make content accessible to a wider audience of mainly unknown individuals, and resemble a broadcasting platform rather than a platform in which content is restricted to people who have been accepted as "contacts", "followers" or "friends".

Given this difference in the public accessibility of platform content, it seems logical to assume that SNSs such as Facebook or Snapchat are more apt at providing relief from FOMO than, for example, video sharing platforms such as Youtube or microblogging services such as Twitter because the former provide greater relief from anxieties surrounding what friends and family are doing.

Indeed, platforms such as Facebook or Instagram are more personal SNS that enable teens to limit content accessibility to the desired public (e.g., friends or friends-of-friends). As a result, these SNS may be especially attractive venues for teens with a high FOMO because it lets them know what people in their primary affiliative groups are thinking and doing. We explore this assumption by asking the following research question:

Research Question. *Is FOMO a stronger predictor of the use of more private social media platforms (that connect mostly to offline networks) than more publicly accessible social media platforms (that connect mostly to online networks)?*

2.3. FOMO and Problematic Social Media Use (PSMU)

When social media use is excessive, it can become problematic. Several studies have addressed problematic social media use (PSMU) [34–36]. There is an ongoing debate in the literature around the differences between problematic social media use and a possible social media behavioral addiction [4,37]. An in-depth discussion of this debate goes beyond the scope of this work. In the current study, however, we use the term problematic social media use, which we define as an unhealthy excessive form of social media use, characterized by a lack of control over the behavior, and continued behavior despite adverse life consequences. Our focus is on revealing the factors that predict to problematic social media use in a general population of teenagers (i.e., the aim is not to diagnose or identify pathological cases).

As mentioned before, one of the aims of this study is to explore if teenagers with a greater FOMO report a higher levels of PSMU. Previous studies suggest that this is the case [38–43], and suggest that those who experience FOMO may try to relieve their anxiety by checking up on other people on social media. Ironically, however, the more people check their social media accounts, however, the more they may find events they are missing out on. Using social media to reduce the anxiety may end up to be another source of FOMO. Therefore this vicious circle may reinforce itself, gradually turning social media use into problematic social media use. Hence we expect:

Hypothesis 2. *Teens who experience greater FOMO, report higher PSMU.*

2.4. FOMO and Phubbing

A final study purpose is to focus on FOMO as a predictor of one particular form of problematic social media use, which is the use of social media during conversations with co-present others. This practice is termed "phubbing" (derived from phone + snubbing), which refers to "the act of snubbing someone in a social setting by concentrating on one's phone instead of talking to the person directly" [44,45]. Experimental studies show that phubbing negatively impacts relational outcomes such as impression formation [46].

Recent findings show that people prefer to use smartphones when going online [47]. Smartphones allows us to be in contact with our affiliation groups on social media, everywhere we are. Therefore, we assume that if people experience anxiety, they may temporary try to reduce it by accessing their social media accounts on their smartphones [48]. It is likely that those high in FOMO, who use social media to address their anxiety, may overuse social media on their smartphones in such a way that it intersects with their offline social interactions, leading them to phub their offline interaction partners.

Hence, the last aim of this study is to explore whether teens with a greater FOMO report to engage in phubbing behavior more frequently, and whether the latter relationship is mediated by PSMU:

Hypothesis 3a. *Teens with a greater FOMO, are more likely to use social media during conversations with co-present others (cf. "phubbing").*

Hypothesis 3b. *PSMU mediates the former relationship.*

3. Method

3.1. *Sample and Procedure*

In Flanders, a consortium of non-profit organizations collaborates bi-annually on a large-scale survey project that examines the state of affairs of digital media ownership and use of Flemish youths. Apart from a large set of recurring questions, every edition of the survey includes a number of questions on topics that are considered relevant at the time.

The data gathered for the current study were part of the 2016 research project [49]. An omnibus survey was administered to the high school pupils of 11 geographically dispersed high schools in Flanders, Belgium. Using the information made available by the ministry of education, quota sampling was used to select schools, and—within the schools—years and classrooms. This procedure resulted in a final sample that is representative for the population in terms of gender, age and school track (see Van Waeg, D'Hanens, Dooms & Naesens [49] for further details).

Within each school, a local collaborator (e.g., the school's information and communications technology coordinator) organized the survey administration process, according to a set of instructions provided by the project leaders. The survey was administered online, but to avoid self-selection bias, the data collection took part during school hours, in the computer rooms of the schools. Unfortunately, no response rates were registered. However, the local collaborators stated that few pupils did not receive permission to participate. In total, the responses of 3291 pupils were gathered. The project leaders subjected these responses to a rigorous data cleaning procedure, leading to removal of 452 responses that were either substantially incomplete, either contained multiple invalid responses to validation screening items. This procedure resulted in a final sample of 2663 pupils (57.1% girls; M_{age} = 14.87, SD = 1.67). This final dataset was distributed by the consortium to the collaborating researchers for further analysis.

Informed consent was collected from both the participating teenagers and their parents. Given the large sample-size, an opt-out procedure was used for collecting consent from parents. The university's institutional review board approved the study.

3.2. *Measures*

3.2.1. Breadth of Social Media Platforms Used

Based on interviews with young persons, a list of 25 frequently used social media applications was constructed. We adhered to Kaplan and Haenlein's [16] definition of social media, which includes all platforms in which users can generate content that is (semi-)publicly available to others. The latter definition excludes platforms that focus exclusively on instant messaging (e.g., Whatsapp, Facebook Messenger). The list of included platforms can be consulted in Table 1. The breadth of social media use was assessed by asking for each platform whether the teenager had an active account (1 = yes, 0 = no), and then summing the total number of active accounts per participant.

Table 1. Scale items, means and standard deviations.

	Fear-of-Missing-Out (FOMO)		
	Items	**M**	**SD**
1	I fear my friends have more rewarding experiences than me	2.33	1.11
2	It is important that I understand my friends' "inside jokes"	3.09	1.05
3	It bothers me when I miss an opportunity to meet up with friends	4.16	0.90
4	When I go on summer camp or vacation, I continue to keep tabs on what my friends are doing	2.66	1.14
	Problematic Social Media Use (PSMU)		
	Items	**M**	**SD**
1	How frequently do you find it difficult to quit using social media?	2.89	1.19
2	How frequently do others (e.g., your parents or friends) tell you that you should spend less time on social media?	2.72	1.28
3	How frequently do you prefer using social media over spending time with others (e.g., with friends or family)?	1.89	0.97
4	How frequently do you feel restless, frustrated or irritated when you can't access social media?	2.33	1.16
5	How frequently do you do your homework poorly because you prefer being on social media?	2.51	1.17
6	How frequently do you use social media because you feel unhappy?	2.31	1.23
7	How frequently do you lack sleep because you spent the night using social media?	2.44	1.35
	Phubbing		
	Items	**M**	**SD**
1	How frequently do you use your mobile phone during a conversation in a bar or restaurant?	2.39	0.99
2	How frequently are you engaged with your phone during a conversation?	2.13	0.96
3	How frequently do you check social media on your phone during a personal conversation?	1.89	0.92

3.2.2. Depth of Social Media Platforms Used

The depth of social media use was measured by assessing for each active platform how frequently it was used (1 = less than once per week, 5 = multiple times per day). Questions with respect to the usage frequency of a platform were only answered by participants who had an active account for the platform. As visible in Table 2, a substantial number of platforms was used by (very) few participants. We opted to only include those platforms who were used by at least 5% of the sample. The analyses for Hypothesis 1a, concerning FOMO as a predictor of platform usage frequency (see Tables 3 and 4) are performed on the basis of the subsample of users of each platform.

Table 2. Percentage of teenagers with an account on various social media platforms and average frequency of use among account holders (1 = less than once/week, 5 = multiple times/day).

Social Media Platform	N	% of Total Sample	Average Usage Frequency		Less than Once per Week	Once per Week	Multiple Times per Week	Daily	Multiple Times per Day
			M	*SD*	%	%	%	%	%
Facebook	2360	89%	4.49	0.87	1.4	3.6	6.4	22.2	66.5
Snapchat	1937	73%	4.36	1.00	2.4	4.5	10.1	20.5	62.5
Instagram	1680	63%	4.36	0.97	1.5	4.4	15.7	31.8	46.6
YouTube	1596	60%	4.17	0.95	2.1	4.4	9.7	22.3	61.4
Google+	925	35%	2.67	1.40	28.2	21.5	19.8	16.4	14.1
Twitter	582	22%	3.63	1.35	8.8	14.9	19.4	18.6	38.3
Swarm	510	19%	4.26	1.09	3.7	5.5	10.8	20.6	59.4
We Heart It	329	12%	3.42	1.34	10.6	16.4	21.9	22.2	28.9
Pinterest	324	12%	2.6	1.34	28.1	21.6	24.4	14.5	11.4
Tumblr	298	11%	3.52	1.35	9.4	16.4	21.1	18.8	34.2
Vine	232	9%	3.12	1.38	15.9	19.8	23.3	18.5	22.4
Foursquare	172	6%	3.03	1.72	34.3	8.7	9.9	13.4	33.7
Tinder	120	5%	2.52	1.51	36.7	20	15.8	9.2	18.3
Kiwi	117	4%	3	1.58	25.6	18.8	13.7	13.7	28.2
Ask.fm	92	3%	3.6	1.60	20.7	6.5	12	14.1	46.7
Runkeeper	72	3%	2.17	1.10	31.9	34.7	23.6	4.2	5.6
Reddit	60	2%	3.07	1.48	20	20	18.3	16.7	25
Happening	48	2%	2.65	1.42	29.2	20.8	20.8	14.6	14.6
Vimeo	32	1%	2.91	1.61	34.4	6.3	15.6	21.9	21.9
Strava	25	1%	2.6	1.44	28	28	16	12	16
LinkedIn	24	1%	2.08	1.38	50	16.7	20.8	12.5	/
Periscope	15	1%	3.07	1.28	13.3	20	26.7	26.7	13.3
Endomondo	11	0%	2.73	1.74	36.4	18.2	9.1	9.1	27.3
Ello	8	0%	1.5	1.41	87.5	/	/	/	12.5
Meerkat	6	0%	2.33	2.07	66.7	/	/	/	33.3

Table 3. Gender, age, school track and Fear-of-Missing-Out (FOMO) as predictors of the frequency of Facebook, Snapchat, Instagram, Youtube, Google Plus and Twitter.

	Facebook			Snapchat			Instagram			Youtube			Google Plus			Twitter		
	PE	SE	Wald	PE	SE	Wald	PE	SE	Wald	PE	SE	Wald	PE	SE	Wald	PE	SE	Wald
Gender (boy)	−0.50	0.09	32.55 ***	−0.68	0.09	52.79 ***	−0.61	0.10	35.85 ***	0.72	0.10	56.21 ***	0.18	0.12	2.23	−0.25	0.15	2.58
Gender (girl)	a																	
Age	0.15	0.03	28.1 ***	0.02	0.03	0.30	0.12	0.03	14.36 ***	−0.01	0.03	0.14	−0.09	0.04	6.42 *	0.02	0.05	0.15
School track (voc)	0.41	0.14	8.72 **	0.40	0.14	8.00 **	−0.34	0.14	5.75 *	0.54	0.15	13.58 ***	0.51	0.17	8.79 **	0.36	0.25	2.18
School track (s-voc)	0.28	0.12	5.67 *	0.35	0.12	8.88 **	−0.01	0.12	0.00	−0.01	0.12	0.00	0.40	0.15	6.84 **	0.76	0.18	19.06 ***
School track (ac)	a																	
FOMO	0.48	0.07	55.09 ***	0.28	0.07	16.89 ***	0.34	0.07	22.48 ***	0.18	0.07	7.08 **	0.04	0.09	0.22	0.15	0.11	2.02
Pearson GOF	$X^2(1821) = 1635.34$, $p = 1.00$			$X^2(1731) = 1842.31$, $p = 0.031$			$X^2(1643) = 1716.37$, $p = 0.102$			$X^2(1623) = 1621.94$, $p = 0.503$			$X^2(1335) = 1370.00$, $p = 0.247$			$X^2(1083) = 1131.58$, $p = 0.148$		
−2LL GOF	$X^2(5) = 150.10$, $p < 0.001$			$X^2(5) = 88.07$, $p < 0.001$			$X^2(5) = 79.19$, $p < 0.001$			$X^2(5) = 75.47$, $p < 0.001$			$X^2(5) = 17.20$, $p = 0.004$			$X^2(5) = 29.41$, $p < 0.001$		
Nagelkerke R^2	0.07			0.05			0.05			0.05			0.02			0.05		

* $p < 0.05$, ** $p < 0.01$, *** $p < 0.001$, Note 1: PE = parameter estimate, SE = standard error, Wald = Wald test statistic, voc = vocational, s-voc = semi-vocational, ac = academic, GOF = goodness-of-fit, a = reference category.

Table 4. Gender, age, school track and Fear-of-Missing-Out (FOMO) as predictors of the frequency of Swarm, We Heart It, Pinterest, Tumlbr, Vine, Foursquare and Tinder.

	Swarm			We Heart It			Pinterest			Tumblr			Vine			Foursquare			Tinder		
	PE	SE	Wald	PE	SE	Wald	PE	SE	Wald	PE	SE	Wald	PE	SE	Wald	PE	SE	Wald	PE	SE	Wald
Gender (boy)	−0.48	0.19	6.58 **	−1.41	0.58	5.87 *	−0.59	0.29	4.18 *	−0.41	0.29	2.01	0.19	0.24	0.64	−0.04	0.29	0.02	−0.11	0.34	0.11
Gender (girl)	a																				
Age	0.21	0.06	11.25 *	−0.12	0.07	2.69	−0.03	0.07	0.16	−0.03	0.07	0.16	−0.13	0.08	2.48	0.03	0.11	0.10	−0.17	0.11	2.36
School track (voc)	−0.58	0.25	5.34 *	0.65	0.31	4.36 *	−0.10	0.27	0.15	−0.50	0.33	2.30	−0.21	0.36	0.33	0.25	0.37	0.46	0.75	0.48	2.45
School track (s-voc)	0.36	0.22	2.78	0.01	0.24	0.00	−0.17	0.25	0.43	0.07	0.25	0.08	0.05	0.29	0.03	0.33	0.34	0.93	0.48	0.42	1.33
School track (ac)	a																				
FOMO	0.16	0.13	1.49	0.24	0.14	2.86	0.19	0.17	1.28	0.29	0.15	3.77 *	0.37	0.18	4.22*	0.47	0.21	5.26 *	0.04	0.23	0.03
Pearson GOF	$X^2(915) = 856.28$, $p = 0.917$			$X^2(571) = 607.49$, $p = 0.141$			$X^2(619) = 627.27$, $p = 0.400$			$X^2(619) = 620.67$, $p = 0.474$			$X^2(599) = 616.26$, $p = 0.304$			$X^2(475) = 488.52$, $p = 0.324$			$X^2(371) = 373.34$, $p = 0.456$		
−2LL GOF	$X^2(5) = 28.53$, $p < 0.001$			$X^2(5) = 12.53$, $p = 0.028$			$X^2(5) = 6.24$, $p = 0.283$			$X^2(5) = 689.76$, $p = 0.123$			$X^2(5) = 8.29$, $p = 0.141$			$X^2(5) = 7.47$, $p = 0.188$			$X^2(5) = 4.26$, $p = 0.513$		
Nagelkerke R2	0.06			0.04			0.02			0.03			0.04			0.05			0.04		

* $p < 0.05$, ** $p < 0.01$, *** $p < 0.001$, Note 1: PE = parameter estimate, SE = standard error, Wald = Wald test statistic, voc = vocational, s-voc = semi-vocational, ac = academic, GOF = goodness-of-fit, a = reference category. Note 2: The results for We Heart It, Pinterest and Tinder have to be interpreted with caution as the assumption of proportional odds was violated.

3.2.3. Private Versus Public Accessibility of Social Media Platforms Used

With respect to the private versus public accessibility of platforms, we consider *Facebook* and *Snapchat* as social media platforms on which content is generally less publicly accessible (i.e., content is oftentimes shielded off to a public of "approved" contacts), and *Youtube* and *Twitter* as social media platforms on which content is generally publicly accessible (i.e., content is usually accessible to everyone who visits the platform).

3.2.4. Fear of Missing Out (FOMO)

The omnibus format of the survey implied a constraint on the number of items we could use. We chose to select four items from Przybylski et al.'s [8] 10-item FOMO-scale, as this scale had been pre-validated by the authors. In Przybylski et al.'s study, the ten scale items loaded on one factor, and were internally consistent. In the absence of information on the factor loadings of the individual items in the original study, we chose to select a subset of four items that reflect the diversity of the original scale items well. Those items were: "It bothers me when I miss an opportunity to meet up with friends", "I fear my friends have more rewarding experiences than me", "When I go on vacation or summer camp, I continue to keep tabs on what my friends are doing", and "It is important that I understand my friends "inside jokes"". The items were measured on a 5-point Likert-scale (1 = completely disagree; 5 = completely agree).

A well-known risk of using a diverse set items to construct a short scale, is that internal consistency may be jeopardized [50]. Indeed, although an exploratory factor analysis revealed that the four items loaded onto one factor, with all factor loadings above 0.55, the total variance explained by the factor (42%) was below the advised 60% threshold, and the overall Kaiser-Meier-Olkin measure (0.65) indicated mediocre sampling adequacy. A further examination of the scale's reliability, confirmed that the internal consistency of the scale was weak ($\alpha = 0.56$), and revealed that it could not be further improved via item selection, as the highest inter-item correlation was 0.36 ($p < 0.001$). Appendix A shows the inter-item correlation matrix. Means and standard deviations can be consulted in Table 1.

A solution to the issue of low internal consistency, is to perform analyses with individual scale items, rather than with a scale variable. For the current study, however, such procedure would imply an inflation of results—particularly when answering Hypothesis 1a, which reduces the comprehensibility of the study findings. The alternative is to continue with a sub-optimal measure, knowing that the main risk of using a scale-measure that suffers from a weak Cronbach alpha, is underestimation of the real relationship [51]. In the context of the current study, we opted for the latter solution for reasons of comprehensibility, and thus work with the scale variable to answer Hypothesis 1. The risk of an underestimation of the real relationship should be kept in mind, however, when interpreting the results. For Hypotheses 2, 3 and 4, we report both the results using the FOMO scale variable and the individual scale items.

3.2.5. Problematic Social Media Use (PSMU)

Problematic social media use was assessed using an adapted version of the C-VAT instrument [52], which is a scale based on the CIUS-scale that was developed and validated by Meerkerk, Van den Eijnden et al. [53] and Meerkerk [54]. The adapted version addresses social media use rather than videogaming. The items were measured on a 5 point Likert-scale ($\alpha = 0.82$). The scale items, their means and standard deviations, and their factor loadings can be consulted in Table 1.

3.2.6. Phubbing Behavior

At the time of constructing the questionnaire, we were unaware of scales measuring phubbing behavior. Hence, we measured phubbing behavior with three self-constructed items: "How frequently do you use your mobile phone during a conversation in a bar or restaurant?", "How frequently are you engaged with your phone during a conversation?", and "How frequently do you check social media on your phone during a personal conversation?". The items were measured on a 5-point Likert scale, ranging from 1 (never) to 5 (almost all the time; $\alpha = 0.77$). The scale items, their means and standard deviations can be consulted in Table 1.

3.2.7. Control variables

Gender (1 = boy, 2 = girl), age and school track (1 = vocational, 2 = semi-vocational, 3 = academic) were included as control variables in the linear regression analyses.

3.3. Analyses

Hypothesis 1a states that teens who have a greater FOMO use social media platforms more frequently. We used ordinal regression analysis in to test this hypothesis because the frequency of use-measures have ordinal response scales. In the analyses with the frequency of use of Snapchat, We Heart it, Pinterest and Tinder as the dependent variables, the assumption of proportional odds was violated; this occurs more frequently in large samples, because minor violations of the parallel lines test may already be statistically significant [55]. Nonetheless, we advise to interpret these results with caution.

Hypothesis 1b states that FOMO positively predicts the breadth of social media use. The "breadth of social media use" variable was operationalized by counting the number of active social media accounts that teens have (min = 0, max = 25). We used multiple linear regression analysis to test the hypothesis, after assessing that the standardized residuals of the variable were normally distributed (and thus that the assumption of normality was not violated: because measurements gathered in large samples typically have very small standard errors, it is advised to assess normality on the basis of the absolute values of skewness and kurtosis rather than on Z-scores of skewness and kurtoses. Advised critical values for skewness, respectively kurtosis in large samples are 2, respectively 7 [56]. Using these guidelines, the skewness (1.22) and kurtosis (5.95) values of the residuals indicated that the assumption of normality for regression analysis was sufficiently met).

To explore our research question on the comparative strength of the correlations between FOMO and private platforms on the one hand, and between FOMO and public platforms on the other, we first calculated the correlations, and next compared the strength of these correlations using Steiger's Z-test [57] in Lee and Preacher's [58] web-based software. The Steiger Z-test operates on the basis of Pearson correlations between two dependent correlations with one variable in common. Because the correlations have to be drawn from the same sample, we first recoded the 'frequency of platform use' variables so that persons without an active account received the lowest usage score (rather than a missing value). This recoding procedure ensured that there were 2663 responses for each variable. Next, we calculated the Pearson correlation coefficients, which form the input for the Steiger's Z-test. The reader may notice that the Pearson correlation test is a parametric test, whereas the "frequency of platform use" variables are ordinal. However, the variables met the standard guidelines for skewness and kurtosis in large samples [56], and the Pearson correlation coefficients and the Spearman rho correlation coefficients were highly similar (i.e., for only two out of ten correlations the difference between the Pearson and the Spearman correlation coefficient exceeded a value of 0.03).

In social science research, scale variables are oftentimes treated as interval variables, based on the idea that the sets of items that comprise each scale form an index that represents an underlying latent factor [59]. The required assumptions for parametric testing were met. Hence, to examine Hypotheses 2 and 3, we fitted a mediation model using model 4 of Hayes' [60]. Process macro for SPSS with FOMO as the independent variable, PSMU as the mediator and phubbing behavior as the dependent variable. The indirect effect was estimated for 5000 bootstrap samples with a 95% bias-corrected confidence interval.

4. Results

4.1. Descriptives

Before addressing the hypotheses and research questions, we briefly report some descriptive statistics for the media use variables. The means and standard deviations for the items of the FOMO-scale, the PSMU-scale and the phubbing scale can be consulted in Table 1.

For 25 social media platforms, we asked the teenagers in our sample whether they had an active account, and if so, how frequently they use it. In terms of active account ownership, Facebook (89% of teens with an active account), Snapchat (73%), Instagram (63%) and Youtube (60%) are the most popular social media platforms. The teenagers in our sample had on average 4.35 (Median = 4, Mode = 4, Min = 0, Max = 25) active social media accounts. The standard deviation (SD = 2.29) reveals that there is substantial variability between teenagers. Most teens who have an active account on Facebook, Snapchat, Instagram and Youtube, reported using the platform more than once per day (see Table 2). There are other social media platforms that are frequently used, such as the location-sharing platform Swarm (M = 4.26, SD = 1.09), but these oftentimes have small user bases (e.g., only 19% of teens has an active Swarm account).

The teenagers in our sample on average had a fairly neutral FOMO score (M = 3.06, SD = 0.69). Using a multiple regression analysis, we explored whether FOMO was predicted by gender, age and school track. Our analysis showed that girls ($ß = 0.08$, $p < 0.001$) reported a higher FOMO, whereas age ($ß = 0.03$, $p = 0.109$) and school track ($ß = -0.01$, $p = 0.800$) were no significant predictors, $R^2 = 0.01$, $F(3.2659) = 5.96$, $p < 0.001$).

4.2. FOMO as a Predictor of the Depth and Breadth of Social Media Use

Hypotheses 1a and 1b concern FOMO as a predictor of the depth and breadth of social media use. We tested Hypothesis 1a using ordinal regression analysis, with gender, age, school track and FOMO as the predictor variables, and the frequency of use of each respective social media platform that was used by 5% of the sample or more as the dependent variable.

Tables 3 and 4 show the results. After controlling for gender, age and school track, FOMO positively predicted the use of the four most popular social media platforms: Facebook, Snapchat, Instagram and Youtube, as well as the frequency of using foursquare, Tumblr and Vine. These findings lend partial support to our hypothesis. While FOMO appears to be a modest predictor of the most common social media platforms, as well as of platforms that are used more rarely, it was not a consistent predictor of social media platform use.

With respect to the breadth of social media use (Hypothesis 1b), a multiple linear regression analysis with gender, age, school track and FOMO as predictors, revealed that gender ($ß = 0.08$, $p < 0.001$), age ($ß = 0.20$, $p < 0.001$), school track ($ß = -0.05$, $p = 0.006$) and FOMO ($ß = 0.14$, $p < 0.001$; $R^2 = 0.08$, $F(4.2658) = 57.27$, $p < 0.001$) were significant, positive predictors of the number of active social media accounts that teenagers have (H1b supported).

4.3. FOMO in Relation to the Public Accessibility of Platforms

We posited that FOMO would be a stronger predictor of social media use when the social media platform examined is a more private platform than when it as a more public platform (RQ1), because more private platforms such as Facebook or Snapchat connect teenagers more strongly to their offline ties, which can be considered the dominant affiliative group on which they want to keep tabs. We calculated Steiner's Z to statistically compare the correlations between FOMO and Facebook, respectively Snapchat use on the one hand, and between FOMO and YouTube, respectively, and Twitter on the other hand (see Tables 5 and 6).

The findings show that the correlations between FOMO and Facebook ($r = 0.16$, $p < 0.001$), respectively Snapchat use ($r = 0.17$, $p < 0.001$), are significantly stronger than the correlations between

FOMO and YouTube ($r = 0.00$, $p = 0.921$), respectively Twitter use ($r = 0.06$, $p = 0.002$), thus lending support to our research question.

Table 5. Correlations between FOMO and frequency of use of less publicly accessible platforms versus more publicly accessible platforms.

Pearson's r	Facebook	Snapchat	YouTube	Twitter
Snapchat	0.48 ***	1		
Youtube	0.13 ***	0.04 *	1	
Twitter	0.15 ***	0.19 ***	0.18 ***	1
FOMO	0.16 ***	0.17 ***	0.00	0.06 ***

* $p < 0.05$, *** $p < 0.001$, Note 1: For these analyses, participants with no active account on the platform were assigned a value of '0' on usage frequency to ensure that the analyses were performed on the same sample size. Note 2: We used Pearson's correlation coefficient, to enable the calculation of a Steiger Z value (see the subsequent set of analyses in Table 6). Note 3: The normality assumption was not violated.

Table 6. Comparison of Pearson correlation strength between FOMO and more private platforms versus FOMO and more public platforms.

Steiner's Z ($r_{FOMO,\ column\ var}$ vs. $r_{FOMO,\ row\ var}$)	Facebook	Snapchat	YouTube	Twitter
Snapchat	−0.41			
Youtube	6.37 ***	6.38 ***		
Twitter	4.18 ***	4.62 ***	−2.30 *	

* $p < 0.05$, *** $p < 0.001$.

4.4. FOMO as a Predictor of PSMU and Phubbing Behavior

Hypotheses 2 stated that FOMO positively predicts PSMU and Hypothesis 3a stated that FOMO positively predicts phubbing behavior. Hypothesis 3b stated that PSMU mediates the relationship between FOMO and phubbing behavior. We tested these hypotheses by estimating a mediation model. The results are depicted in Figure 1. All hypotheses were supported. FOMO has a direct, positive predictor of both PSMU ($ß = 0.40$, $p < 0.001$) and phubbing behavior ($ß = 0.20$, $p < 0.001$). When PSMU is accounted for, the relationship between FOMO and phubbing behavior weakens considerably. The indirect effect is significant ($ß = 0.16$, $p < 0.001$).

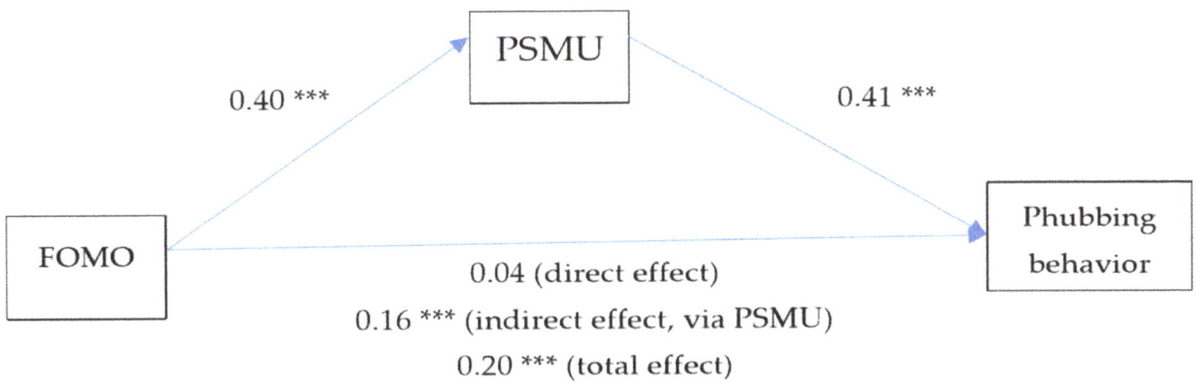

Figure 1. Mediation model of the relationship between FOMO, PSMU and phubbing behavior (*** $p < 0.001$). FOMO: Fear-of-missing-out; PSMU: problematic social media use.

Given that the internal consistency of the FOMO scale was unsatisfactory, we performed the mediation analysis on the individual items of the FOMO scale (see Table 7). For three items, the mediation analysis resulted in a similar results pattern. For the item "It bothers me when I miss an opportunity to meet with friends", however, the direct relationship with PSMU was much weaker (albeit still significant; $ß = 0.05$, $p = 0.008$), and the direct relationship with phubbing behavior was negative ($ß = -0.04$, $p = 0.011$).

Table 7. Mediation analysis results for the individual items of the FOMO scale and the FOMO scale variable.

	a	b	c	c′	Indirect Effect Estimate
FOMO (4-item scale)	0.40 ***	0.41 ***	0.04	0.20 ***	0.16 [0.14; 0.19]
Individual items					
I fear my friends have more rewarding experiences than me	0.21 ***	0.42 ***	0.00	0.09 ***	0.09 [0.07; 0.10]
It is important that I understand my friends' "inside jokes"	0.15 ***	0.43 ***	−0.01	0.05 ***	0.06 [0.05; 0.08]
It bothers me when I miss an opportunity to meet up with friends	0.05 **	0.43***	−0.04 *	−0.02	0.02 [0.00; 0.04]
When I go on summer camp or vacation, I continue to keep tabs on what my friends are doing	0.22 ***	0.38 ***	0.09 ***	0.18***	0.09 [0.07; 0.10]

* $p < 0.05$, ** $p < 0.01$, *** $p < 0.001$. Notes: a = effect of FOMO on PSMU. b = effect of PSMU on phubbing. c = effect of FOMO on phubbing. c′= total effect of FOMO on phubbing.

5. Discussion

Drawing from the results of a survey study among 2663 Flemish teenagers, the aims of this study were fourfold: (1) to examine FOMO as a predictor of the depth and breadth of social media use; (2) to examine whether FOMO relates more strongly to the use of more private social media platforms than more public platforms; (3) to test whether FOMO predicts PSMU and (4) whether FOMO predicts, both directly and indirectly via PSMU, phubbing behavior.

With respect to the breadth of social media use (Hypothesis 1b), we found support for the hypothesis that teens who have a greater FOMO use a wider variety of social media platforms. With respect to the depth of social media use, the study findings partially support the hypothesis that teenagers with a higher FOMO use social media more frequently (Hypothesis 1a), as FOMO was identified as a predictor for the frequency of use of some, but not all social media platforms examined. We did find a consistent relationship with the usage frequency of the four most used platforms: Facebook, Snapchat, Instagram and YouTube. This finding suggests that the relationship between FOMO and the frequency of use of these popular platforms is generalizable to the population of at least Flemish teenagers. These findings also support the findings of earlier work that characterize FOMO as an intrapersonal characteristic that predicts the use of Facebook [28,29] and Instagram [30,31].

The relationships found between FOMO and the frequency of using less popular social media platforms such as Foursquare, Tumblr and Vine are more difficult to interpret, as these social media platforms differ considerably from each other in what they afford the user to do: Foursquare is a location-based social network site, Tumblr is a blogging service, and Vine let users share short videoclips. Future research may explore the relationship between FOMO and the use of these particular platforms more in-depth via the use of interviews with teenagers, as greater insight into their personal experiences with these platforms and their anxieties concerning missing out may shed new light on what makes these particular platforms attractive.

As mentioned above, a pertinent question is whether the social gratification provided by social media use sooths or aggravates the anxieties of teenagers; after all, studies on social comparison on social media platforms [61] suggest that exposure to other people's social media accounts may make the experience of missing out on rewarding experiences even greater. A limitation of our study is its correlational nature, which prevents from making claims concerning the potential bi-directional causality of the relationship between FOMO and social media use. Future research may address this question via the use of longitudinal study designs that enable the modelling of cross-lagged path models.

It is essential for our understanding of FOMO to unravel how it resemblances, but also differs from other, associated personality factors. One factor that has been identified in the extant literature and that appears relevant to consider, is sociotropy [62], which refers to an insatiable need for belongingness to others, visible in an over-reliance on approval from others, which can go at the expense of personal autonomy. In recent work, sociotropy is linked to the ritualistic monitoring of, oftentimes multiple social media platforms [63]. Future research may explore how the fear of negative feedback or rejection that is typical for sociotropic individuals aligns with a fear of missing out.

We questioned whether FOMO would be a stronger predictor of more private social media platforms such as Facebook or Snapchat than of more public platforms such as YouTube and Twitter (RQ1). Our exploratory analysis suggests this is indeed the case. This is unsurprising, given that FOMO itself has been conceptualized and operationalized in the current study as a fear to miss out on what friends are thinking and doing, and information about these friends can be found mostly on platforms that connect to people who are part of one's offline network. Nonetheless the stronger relationship between FOMO and these private platforms, we need to remark that FOMO still remains a weak, yet significant predictor of some more publicly accessible platforms (e.g., Tumblr). A pertinent question is what still drives those higher on FOMO to use the latter platforms, then. As mentioned above, qualitative research seems relevant to further expand on the affordances in which various social media platforms resemble or differ from one another, and how these affordances are perceived, valued and acted upon by those with a higher versus lower FOMO.

FOMO was found to predict PSMU (Hypothesis 2), a result that aligns with the findings from other recent studies which showed that greater FOMO is associated with more problematic internet and smartphone use [40,64,65]. Moreover, FOMO was also associated with phubbing behavior (Hypothesis 3a), consistently with previous research that showed a similar pattern of associations [44]. Interestingly, our results showed that the relationship between FOMO and phubbing behavior was mediated by PMSU (cf. Hypothesis 3b), accordingly to the proposed conceptual model by Chotpitayasunondh & Douglas [44], which found that FOMO was a positive predictor of smartphone addiction, and that smartphone addiction predicted smartphone behavior. Thus, adolescents who are high in their fear of missing out are more likely to overuse the social media and smartphones, which in turns leads them to phub their offline interaction partners [66]. Scholars in the field of problematic media use research advocate to invest greater effort into the study of the pathways that lead to problem behavior [6]. Our study findings represent such an effort, as they reveal that FOMO is an intra-personal characteristic that leads to phubbing behavior by inducing excessive, uncontrolled social media use.

The findings reported in this study are generalizable as they stem from a large-scale survey study that was administered to representative sample of Flemish teenagers. There are a number of limitations to the current study, however. We used a shortened, four item version of the FOMO-scale developed by Przybylski et al. [8] to assess teenagers' FOMO. The internal consistency of the scale was unsatisfactory, which increases the risk of underestimating the real relationship (see Schmitt [51]). The low internal consistency for our scale illustrates the importance for research in this field to use complete and validated scales—for the reason of making reliable claims about one's study, and for enabling valid comparisons between studies.

In light of the unsatisfactory internal consistency of our FOMO-scale, we tested Hypotheses 2 and 3 using both the scale variable and the individual items. This analysis revealed that for one item the relationship with phubbing behavior was reversed: The more teens agreed to feel bothered when missing an opportunity to meet with friends (i.e., indicative of a greater fear-of-missing-out), the less they report phubbing their interaction partner during a face-to-face interaction. This finding indicates that some teenagers attach great importance to face-to-face interactions with friends, leading them to prioritize these interactions over smartphone interactions. This finding suggests that it is relevant to further investigate how FOMO relates to relational behavior, not only online (in the form of social media use), but also offline.

Second, our study used a narrow definition of social media [16], which excludes mobile messaging applications. It is likely that those with a greater FOMO also heavily rely on the use of these messengers to soothe their anxieties about what others in their social networks are doing. The latter applications are different from social media, however, in that they are oftentimes used for small-group communication, and therefore are more dialogical in nature [67]. It is more difficult—if not impossible—to "lurk" in dyadic and small-group conversations, as they generally rely on a certain degree of reciprocity. With respect to FOMO, this difference in the interactional affordances of social media platforms and (mobile) instant messengers raises interesting questions. It may be the case that people with a high FOMO are particularly attracted to social media because they can lurk on these platforms without risking a label of "voyeur", and without having to engage in reciprocal disclosures about themselves. As mentioned above, it seems relevant to explore the difference between FOMO and sociotropy [62] in this context, as active disclosures on social media platforms and messaging platforms may provide sociotropic individuals with a means to gather the social approval they long for, while those with a high FOMO may seek information about other people's experiences without necessarily wanting to engage in interactions with them. Future research may explore this.

In short, this study is valuable because it provides generalizable findings on the relationships between FOMO, social media use, PSMU and phubbing behavior among teenagers. As such, it can serve as a starting ground for future research. This research needs to look into the pathways via which FOMO leads to particular forms of (problematic) media use, and how these pathways are similar to or different from other pathways.

6. Conclusions

To conclude, and on the basis of the findings presented in this article, FOMO is an important factor explaining teenagers' social media use. The present study found support for the hypothesis that teens who have a greater FOMO use a wider variety of social media platforms. Also, the present study found partially support for the hypothesis that teenagers with a higher FOMO use social media more frequently: FOMO was identified as a predictor for the frequency of use of some, but not all social media platforms examined. In particular, there was a consistent relationship between FOMO and the usage frequency of Facebook, Snapchat, Instagram and YouTube. Moreover, FOMO was found to predict PSMU. This result aligns with the findings from other recent studies which showed that greater FOMO is associated with more problematic internet and smartphone use [40,64,65]. Finally, FOMO was associated with phubbing behavior. Our results additionally showed that the relationship between FOMO and phubbing behavior was mediated by PSMU. Teens who are high in their fear of missing out are more likely to overuse the social media and smartphones, which in turns may lead them to phub their offline interaction partners [66].

Author Contributions: V.F. and M.V.A. performed analyses and wrote initial drafts of the manuscript. A.J.v.R., G.L.C., and L.D.M. proofread drafts, contributed ideas and edited the various versions.

Appendix A

Table A1. Intercorrelation matrix of items measuring the Fear-of-Missing-Out (FOMO).

Items FOMO Scale	1	2	3	4
I fear my friends have more rewarding experiences than me	1	0.36 ***	0.17 ***	0.26 ***
It is important that I understand my friends' "inside jokes"		1	0.25 ***	0.21 ***
It bothers me when I miss an opportunity to meet up with friends			1	0.15 ***
When I go on summer camp or vacation, I continue to keep tabs on what my friends are doing				1

*** $p < 0.001$.

References

1. Moreno, M.A.; Jelenchick, L.; Koff, R.; Eikoff, J.; Diermyer, C.; Christakis, D.A. Internet use and multitasking among older adolescents: An experience sampling approach. *Comput. Hum. Behav.* **2012**, *28*, 1097–1102. [CrossRef]
2. Billieux, J.; Schimmenti, A.; Khazaal, Y.; Maurage, P. Are we overpathologizing everyday life? A tenable blueprint for behavioral addiction research. *J. Behav. Addict.* **2015**, *4*, 119–123. [CrossRef] [PubMed]
3. Bean, A.M.; Nielsen, R.K.; Van Rooij, A.J.; Ferguson, C.J. Video game addiction: The push to pathologize video games. *Prof. Psychol. Res. Pract.* **2017**, *48*, 378–389. [CrossRef]
4. Kardefelt-Winther, D.; Heeren, A.; Schimmenti, A.; Van Rooij, A.; Maurage, P.; Carras, M.; Edman, J.; Blaszczynski, A.; Khazaal, Y.; Billieux, J. How can we conceptualize behavioral addiction without pathologizing common behaviours? *Addiction* **2017**, *112*, 1709–1715. [CrossRef] [PubMed]
5. Van Rooij, A.J.; Daneels, R.; Liu, S.; Anrijs, S.; Van Looy, J. Children's motives to start, continue, and stop playing video games: Confronting popular theories with real-world observations. *Curr. Addict. Rep.* **2017**, *4*, 323–332. [CrossRef]
6. Billieux, J. Problematic use of the mobile phone: A literature review and a pathways model. *Curr. Psychiatry Rev.* **2012**, *8*, 299–307. [CrossRef]
7. Billieux, J.; Maurage, P.; Lopez-Fernandez, O.; Kuss, D.J.; Griffiths, M.D. Can disordered mobile phone use be considered a behavioral addiction? An update on current evidence and a comprehensive model for future research. *Curr. Addict. Rep.* **2015**, *2*, 156–162. [CrossRef]
8. Przybylski, A.K.; Murayama, K.; DeHaan, C.R.; Gladwell, V. Motivational, emotional, and behavioral correlates of fear of missing out. *Comput. Hum. Behav.* **2013**, *29*, 1841–1848. [CrossRef]
9. Deci, E.L.; Ryan, R.M. *Intrinsic Motivation and Self-Determination in Human Behavior*; Plenum Press: New York, NY, USA, 1985.
10. Oulasvirta, A.; Rattenbury, T.; Ma, L.; Raita, E. Habits make smartphone use more pervasive. *Personal Ubiquitous Comput.* **2012**, *16*, 105–114. [CrossRef]
11. LaPlante, D.A.; Nelson, S.E.; Gray, H.M. Breadth and depth involvement: Understanding Internet gambling involvement and its relationship to gambling problems. *Psychol. Addict. Behav.* **2014**, *28*, 396. [CrossRef] [PubMed]
12. Abel, P.J.; Buff, C.L.; Burr, S.A. Social media and fear of missing out: Scale development and assessment. *J. Bus. Econ. Res.* **2016**, *14*, 34–44. [CrossRef]
13. Simon, J. Love: Addiction or road to self-realization, a second look. *Am. J. Psychoanal.* **1982**, *42*, 253–263. [CrossRef] [PubMed]
14. Baumeister, R.F.; Leary, M.R. The need to belong: Desire for interpersonal attachments as a fundamental human motivations. *Psychol. Bull.* **1995**, *117*, 497–529. [CrossRef] [PubMed]
15. Boyd, D.; Ellison, N.B. Social network sites: Definition, history and scholarship. *J. Comput. Mediat. Commun.* **2008**, *13*, 210–230. [CrossRef]
16. Kaplan, A.M.; Haenlein, M. Users of the world, unite! The challenges and opportunities of Social Media. *Bus. Horiz.* **2010**, *53*, 59–68. [CrossRef]
17. Clayton, R.B.; Leshner, G.; Almond, A. The extended iself: The impact of iphone separation on cognition, emotion and physiology. *J. Comput. Mediat. Commun.* **2015**, *20*, 119–135. [CrossRef]
18. Kruger, D.J.; Djerf, J.M. High ringxiety: Attachment anxiety predicts experiences of phantom cell phone ringing. *Cyberpsychol. Behav. Soc. Netw.* **2016**, *19*, 56–59. [CrossRef] [PubMed]
19. Belk, R.W. Possession and the extended self. *J. Consum. Res.* **1988**, *15*, 139–168. [CrossRef]
20. Tandor, E.C.; Ferrucci, P.; Duffy, M. Facebook use, envy, and depression among college students: Is facebooking depressing? *Comput. Hum. Behav.* **2014**, *43*, 139–146. [CrossRef]
21. Casale, S.; Rugai, L.; Fioravanti, G. Exploring the role of positive metacognitions in explaining the association between the fear of missing out and social media addiction. *Addict. Behav.* **2018**, *85*, 83–87. [CrossRef] [PubMed]
22. Katz, E. Mass communications research and the study of popular culture: An editorial note on a possible future for this journal. *Stud. Public Commun.* **1959**, *2*, 1–6.
23. Katz, E.; Blumler, J.G. *The Uses of Mass Communications: Current Perspectives on Gratifications Research*; Sage Publications: Beverly Hills, CA, USA, 1974.

24. Ajzen, I. The theory of planned behavior. *Organ. Behav. Hum. Decis. Process.* **1991**, *50*, 179–211. [CrossRef]
25. Lee, E.; Lee, J.A.; Moon, J.H.; Sung, Y. Pictures speak louder than words: Motivations for using Instagram. *Cyberpsychol. Behav. Soc. Netw.* **2015**, *18*, 552–556. [CrossRef] [PubMed]
26. Sheldon, K.M.; Abad, N.; Hirsch, C. A two-process view of Facebook use and relatedness need-satisfaction: Disconnection drives us and connection rewards it. *J. Personal. Soc. Psychol.* **2011**, *100*, 766–775. [CrossRef] [PubMed]
27. Sheldon, P.; Bryant, K. Instagram: Motives for its use and relationship to narcissism and contextual age. *Comput. Hum. Behav.* **2015**, *58*, 89–97. [CrossRef]
28. Beyens, I.; Frison, E.; Eggermont, S. "I don't want to miss a thing": Adolescents' fear of missing out and its relationship to adolescents' social needs, Facebook use, and Facebook related stress. *Comput. Hum. Behav.* **2016**, *64*, 1–8. [CrossRef]
29. Błachnio, A.; Przepiórka, A. Facebook Intrusion, fear of missing out, narcissism, and life satisfaction: A cross-sectional study. *Psychiatry Res.* **2018**, *259*, 514–519. [CrossRef] [PubMed]
30. Barry, C.T.; Reiter, S.R.; Anderson, A.C.; Schoessler, M.L.; Sidoti, C.L. "Let me take another selfie": Further examination of the relation between narcissism, self-perception, and Instagram posts. *Psychol. Popul. Media Cult.* **2017**. [CrossRef]
31. Salim, F.; Rahardjo, W.; Tanaya, T.; Qurani, R. Are self-presentation of instagram users influenced by friendship-contingent self-esteem and fear of missing out? *Makara Hubs Asia* **2017**, *21*, 70–82. [CrossRef]
32. Bayer, J.B.; Ellison, N.B.; Schoenebeck, S.Y.; Falk, E.B. Sharing the small moments: Ephemeral social interaction on Snapchat. *Inf. Commun. Soc.* **2016**, *19*, 956–977. [CrossRef]
33. Alhabash, S.; Ma, M. A tale of four platforms: Motivations and uses of Facebook, Twitter, Instagram, and Snapchat among college students? *Soc. Media Soc.* **2017**, *3*, 1–13. [CrossRef]
34. Caplan, S. Relations among loneliness, social anxiety, and problematic internet use. *Cyberpsychol. Behav.* **2006**, *10*, 234–242. [CrossRef] [PubMed]
35. Milani, L.; Osualdella, D.; Di Blasio, P. Quality of interpersonal relationships and problematic internet use in adolescents. *CyberPsychol. Behav.* **2009**, *12*, 681–684. [CrossRef] [PubMed]
36. Chakraborty, K.; Basu, D.; Vijaya, K. Internet Addiction: Consensus, Controversies and the Way Ahead. *East Asian Arch Psychiatry.* **2010**, *20*, 123–132. [PubMed]
37. Griffiths, M.D.; Kuss, D.J. Adolescent Social Media Addiction (revised). *Educ. Health* **2017**, *35*, 49–52.
38. Buglass, S.L.; Binder, J.F.; Betts, L.R.; Underwood, J.D. Motivators of online vulnerability: The impact of social network sites use and FOMO. *Comput. Hum. Behav.* **2017**, *66*, 248–255. [CrossRef]
39. Fuster, H.; Chamarro, A.; Oberst, U. Fear of missing out, online social networking and mobile phone addiction: A latent profile approach. *Revista de Psicologia Ciències de l'Educació i de l'Esport* **2017**, *35*, 23–30.
40. Oberst, U.; Wegmann, E.; Stodt, B.; Brand, M.; Chamarro, A. Negative consequences from heavy social networking in adolescents: The mediating role of fear of missing out. *J. Adolesc.* **2017**, *55*, 51–60. [CrossRef] [PubMed]
41. Wegmann, E.; Oberst, U.; Stodt, B.; Brand, M. Online-specific fear of missing out and Internet-use expectancies contribute to symptoms of Internet-communication disorder. *Addict. Behav. Rep.* **2017**, *5*, 33–42. [CrossRef] [PubMed]
42. Elhai, J.D.; Levine, J.C.; Alghraibeh, A.M.; Alafnan, A.A.; Aldraiweesh, A.A.; Hall, B.J. Fear of missing out: Testing relationships with negative affectivity, online social engagement, and problematic smartphone use. *Comput. Hum. Behav.* **2018**, *89*, 289–298. [CrossRef]
43. Scott, H.; Woods, H.C. Fear of missing out and sleep: Cognitive behavioural factors in adolescents' nighttime social media use. *J. Adolesc.* **2018**, *68*, 61–65. [CrossRef] [PubMed]
44. Chotpitayasunondh, V.; Douglas, K.M. How "phubbing" becomes the norm: The antecedents and consequences of snubbing via smartphone. *Comput. Hum. Behav.* **2016**, *63*, 9–18. [CrossRef]
45. Kenny, M. Cell Phones, College Students, and Conversations: Exploring Mobile Technology Use during Face-to-Face Interactions. Bachelor's Thesis, The Florida State University, Tallahassee, FL, USA, 2016.
46. Vanden Abeele, M.M.V.; Antheunis, M.L.; Schouten, A.P. The effect of mobile messaging during a conversation on impression formation and interaction quality. *Comput. Hum. Behav.* **2016**, *62*, 562–569. [CrossRef]
47. Ofcom. *The Communications Market Reports*; Ofcom: Warrington, UK, 2015.

48. Kuss, D.J.; Kanjo, E.; Rumsey-Crook, M.; Kibowski, F.; Wang, G.Y.; Sumich, A. Problematic mobile phone use and addiction across generations: The roles of psychopathological symptoms and smartphone use. *J. Technol. Behav. Sci.* **2018**, *3*, 141–149. [CrossRef] [PubMed]
49. Van Waeg, S.; D'hanens, K.; Dooms, V.; Naesens, J. Onderzoeksrapport Apestaartjaren 6/Research Report Apestaartjaren 6. Available online: www.apestaartjaren.be/onderzoek/apestaartjaren-6 (accessed on 17 August 2018).
50. Tavakol, M.; Dennick, R. Making sense of Cronbach's alpha. *Int. J. Med. Educ.* **2011**, *2*, 53. [CrossRef] [PubMed]
51. Schmitt, N. Uses and Abuses of Coefficient Alpha. *Psychol. Assess.* **1996**, *4*, 350–353. [CrossRef]
52. Van Rooij, A.J.; Ferguson, C.J.; Van de Mheen, D.; Schoenmakers, T.M. Time to abandon Internet Addiction? Predicting problematic Internet, game, and social media use from psychosocial well-being and application use. *Clin. Neuropsychiatry* **2017**, *14*, 113–121.
53. Meerkerk, G.; Van den Eijnden, R.J.J.M; Vermulst, A.A.; Garretsen, H.F.L. The Compulsive Internet Use Scale (CIUS): Some psychometric properties. *Cyberpsychol. Behav.* **2009**, *1*, 1–6. [CrossRef] [PubMed]
54. Meerkerk, G.; Pwned by the Internet. Explorative research into the causes and consequences of compulsive internet use. Ph.D. Thesis, Erasmus University, Rotterdam, The Netherlands, 2007.
55. Williams, R. Generalized ordered logit/partial proportional odds models for ordinal dependent variables. *Stata J.* **2006**, *6*, 58.
56. Kim, H. Statistical notes for clinical researchers: Assessing normal distribution (2) using skewness and kurtosis. *Restor. Dent. Endod.* **2013**, *38*, 52–54. [CrossRef] [PubMed]
57. Steiger, J.H. Tests for comparing elements of a correlation matrix. *Psychol. Bull.* **1980**, *87*, 245–251. [CrossRef]
58. Lee, I.A.; Preacher, K.J. Calculation for the Test of the Difference between Two Dependent Correlations with One Variable in Common (Computer Software). Available online: http://quantpsy.org (accessed on 2 October 2018).
59. Allen, I.E.; Seaman, C.A. Likert scales and data analyses. *Qual. Prog.* **2007**, *40*, 64–65.
60. Hayes, A.F. *Introduction to Mediation, Moderation, and Conditional Process. Analysis*; Guilford Press: New York, NY, USA, 2013.
61. Fox, J.; Moreland, J.J. The dark side of social networking sites: An exploration of the relational and psychological stressors associated with Facebook use and affordances. *Comput. Hum. Behav.* **2015**, *45*, 168–176. [CrossRef]
62. Beck, A.T. Cognitive therapy of depression: New perspectives. In *Treatment of Depression: Old Controversies and New Approaches*; Clayton, P.J., Barrett, J.E., Eds.; Raven Press: New York, NY, USA, 1983; pp. 265–290.
63. Orchard, L.J.; Fullwood, C.; Galbraith, N.; Morris, N. Individual differences as predictors of social networking. *J. Comput. Mediat. Commun.* **2014**, *19*, 388–402. [CrossRef]
64. Elhai, J.D.; Levine, J.C.; Dvorak, R.D.; Hall, B.J. Fear of missing out, need for touch, anxiety and depression are related to problematic smartphone use. *Comput. Hum. Behav.* **2016**, *63*, 509–516. [CrossRef]
65. Stead, H.; Bibby, P.A. Personality, fear of missing out and problematic internet use and their relationship to subjective well-being. *Comput. Hum. Behav.* **2017**, *76*, 534–540. [CrossRef]
66. Roberts, J.A.; David, M.E. My life has become a major distraction from my cell phone: Partner phubbing and relationship satisfaction among romantic partners. *Comput. Hum. Behav.* **2016**, *54*, 134–141. [CrossRef]
67. Ling, R.; Lai, C. Microcoordination 2.0: Social Coordination in the Age of Smartphones and Messaging Apps. *J. Commun.* **2016**, *66*, 834–856. [CrossRef]

Permissions

All chapters in this book were first published by MDPI; hereby published with permission under the Creative Commons Attribution License or equivalent. Every chapter published in this book has been scrutinized by our experts. Their significance has been extensively debated. The topics covered herein carry significant findings which will fuel the growth of the discipline. They may even be implemented as practical applications or may be referred to as a beginning point for another development.

The contributors of this book come from diverse backgrounds, making this book a truly international effort. This book will bring forth new frontiers with its revolutionizing research information and detailed analysis of the nascent developments around the world.

We would like to thank all the contributing authors for lending their expertise to make the book truly unique. They have played a crucial role in the development of this book. Without their invaluable contributions this book wouldn't have been possible. They have made vital efforts to compile up to date information on the varied aspects of this subject to make this book a valuable addition to the collection of many professionals and students.

This book was conceptualized with the vision of imparting up-to-date information and advanced data in this field. To ensure the same, a matchless editorial board was set up. Every individual on the board went through rigorous rounds of assessment to prove their worth. After which they invested a large part of their time researching and compiling the most relevant data for our readers.

The editorial board has been involved in producing this book since its inception. They have spent rigorous hours researching and exploring the diverse topics which have resulted in the successful publishing of this book. They have passed on their knowledge of decades through this book. To expedite this challenging task, the publisher supported the team at every step. A small team of assistant editors was also appointed to further simplify the editing procedure and attain best results for the readers.

Apart from the editorial board, the designing team has also invested a significant amount of their time in understanding the subject and creating the most relevant covers. They scrutinized every image to scout for the most suitable representation of the subject and create an appropriate cover for the book.

The publishing team has been an ardent support to the editorial, designing and production team. Their endless efforts to recruit the best for this project, has resulted in the accomplishment of this book. They are a veteran in the field of academics and their pool of knowledge is as vast as their experience in printing. Their expertise and guidance has proved useful at every step. Their uncompromising quality standards have made this book an exceptional effort. Their encouragement from time to time has been an inspiration for everyone.

The publisher and the editorial board hope that this book will prove to be a valuable piece of knowledge for researchers, students, practitioners and scholars across the globe.

List of Contributors

Hui Jiang
Center for Health Behaviours Research, School of Public Health and Primary Care, The Chinese University of Hong Kong, Hong Kong, China

Phoenix Kit-han Mo and Joseph T. F. Lau
The Chinese University of Hong Kong Shenzhen Research Institute, Shenzhen 518057, China
Center for Health Behaviours Research, School of Public Health and Primary Care, The Chinese University of Hong Kong, Hong Kong, China

Ji-Bin Li
Department of Clinical Research, State Key Laboratory of Oncology in South China, Collaborative Innovation Center for Cancer Medicine, Sun Yat-sen University Cancer Center, Guangzhou 510060, China

Young-Mi Ko
Mental Health Research Institute, National Center for Mental Health, Seoul 04933, Korea

Sungwon Roh
Department of Psychiatry, Hanyang University, College of Medicine, Seoul 04763, Korea

Tae Kyung Lee
Department of Mental Health, ChunCheon National Hospital, ChunCheon City 24409, Korea

Sina Ostendorf and Elisa Wegmann
Department of General Psychology: Cognition and Center for Behavioral Addiction Research (CeBAR), University of Duisburg-Essen, 47057 Duisburg, Germany

Matthias Brand
Department of General Psychology: Cognition and Center for Behavioral Addiction Research (CeBAR), University of Duisburg-Essen, 47057 Duisburg, Germany
Erwin L. Hahn Institute for Magnetic Resonance Imaging, 45141 Essen, Germany

Kuan-Ying Hsieh
Department of Child and Adolescent Psychiatry, Kaohsiung Municipal Kai-Syuan Psychiatric Hospital, Kaohsiung 80276, Taiwan
Graduate Institute of Medicine, College of Medicine, Kaohsiung Medical University, Kaohsiung 80708, Taiwan
Department of Psychiatry, Children's Hospital and Regional Medical Center, Seattle, WA 98195, USA

Yi-Hsin Yang
Graduate Institute of Medicine, College of Medicine, Kaohsiung Medical University, Kaohsiung 80708, Taiwan
School of Pharmacy, Kaohsiung Medical University, Kaohsiung 80708, Taiwan

Kun-Hua Lee
Department of Educational Psychology and Counseling, National Tsing Hua University, Hsin-Chu City 30013, Taiwan

Cheng-Fang Yen
Graduate Institute of Medicine, College of Medicine, Kaohsiung Medical University, Kaohsiung 80708, Taiwan
Department of Psychiatry, Kaohsiung Medical University Hospital, Kaohsiung 80708, Taiwan
Department of Psychiatry, School of Medicine and Graduate Institute of Medicine, College of Medicine, Kaohsiung Medical University, Kaohsiung 80708, Taiwan

Antonio-José Moreno-Guerrero, Gerardo Gómez-García, Jesús López-Belmonte and Carmen Rodríguez-Jiménez
Department of Didactics and School Organization, University of Granada, 18071 Granada, Spain

Soo-Hyun Paik, Hyun Cho, Ji-Won Chun and Jo-Eun Jeong
Department of Psychiatry, Seoul St. Mary's Hospital, The Catholic University of Korea, Seoul 06591, Korea

Hiu Yan Wong, Hoi Yi Mo, Mung Ni Monica Chan, Wai Man Lau, Tsz Kwan Chui and Chung-Ying Lin
Department of Rehabilitation Sciences, The Hong Kong Polytechnic University, Hung Hom, Hong Kong

Marc N. Potenza
Departments of Psychiatry and Neuroscience and the Child Study Center, School of Medicine, Yale University, New Haven, CT 06511, USA
Connecticut Council on Problem Gambling, Wethersfield, CT 06109, USA
Connecticut Mental Health Center, New Haven, CT 06519, USA

Amir H. Pakpour
Social Determinants of Health Research Center, Research Institute for Prevention of Non-Communicable Diseases, Qazvin University of Medical Sciences, Qazvin 3419759811, Iran
Department of Nursing, School of Health and Welfare, Jönköping University, 55511 Jönköping, Sweden

Lijun Chen and Xiaoliu Jiang
Department of Psychology, School of Humanities and Social Sciences, Fuzhou University, Fuzhou 350108, China

Songli Mei
School of Public Health, Jilin University, Changchun 130021, China

Jingxin Chai
Hepin Street, Dongcheng District, Beijing Center for Disease Prevention and Control, Beijing 100013, China

Shi-Bin Wang
Guangdong Mental Health Center, Guangdong General Hospital and Guangdong Academy of Medical Sciences, Guangzhou 510120, China

Chee H. Ng
Department of Psychiatry, University of Melbourne, Melbourne, VIC 3050, Australia

Gabor S. Ungvari
Division of Psychiatry, Notre Dame university Australia, Fremantle, WA 6160, Australia
Graylands Hospital, Claremont, WA 6010, Australia

Yu-Tao Xiang
Unit of Psychiatry, Faculty of Health Sciences, University of Macau, Avenida da Universidade, Taipa, Macau, China

Amandine Luquiens
Hôpital Paul Brousse, APHP Villejuif, France
Université Paris-Saclay, 94800 Villejuif, France
CMAP, Ecole Polytechnique, 91128 Palaiseau Cedex, France
Université Paris-Sud membre de Université Paris-Saclay, UVSQ, CESP, INSERM, 94800 Villejuif, France
Addictions Department, Nîmes University Hospital, 30000 Nîmes, France

Amine Benyamina
Hôpital Paul Brousse, APHP Villejuif, France
Université Paris-Saclay, 94800 Villejuif, France

Stéphane Gaïffas
CMAP, Ecole Polytechnique, 91128 Palaiseau Cedex, France
LPSM UMR 8001, Université Paris Diderot, 8001 Paris, France

Aline Dugravot and Henri Panjo
Université Paris-Sud membre de Université Paris-Saclay, UVSQ, CESP, INSERM, 94800 Villejuif, France

Emmanuel Bacry
CMAP, Ecole Polytechnique, 91128 Palaiseau Cedex, France
CEREMADE UMR 7534 CNRS, Université Paris-Dauphine PSL, 75765 Paris Cedex 16, France

Ki Hyeon Kwak, Hyun Chan Hwang, Sun Mi Kim and Doug Hyun Han
Department of Psychiatry, Chung Ang University Hospital, 102 Heuk seok ro, Dongjak gu, Seoul 06973, Korea

Yeon-Jin Kim
Department of Psychiatry, SMG-SNU Boramae Medical Center, Seoul 07061, Korea

Hye Min Jang and Donghwan Lee
Department of Statistics, Ewha Womans University, Seoul 03760, Korea

Youngjo Lee
Department of Statistics, Seoul National University, Seoul 08826, Korea

Dai-Jin Kim
Department of Psychiatry, Seoul St. Mary's Hospital, The Catholic University of Korea College of Medicine, Seoul 06591, Korea

María Luisa Ballestar-Tarín
Nursing Department, Facultat d'Infermeria I Podologia, Universitat de València, 46010 Valencia, Spain

Conchín Simó-Sanz and Elena Chover-Sierra
Nursing Department, Facultat d'Infermeria I Podologia, Universitat de València, 46010 Valencia, Spain
Hospital General, Universitario de Valencia, 46014 Valencia, Spain

Carlos Saus-Ortega
Nursing Department, Facultat d'Infermeria I Podologia, Universitat de València, 46010 Valencia, Spain
Nursing School La Fe, Universitario de Valencia, 46026 Valencia, Spain

Carmen Casal-Angulo
Nursing Department, Facultat d'Infermeria I Podologia, Universitat de València, 46010 Valencia, Spain
Emergencies Service, Extra-hospital, 46010 Valencia, Spain

Antonio Martínez-Sabater
Nursing Department, Facultat d'Infermeria I Podologia, Universitat de València, 46010 Valencia, Spain
Hospital Clínico, Universitario de Valencia, 46010 Valencia, Spain

Xinchen Fu, Ru-De Liu and Fangkai Jin
Beijing Key Laboratory of Applied Experimental Psychology, National Demonstration Center for Experimental Psychology Education (Beijing Normal University), Faculty of Psychology, Beijing Normal University, Beijing 100875, China

Jingxuan Liu
Department of Psychology and Neuroscience, Duke University, Durham, NC 27708, USA

Yi Ding
Graduate School of Education, Fordham University, New York, NY 10023, USA

Jia Wang
Teachers' College, Beijing Union University, Beijing 100011, China

Rui Zhen
Institute of Psychological Sciences, College of Education, Hangzhou Normal University, No. 2318 Yuhangtang Road, Hangzhou 311121, China

Jui-Kang Tsai
Department of Psychiatry, Kaohsiung Armed Forces General Hospital, Kaohsiung 80284, Taiwan
Department of Nursing, Meiho University, Pingtung 91202, Taiwan

Wei-Hsin Lu
Department of Psychiatry, Ditmanson Medical Foundation Chia-Yi Christian Hospital, Chia-Yi City 60002, Taiwan
Department of Senior Citizen Service Management, Chia Nan University of Pharmacy and Science, Tainan 71710, Taiwan

Ray C. Hsiao
Department of Psychiatry and Behavioral Sciences, University of Washington School of Medicine, Seattle, WA 98105, USA
Department of Psychiatry, Children's Hospital and Regional Medical Center, Seattle, WA 98105, USA

Huei-Fan Hu
Department of Psychiatry, Tainan Municipal Hospital (managed by Show Chwan Medical Care Corporation), Tainan 70173, Taiwan

Dmitri Rozgonjuk
Institute of Psychology, University of Tartu, Tartu 50409, Estonia
Department of Psychology, University of Toledo, Toledo, OH 43606, USA

Kristiina Saal and Karin Täht
Institute of Psychology, University of Tartu, Tartu 50409, Estonia

Christian Montag and Bernd Lachmann
Department of Molecular Psychology, Institute of Psychology and Education, Ulm University, 89081 Ulm, Germany

Marc Herrlich
Serious Games Engineering, TU Kaiserslautern, 67663 Kaiserslautern, Germany

Katharina Zweig
Algorithm Accountability Lab, TU Kaiserslautern, 67663 Kaiserslautern, Germany

Vittoria Franchina and Gianluca Lo Coco
Department of Psychology and Educational Sciences, University of Palermo, 90133 Palermo, Italy

Mariek Vanden Abeele
Tilburg School of Humanities and Digital Sciences, Tilburg University, 5037AB Tilburg, The Netherlands

Lieven De Marez
imec-mict-UGent, Department of Communication Sciences, Ghent University, 9000 Ghent, Belgium

Antonius J. van Rooij
imec-mict-UGent, Department of Communication Sciences, Ghent University, 9000 Ghent, Belgium
Department of Youth & Risky Behavior, Trimbos Institute, 3521 VS Utrecht, The Netherlands

Index

www.ingramcontent.com/pod-product-compliance
Lightning Source LLC
LaVergne TN
LVHW060533210926
848485LV00005B/1192
* 9 7 8 1 6 4 6 4 7 5 8 6 5 *